# MASLD, NAFLD & NASH
## The Definitive Guide for Patients with Fatty Liver Disease

Prof David EJ Jones OBE &
Dr Vanessa C Linnett

*Lynup Medica*

MASLD, NAFLD & NASH: The Definitive Guide for Patients

Copyright © 2024 David EJ Jones & Vanessa C Linnett
**Lynup Medica Ltd**

All rights reserved.

ISBN: 9798343197976

# DEDICATION

This book is dedicated to all the patient groups, and liver disease patients, who work so hard to help each other. They are an inspiration. Enormous thanks go to Matthew and Thomas for all the thoughts and suggestions, and for their tolerance as we have embarked on this journey.

MASLD, NAFLD & NASH: The Definitive Guide for Patients

# CONTENTS

|  | This Guide and How to Use It | 1 |
|---|---|---|
| 1 | Introduction to the Liver | 6 |
| 2 | Introduction to MASLD | 23 |
| 3 | The Causes of MASLD | 35 |
| 4 | Diagnosing and Monitoring MASLD | 66 |
| 5 | Treating MASLD 1: Introduction | 97 |
| 6 | Treating MASLD 2: Diet | 103 |
| 7 | Treating MASLD 3: Exercise | 125 |
| 8 | Treating MASLD 4: Drug Treatment | 141 |
| 9 | Treating MASLD 5: Cirrhosis Management | 156 |
| 10 | Treating MASLD 6: Transplantation | 167 |
| 11 | Symptoms in MASLD | 186 |
| 12 | Living With MASLD | 207 |
| 13 | MASLD in Children | 224 |
| 14 | The Future | 233 |
|  | Appendix 1: A Dictionary of MASLD (with Index) | 243 |
|  | Appendix 2: The Newcastle Approach to Fatigue | 286 |
|  | Appendix 3: Micronutrients | 291 |

# THIS GUIDE AND HOW TO USE IT
## 2ND EDITION

David Jones has been managing adult liver disease for over 30 years at the Freeman Hospital in Newcastle upon Tyne in the UK. His great interest has always been in the way liver disease changes the lives of patients; the symptoms and their impact on quality of life (in particular the fatigue that bedevils so many patients with liver disease); the frustration that many patients feel at the challenge of getting access to up to date treatment in diseases often underestimated by the general medical community (the more so at a time when treatment options are developing rapidly). One of his missions in liver disease, working with the patient groups such as LIVErNORTH who do so much to support patients, has been to help patients and their families understand their disease, and the way that it affects them, better. A thing that has always surprised him is the lack of easily accessible books explaining liver disease, aimed at patients and families, that could be recommended in the clinic.

In 2019, when he began the first book in this series on PBC it was easier to buy a PBC T-shirt than a book explaining the disease! After a working lifetime of talking about the disease in ways that people (hopefully) understand, he always intended to write that book. The book ("PBC; The Definitive Guide for Patients with Primary Biliary Cholangitis) was published in 2020 and the feedback from patients and their families was really positive. It suggested that the book was a real help and filled a long-standing gap. The success of that book, and the ongoing sense of the need for better information to increase awareness about other liver diseases, led him to write the next two books in this series, covering autoimmune hepatitis and primary sclerosing cholangitis.

When the manuscript for the PBC Definitive Guide was half-completed, the world changed with the COVID-19 pandemic. Although the patients that he managed did not appear to be particularly disproportionately impacted (other than when people had end-stage cirrhosis), there was a more subtle consequence. The needs of the emergency clinical service meant that even the best elective clinical services struggled to deliver the same level of care as before to their chronic liver disease patients. The need for patients to be in control of their own destiny, to be able to understand and manage their disease themselves as much as possible, became clear. This made the need for books like these more pressing than ever.

Vanessa Linnett originally trained as a physician before qualifying as an anaesthetist and intensive care consultant. She works at the Queen Elizabeth Hospital in Gateshead in the North East of England. Her work with people often from very deprived communities led to her developing a deep interest in the role played by poor nutrition in adverse health outcomes. As a result of this she has had a long-standing interest in how dietary changes can make a big difference to poor health. Helping people to help themselves. This area of interest naturally led to a focus on obesity and its sequelae such as MASLD.

What people who bought the previous books in the series have told us is that what was most valuable about them was the really practical advice they gave to people about how they could do things, and approach clinicians, in ways that really helped them to improve their condition and reduce its impacts. Put simply, they empowered people. The mantra that has been used in all of the books in the series is "own the problem, own the solution". What we mean by this is that there can be a natural tendency for people with a chronic disease to feel sorry for themselves, putting all their problems down to bad luck and a failure of the system to have better ways to treat them. In fact, in most liver disease, a significant part of the solution lies in the hands of patients themselves, to take steps that will result in improvement in their disease. In PBC, AIH and PSC this was true around seeking better care from healthcare systems, and was certainly true about reducing the impact of symptoms such as fatigue. MASLD takes this aspect of management to a whole new level. In conditions such as PBC, AIH and PSC the fundamental issue is change in the way the immune system works; change which results in liver injury. This aspect of the disease lies beyond the control of patients. Mitigating its impacts can be improved, but the underlying issue can't. Whereas, in MASLD, in contrast, almost every aspect of the disease can be controlled by patients themselves. It truly is the disease where the mantra of owning the problem and owning the solution comes into its own. Owning the problem is all about understanding why things are the way they are, accepting why the problems have arisen and then using that information to make it better.

We took the decision to write a second edition of the book in 2024 for two reasons. The first is, as we will cover in some detail, the decision to change the name of the disease from non-alcoholic fatty liver disease (NAFLD) and its higher risk inflammatory variant non-alcoholic steatohepatitis (NASH) to metabolic dysfunction-associated steatotic liver disease (MASLD) and metabolic dysfunction-associated steatohepatitis (MASH). There were two drivers for this name change. The first was that defining a disease in terms of what didn't cause it (alcohol in this case) was always a little counter intuitive. The second driver was the stigma perceived by patients in relation to inclusion of the word "alcohol" (even though it was an exclusion of alcohol rather than an implication that it played a role) and the word "fatty" (steatotic means the same thing, although it is perhaps a slightly less "blunt" term). This movement to change the name was something of a "déjà vu moment" for us as we were heavily involved in the move to change the name of primary biliary cirrhosis to primary biliary cholangitis a number of years ago (although that name change involved a very deliberate retention of the abbreviation of PBC). Name changes can, however good the rationale behind them, cause confusion, all the more so if there is an abbreviation change as well. We will address this throughout the book to help people who may be confused by the terminology to adapt to the new naming.

The second reason for writing a second edition of the book was the fundamentally important step of the licensing of the first drug for the treatment of MASLD, resmetirom, in spring 2024. We discussed this drug in the first edition of the book, describing it as one of the emerging treatments that showed real promise. That promise has been realised (although it is important to keep in mind that although it is effective it is no cure for MASLD). Experience in other liver disease areas such as hepatitis C and PBC is that the approval of the first new drug in a disease is often followed rapidly by others, leading to treatment options for patients and a rapid acceleration of progress. It is interesting to note that a number of the other drugs described as promising in the first edition have not delivered on that promise and have faded away. We will discuss later in the book what this means for our understanding of drug development and its challenges in MASLD. These "promising but ultimately disappointing" drugs have been replaced by a further set. Time will tell which direction their development goes in.

Before starting on the story of MASLD, we thought it would be helpful to outline the different ways in which you can approach this book. We wrote it with the intention, as was the case with the previous volumes in the series, that people read it as a whole from beginning to end; to tell a story. We have deliberately not referenced specific pieces of the scientific literature as this hinders the readability, and the source material is not readily available to the public. We have, however, attempted to include all current thinking. We hope you, the reader, find it both interesting and helpful. Although the book is mainly aimed at patients, we strongly suggest that you get spouses and relatives to also read it. It will help them understand you and the challenges that you face. It will also be helpful to doctors, nurses and researchers who are coming into MASLD for the first time. In deciding on our approach, it was very clear that there is a balance to be struck between giving all the information that many people want, and avoiding making the book feel either over technical and daunting or "dumbed down". For this reason, at the beginning of most chapters we have included a **Two Minute Version** which summarises the key information in that chapter. The early chapters introducing the liver and MASLD itself provide important background that will help you understand the later chapters that explain how to treat the disease better. Where there is repetition between chapters it is intentional as we are building the story as we go along, and it is important to reinforce certain concepts. If a particular chapter is too much for you then please do read its two minute version before moving on. Alternatively, just reading all the two minute versions in sequence would give you a better knowledge and understanding of MASLD than 90% of doctors!

It is said that a medical student learns, in their first year at university, more new words than a foreign language student does. This means that a number of technical terms are used ("medical jargon" if you like). These terms are introduced in the text the first time they are used and are explained in more detail in an appendix which we have called "A Dictionary of MASLD". Do keep referring to this as it will help you follow the story.

Finally, in the appendix we have also outlined our detailed approach to managing fatigue in patients with liver disease. This outlines the approach taken in the clinic in Newcastle that focuses specifically on symptoms in liver disease. The most significant of these is fatigue, to which we take a very practical approach. This appendix outlines this approach. Any doctor could take this and fully replicate our approach to management. Feel free to share it with your doctors.

**There are two final, really important, points. The first is that the book is designed to be an aid to understanding of the disease. It cannot possibly cover all the scenarios that any individual patient might encounter. It is vital, therefore, that any decisions about your disease and its management are made following discussion with your doctor or nurse. If reading this book makes those discussions easier to have, then we have done our job. The book isn't designed to, and cannot possibly be, a replacement for direct clinical care. The second is that we are adult care doctors and don't look after children with MASLD. There are highly dedicated specialised teams who do this. This is a really important global health challenge with increasing numbers of children and young adults developing the condition. All adult hepatologists are increasingly seeing patients who developed significant MASLD in childhood and who, even as young adults, are already experiencing the complications of advanced liver disease. This book is aimed at people interested in adult MASLD and we couldn't, and shouldn't, try to cover the complex issues around childhood disease in detail. Hopefully one day someone more appropriate than us will write just such an introduction to MASLD for the parents of affected children. We felt, however, that it would have been wrong, given the growing health challenge, to ignore the issue of children with MASLD, the problems they face and the issues as they move through into adult clinical services. We have, therefore, included a short chapter entitled "An Introduction to MASLD in Children". It is just that, an introduction and doesn't attempt to be comprehensive.**

***A Note on Terminology:*** In the first edition of the book we included this "Note on Terminology" to help people with the plethora of terms that were used in the field and the confusion that could result. As outlined above, however, the terminology has, in the short term at least, become more complex still and potentially even more confusing (although over time it is to be hoped that the new terminology comes to be accepted and widely used). One area of real confusion in the topic area covered by this book is terminology. In keeping with the change, we have moved entirely to the new terminology. We will use the term metabolic dysfunction-associated steatotic liver disease (MASLD) to encompass the whole spectrum of metabolic liver disease (the spectrum of disease previously encompassed by the term non-alcoholic fatty liver disease (NAFLD) and sometimes described using other, somewhat less precise, terms such as "fatty liver" and "hepatic steatosis"). We will use the term metabolic dysfunction-associated steatohepatitis (MASH) for the more aggressive inflammatory form of the disease previously known as non-alcoholic steatohepatitis (NASH). We have very deliberately used both the new and the old terms in the title of the book for the simple reason that in order to read this explanation as to the meaning of the new terminology people have to realise that we are talking about the same disease but with different names and buy the book in the first place! We will explore the terminology in more detail in **Chapter 2** as it is actually a really important issue.

A final note on terminology relates to the specialist doctors who look after patients with liver disease. Throughout the book we have used the term "hepatologist", which is a specialist in diseases of the liver and biliary tree. Many people in the UK will have specialist care for MASLD provided by a gastroenterologist, who is a specialist in diseases of the gastrointestinal tract (the bowels) and related organs, including the liver, biliary tree and pancreas. We will use the term hepatologist to cover both these related specialties.

# CHAPTER 1: **INTRODUCTION TO THE LIVER**

### *The 2-Minute Version*

- The liver is one of the largest organs in the body, weighing up to 1.5Kg in adult males. It is located in the upper abdomen on the right hand side, tucked under the rib cage which protects it from injury (it is very soft and easily injured by trauma).
- Its structure is simple (millions of identical cells all doing the same thing) but its function is complex (each of those cells does many different things). This complexity of function is why it has proved very difficult to replace it with a machine.
- Amongst the functions of the liver are **processing** of nutrients taken up from the bowel after meals, **making** proteins including those that control blood clotting, **cleaning** the blood to remove toxins (including bilirubin and by-products of the body functions) and **protecting** the rest of the body against bacteria and other organisms that get out of the bowel and into the blood stream.
- The liver plays a major role in metabolism, controlling many of the processes that are critical for the healthy functioning of the body. Many of these relate to the regulation of energy in the body, processing, converting and in some cases storing, nutrients. An example is control of blood sugar levels by **storing** sugar in the form of glycogen. Dysfunction of these energy-regulating processes lies at the heart of MASLD biology and normalising them is at the heart of control and treatment.
- The liver has two types of blood flow into it (the hepatic artery and the portal vein) and one blood flow out (the hepatic vein). It has a second flow out, that of bile, which is made by the liver and drains out of it via the bile duct which eventually drains into the bowel. The bile drainage system allows those things the body wants to get rid of to be drained safely into the bowel. It also carries bile acids (cholesterol-based molecules made by the liver) into the bowel where they play an essential role in making fat in the diet soluble so the body can handle it.
- The portal vein carries blood from the bowel wall into the liver and is the main route for nutrients from the diet to be taken to the liver for processing.
- The liver can be injured by a number of different things, including infections, drugs and the effects of the immune system. It usually recovers completely after an insult as it has an enormous capacity to re-grow after injury.

- If the liver tries to recover whilst injury is still going on scarring can result. If that scarring becomes extensive, whilst regrowth is still happening, then the result is cirrhosis. This can limit the ability of the liver to work, and can cause a pressure rise in the portal vein. This is the cause of varices, bleeding from which is an important complication of cirrhosis. Prevention is better than treatment, which is why it is particularly important to try and control the causes of liver disease throughout its course.
- Liver diseases fall into two broad groups. These are disease of the liver cells themselves (the hepatocytes) and diseases of the bile duct (cholestatic diseases). MASLD represents a spectrum of liver injury from the benign to the significant and is, fundamentally, a disease of direct hepatocyte injury with its potential consequences of scarring and, eventually, and if not treated appropriately, cirrhosis.

MASLD itself, although part of a broader "family" of linked conditions (the metabolic syndrome) that have very wide-ranging impacts, is primarily a disease of the liver. Before you can fully understand the disease, it is important to understand a little about the liver, how it is structured, how it works and how it impacts on people when it does not function normally. The clinical features seen in MASLD, and in particular in MASH where overt liver injury becomes a real issue, all make sense in the context of how it works (or doesn't work) properly.

## **_THE NORMAL LIVER_**

The liver is an organ that plays a critical role in the healthy functioning of the body. It is one, however, that people tend to know next to nothing about. A few years ago a survey suggested that over 80% of people didn't even know where the liver was in the body, let alone how it functioned.

Unfortunately, the one thing that people do tend to know about the liver is that it is injured directly by alcohol. This is something that has, in essence, nothing to do with MASLD. Alcohol can act as a powerful energy source, adding to the nutritional imbalances that lie at the heart of MASLD (as we will explore in **Chapter 3**; think of going to the pub and drinking 4 pints a night of full sugar fizzy drink and what it would do to your health), but the other injury processes seen with alcohol just aren't there. The assumption by many in society (and, all too often sadly, those in the medical professions) that liver disease and excess alcohol are the same thing can be very unhelpful to patients and their families. By the same token, the word "hepatitis" in the term metabolic associated steatohepatitis (the full version of MASH) can also be very unhelpful because of the, again erroneous, association with viral hepatitis.

The liver is a large organ which is located in the upper abdomen on the right-hand side. The abdominal cavity is a body cavity that contains many key organs, in particular the bowel (stomach, small bowel and large bowel) and the liver. The abdominal cavity is separated from the chest cavity above it by the diaphragm, a muscular sheet which actively moves up and down as part of the breathing process. The diaphragm is domed in shape, meaning that the abdominal cavity extends higher up in the body than people tend to imagine. This is particularly relevant in the case of the liver, which is normally entirely located within the dome of the diaphragm and covered by the lower ribs. This coverage by the ribs is, presumably, to provide protection against trauma to what is, in practice, a very soft and vascular organ which can bleed profusely if injured. The liver is roughly triangular in shape and can weigh up to 1.5Kg in men (and proportionately less in women).

The anatomy of the liver reflects its key role in metabolism (itself key in MASLD), and the structure that it needs to perform that role. It is made up of millions of identical liver cells (hepatocytes), each of which undertakes all of the key liver functions. It is, in essence, a simple structure made up of repeating identical cells, all of which have complex function. This contrasts with the kidney, which has a number of very different cell types performing individual functions, which collectively allow regulation of fluid and salt load in the body (a complex structure performing a simple function). One interesting contrast between the liver and the kidney has been the extent to which function of the organ can be replaced by a mechanical device. Dialysis, in all its forms, is long-established as a replacement therapy for kidney disease. There is, however, no equivalent replacement system for liver disease; something which often surprises both patients and trainee doctors. It is the very complexity of liver function, and the need to replace all missing processes, that means that the liver cannot easily be replaced by anything other than a functioning liver (through recovery of the patient's own liver following failure of the liver or, where needed, transplantation). The, in essence, single function of the kidney makes it far easier to replace it with a mechanical system.

The structure of the liver is simple. Blood flows into it and perfuses the hepatocytes which are organised in sheets. Nutrients, oxygen, and toxins are then taken up from the blood and processed by the hepatocytes. This seemingly simple process, and its imbalances, lies at the absolute heart of MASLD which is a disease of direct and indirect injury to these hepatocytes. At the end of the sheets of hepatocytes, the now "cleaned" and de-oxygenated blood leaves the liver via the hepatic vein, joining the inferior vena cava and being returned to the heart for re-oxygenation by the lungs. The liver is unique as an organ in having two sources of blood entering it (in contrast, the kidney has a single blood flow in through the renal artery and a single flow out through the renal vein). These are the hepatic artery and the portal vein. The hepatic artery arises from the celiac artery, thereby sharing blood supply with the upper bowel. It supplies oxygenated blood to the bile duct in its entirety and contributes to the oxygenation of the liver. The second blood flow into the liver, the portal vein, perfuses the hepatocytes with a blood supply which has drained from the bowel wall. Although partially de-oxygenated (the blood has already perfused the bowel and supplied its necessary oxygen) this flow makes an important contribution to overall liver oxygenation. Critically, however, the outflow from the bowel wall forming the inflow into the liver allows the liver to play its critical role of processing nutritional components absorbed from the bowel.

As well as making, modifying and breaking down molecules taken up from the blood, the hepatocytes need to dispose of residual toxins. This they do by transferring them out of the opposite side of the cell to the one exposed to the blood supply, into spaces called the bile canaliculi. All the bile canaliculi join together to form the small and then large bile ducts (like streams joining together to form a river). The fluid passing through them is called bile. Eventually, ducts from the right and left side of the liver connect to form the common bile duct, which joins the bowel in the duodenum (usually just after being joined by the duct draining the pancreas). The by-products of metabolism, and toxins that the body wants to dispose of are, therefore, drained out into the bowel and exit the body in the stool. The small branches of the two blood supplies into the liver (the hepatic artery and portal vein) are bundled together with the branches of the bile duct. This structure, known as the portal tract, is somewhat akin to an electric 3-core cable and acts as a "service network" present throughout the liver.

Bile performs another essential role unrelated to disposal of toxins. Fat in the diet is not water-soluble, meaning that it will not, in its native form, be absorbed from the diet (it forms fat globules amidst the water-based gut fluid). In order to be solubilised it needs to be dispersed by the actions of a detergent. The natural detergents used by the body to solubilise fat are the bile acids; cholesterol based molecules synthesised by the hepatocytes and transported into the bile for drainage into the bowel. The pancreas produces an enzyme, lipase, which breaks down common fats solubilised by bile acids. Lipase is released into the gut in the pancreatic juice via the pancreatic duct, which, as we have discussed, joins the bile duct at the point where the pancreatic duct joins the bowel in the duodenum. The net result is that fat in the diet is made absorbable by the body. Reduced release of either bile acids or lipase results in a failure of absorption of fat from the diet. This state is called fat malabsorption. Normal absorption of fat from the diet is also important to maintain the levels of a number of key vitamins (vitamin A, vitamin D and vitamin K are fat soluble and pass through the bowel if fat droplets are not dispersed). The effects of fat malabsorption are weight loss, oily and foul-smelling stools, and the effects of shortage of fat-soluble vitamins (including night blindness because of vitamin A shortage, bone disease because of vitamin D shortage and clotting abnormality as a result of vitamin K shortage).

One of the critical roles played by the liver is to act as a buffer between the bowel and the circulation. It balances the needs of nutrition with protection of the body as a whole, from the effects of toxic substances ingested in the diet, some of which have been synthesised by the bacteria which are normally present in the bowel or form part of the breakdown products of those bacteria. Often not thought of as a part of the immune system the liver is, in fact, an important contributor to protecting against, in particular, bacterial infections. Many disease states, including MASLD in its more harmful forms, result in the bowel wall becoming "leaky", allowing the normally harmless (indeed beneficial) bowel bacteria to get into the portal vein. Unchecked, they would get into the wider blood circulation causing sepsis. Enormous numbers of macrophages, cells of the body's protective inflammatory/immune system that "eat" and neutralise bacteria (called, in the context of the liver, Kupffer Cells), are present, aligned to the blood vessels of the liver in a position where they can "consume" any bacteria that get as far as the portal venous inflow into the liver tissue. Where the Kupffer Cells are lost, in the setting of acute liver failure, one of the major risks to life is sepsis because bowel bacteria which get into the portal vein after the bowel wall has become leaky are no longer cleared from the blood.

The liver is essential to clear other toxins and by-products of metabolism produced by the other organs of the body, and to make proteins which are important for body functions. An example of the clearance function is bilirubin, the pigment which, if elevated in the blood, is responsible for jaundice. Bilirubin is a by-product of the breakdown of old red blood cells in the spleen (it is normal for red cells to be "recycled" after around 150 days, with the iron being re-used by the body and the structure that it normally sits in, the haem group, being converted into bilirubin for disposal by the liver). The disposal is an active process. The bilirubin is conjugated (in essence "tagged for disposal") and then transported out into the bile. If this process is disrupted through a failure to conjugate bilirubin, or because of a blockage of the flow of bile, then levels of bilirubin build up in the liver cells and leak back into the blood. The yellow colouring of the bilirubin then gives rise to the clinical appearance of jaundice. Levels of bilirubin in the blood can be measured easily, and are one of the clinical tests that are used to monitor liver diseases. Bilirubin is just one of a number of toxic substances that the liver needs to be able to clear. It is, however, the easiest to see and measure. Best thought of as body "poisons", when they build up in liver failure they can give rise to a toxic state (internal poisoning if you like) which is exemplified by hepatic encephalopathy, a state of brain toxicity beginning with confusion and sleep disturbance and leading eventually to coma. Amongst the other functions of the liver that are essential for healthy life are

- **Conversion of glucose into and out of its storage form - glycogen:** This occurs when glucose levels are high in the portal vein after a meal and is in response to insulin released by specialised cells in the pancreas (the Islets of Langerhans). The liver plays a key role in "smoothing out" blood sugar levels from very high peaks after meals to very low in between meals. When the glucose level falls between meals glycogen is broken down again, releasing glucose from the liver (and muscle where glycogen is also present) to boost the dietary-derived level. Patients with failure of their liver often have very abnormal blood glucose levels. These are typically very low because such patients often have a low dietary intake as a result of the low-grade sense of nausea which is common in people with liver disease.

- **Metabolic function:** The term metabolic function refers to the key processes of body metabolism whereby energy is generated to fuel the cells. In addition to the key metabolic function of glucose regulation, many of the body's other key metabolic processes also take place within the hepatocytes. Most of the inborn errors of metabolism (genetic diseases in which specific metabolic processes are abnormal) are thus expressed in the liver. An example is hereditary oxalosis, a genetic disease in which oxalic acid builds up in the blood and causes kidney failure (oxalic acid is also present in high levels in the leaves of rhubarb plants and is the reason why the leaves, in contrast to the stalks, must not be eaten). Although the tissue injury in hyper-oxalosis is entirely to the kidney, the defect causing oxalic acid build-up is exclusively expressed in the liver. Kidney transplant is rapidly followed by loss of the new kidney unless accompanied by liver transplant which corrects the underlying abnormality.
- **Protein synthesis:** Almost all of the proteins that the body makes for release into the circulation are produced in part or entirely by the hepatocytes. These include clotting factors (the proteins needed for the blood to clot) and albumin (a blood protein which is essential for the transport of bilirubin etc in the circulation). Albumin in the circulation also plays a key role in regulating tissue fluid levels, exerting oncotic pressure and drawing fluid from the tissues back into circulation. When albumin levels fall in liver disease it is a major contributor to tissue oedema or swelling, including the collection of fluid in the abdominal cavity (ascites).
- **Immune/inflammatory function:** Although seldom thought of as a key part of the body's protection against infection the liver is, as outlined above, a key component of the immune system. In addition to the "filter" role played by the Kupffer Cells it also produces key protective proteins called defensins which are directly anti-bacterial. The liver is also the site of the breakdown of lymphocytes, key white blood cells, after they have performed their typically anti-viral functions. The importance of the liver in infection control is indicated by the high level of infection risk seen in patients with liver failure.
- **Cholesterol and steroid hormone metabolism:** The liver plays a key role in the control of lipid levels in the body; a role that is integral to the pathogenesis of MASLD and, perhaps less obviously, hepatitis C infection (where the virus gains entry into the hepatocyte through lipoprotein receptors). The liver is responsible for the synthesis of around 80% of the cholesterol made by the body. Something that surprises many people is that the vast majority of our cholesterol is

made by the body, and not taken up from the diet. Cholesterol is a completely normal thing to have in the blood and is, indeed, really important for normal body function. This is something which, again, surprises people given the association between high cholesterol and heart disease. A proportion of the cholesterol made in the liver is converted into bile acids; molecules which, as we have discovered, play an integral role in the absorption of fat from the diet. Bile acids synthesised by the hepatocytes and released into the bile are then taken up again in the ileum (the far end of the small bowel) and returned to the liver via the portal circulation. This "entero-hepatic circulation" means that the vast majority of bile acids are recycled rather than being lost in the stool. It also, however, exposes the bile acid pool to the environment, including the bacteria that normally colonise parts of the bowel. Bile acids can be modified during their passage through the bowel to form secondary and tertiary bile acids with subtly different physical properties to the newly synthesised primary bile acids. In addition to cholesterol metabolism the liver also plays a key role in the breakdown of steroid hormones (hormones which are themselves derived from cholesterol, examples of which include cortisol, oestrogen and testosterone). This can have impacts ranging from failure to break down aldosterone (a hormone that regulates salt and fluid levels in the body, build-up of which leads to fluid retention and ascites) to retention of oestrogen which can lead to development of feminine features such as breast development; something seen in particular in people with alcoholic cirrhosis.

## *LIVER DISEASE: AN OVERVIEW*

Disease of the liver is a common and growing problem in all populations. There are two broad forms of liver disease; those in which the target for injury is the hepatocytes themselves (examples include, obviously, MASLD, as well as viral hepatitis and alcohol-related liver disease), and those where the target for injury is the cells lining the bile duct (the biliary epithelial cells (BEC) or cholangiocytes). MASLD is a disease of injury to the hepatocytes, with the clinical features of the condition arising either directly or indirectly from that injury. BEC injury can also be seen in MASLD patients and, in some people, can contribute to the clinical picture of the disease, including itch and, potentially, fatigue.

In all hepatocellular diseases, clinical problems arise from the combined effects of the injury to hepatocytes and the response of the body to that injury. Depending on the disease type there can also be clinical features related to the non-liver impacts of the underlying disease cause and to the treatment for the disease. In a condition such as alcohol-related liver disease, many of the clinical issues experienced by patients relate to the many effects of alcohol on the organs of the body other than the liver. By the same token, the clinical picture in MASLD is frequently very complex indeed with the cumulative impacts of the liver component, the other aspects of the metabolic syndrome such as type 2 diabetes and cardiac disease and the side-effects of the treatments used for all these components.

When hepato-cellular injury first begins in liver disease there is no clinical impact. This often surprises people. It is a direct result of the "spare capacity" that we have in-built in to our livers to allow the body to cope with the unexpected (a major infection, consuming poisons in the diet, major injury etc). In all these cases, the liver will be needed to "clean up". If the liver were to be overwhelmed every time an event such as this took place it would be highly detrimental. In practice, the liver has about three to four times the capacity it needs to "tick over"; something which has proved very useful in allowing us to surgically remove cancers from the liver and even, as we will discuss in **Chapter 10**, use a section of a healthy person's liver to transplant into a liver disease patient. This prolonged period of low-grade impact without apparent clinical consequences, before more aggressive injury takes hold, is absolutely the pattern in MASLD with early fat deposition in hepatocytes ("simple steatosis") being very common indeed. It is the subsequent development of inflammation in the context of MASH that accelerates liver injury and is the beginning of progressive liver disease.

The liver also has another important property that is crucial in allowing it to cope with disease. It can regenerate following injury. This is achieved through the division of cells (both the hepatocytes themselves and "stem cells" whose sole function is to replenish the liver with cells). In essence, this process is ongoing, giving rise to an increasing number of cells until the liver size needed for the body is achieved. The way the body achieves this is simple and very clever. The cells in the body outside the liver produce a molecule called hepatocyte growth factor that "tells" the cells of the liver to divide and increase their number. Hepatocyte growth factor is, however, broken down by the hepatocytes. When the liver reaches the correct size for the body, the level of breakdown of hepatocyte growth factor by the enlarged liver matches its production by the cells of the body and the stimulus to grow is, in essence, switched off. The capacity of the liver to regrow in this way has undoubted natural survival advantages, as well as properties that we as doctors can make use of. It has, however, one important downside. As we will discuss at length later, if this regeneration takes place in the context of liver scarring it contributes to the development of cirrhosis; the end stage of the progression of liver injury. The prevention of cirrhosis development is a key aspect of the management of MASLD, as it is for all forms of chronic liver disease.

The natural survival advantage resulting from the capacity of the liver to regrow is clear. If hepatocytes are damaged by an infection (such as hepatitis A infection) or, in the context of MASLD, by a combination of cell distortion because of fat deposition within the cell (and then inflammation in MASH), it means that the lost cells can be replaced once the acute event is over, meaning that the liver returns to its full, natural size within a matter of weeks or, at most, months. Without this recovery capacity, each infection or other event that damaged the liver would further reduce the amount of liver reserve until there was insufficient left for life.

The properties that clinicians can take advantage of follow on naturally from the observations made earlier about liver reserve. If a proportion of the liver is removed, either because it has a cancer within it, or it is going to be used as a donor organ for someone needing a liver transplant, the remaining liver will regrow until it returns to its original size (although not the same structure and shape).

Once hepatocyte loss becomes significant, the clinical features of acute liver injury become apparent. Loss of hepatocyte function is one important component of liver injury, and thus liver disease. The other major component is the effects of the body's response to that injury. In practice, the majority of the problems encountered in long-term liver conditions relate more to the nature of this response than to the initial injury process. All initial liver injuries give rise to one or both of two cardinal responses; necrosis of the hepatocytes and apoptosis. Necrosis can be thought of as a traumatic, or disorderly, form of cell death (a messy death). Apoptosis is an orderly form of cell death (a clean death) in which a cell folds in on itself. It packages itself up for disposal if you like. Necrosis is the type of injury associated with burns or acid injury. Apoptosis is the mechanism of injury seen in response to an immune response (clearance of a cell infected by a virus for example). In both situations, there is a negative consequence from the loss of the cell and, if enough liver cells are lost, liver failure. To this, necrosis, but importantly not apoptosis, adds the negative effects of the cells falling apart, releasing irritant cell contents into the local environment. In a skin burn, where necrosis is a key process, much of the pain and reddening of the skin is a direct result of local inflammation worsened by the effects of necrosed cells. If cell injury continues over a long period of time, then a third form of cell injury can come into play; senescence. The role played by this process in MASLD, and its potential as a treatment target, is only just beginning to be understood.

Paradoxically, given that this book is focused on the long-term effects of liver injury, most episodes of such injury actually result in complete recovery. The damaged and dying cells are cleaned up by the macrophages, and the hepatocytes and their stem cells begin to divide and proliferate to replace the cells that have been lost. If the degree of hepatocyte injury becomes too great, then the clinical features of liver failure will begin to emerge. These are, in simple terms, the effects of the loss of the functions of the liver outlined above, especially where change in function level can have short-term effects. These include problems with:

- **Conversion of glucose into and out of its storage form glycogen.** If hepatocyte function is reduced, then this important glucose "buffering" effect is lost. Glucose levels in the blood can rise rapidly after eating (because glycogen isn't being made in the hepatocyte), and then fall sharply between meals. Given that patients with acute liver injury often feel nauseated, and thus can struggle to eat, it is far commoner to see issues around low blood glucose than high.

- **Metabolic function:** This is one of the key areas of impact when liver function is impaired. The capacity of the liver to detoxify, modify and eliminate potentially harmful chemicals is reduced, leading to build up in the body. The most obvious manifestation of this is the build-up of bilirubin, leading to jaundice, a very visual expression of disease. At a general level, the build-up of harmful molecules can cause two important and interlinked problems. The first is to cause impaired function of the brain. This is known as hepatic encephalopathy, and it can complicate liver dysfunction of all types. Encephalopathy usually starts with very subtle changes in personality. These can be so subtle as to only be noticeable by a close family member who knows the patient well. This can be accompanied by alterations in the day/night cycle, with patients being sleepy during the day and wide awake at night. As it worsens there is a more generalised reduction in conscious level with, for example, people drifting off to sleep during conversations. Eventually, unconsciousness and coma can follow. The second toxic state is the effect that harmful chemicals which the liver is no longer able to clear can have on the blood vessels. The blood vessels play an important part in maintaining our blood pressure (and thereby the blood flow to the brain). The heart pumps blood around the body, but there needs to be tone or tension in the arteries to allow the pressure of the heartbeat to push blood around the arteries. In the toxic state of liver failure the arteries are to a degree "poisoned" and can lose their tone. This means that blood pressure falls, and oxygen can fail to reach the tissues. This can have significant effects on the organs of the body not getting adequate levels of oxygen. In addition to the key metabolic function of glucose regulation many of the body's other key metabolic processes also take place within the hepatocytes. Most of the inborn errors of metabolism, genetic diseases in which specific metabolic processes are abnormal, are thus expressed in the liver. An example mentioned previously is hereditary oxalosis.

- **Protein synthesis:** Impaired protein manufacture by the liver manifests itself, in particular, in three important ways. The first is the reduced production of proteins that are important in fighting infection. This contributes to the risk of infections seen in liver failure. The second is through reduced production of albumin which is, as we have discussed, essential for keeping fluid "in the right place" in the body, in particular preventing excessive amounts building up in the tissues. When this effect is lost, we see swelling of tissues such as the ankles and the collection of fluid in the abdomen (ascites). The third effect is through reduced production of clotting factors. These are an important part of the system that leads to blood clotting (along with the platelets, tiny cells in the blood which clump together contributing to clot formation) and are largely made in the liver. Reduced liver function can lead to a rapid decrease (within hours) and an increase in bleeding risk. The other important aspect to protein clotting factors is that their function can be measured in simple blood tests. Warfarin, the blood-thinning tablet, works by blocking the same clotting factors and the tests done to monitor its levels are also, therefore, useful in assessing liver failure.
- **Immune/inflammatory function:** One of the major risks to patients with liver failure is from infection, in particular from bacteria and yeasts which get into the blood. An important source of these is the bowel. As we have discussed, bacteria and yeast are normally prevented from crossing the bowel wall by its "leakproof" properties. These result from the cells of the bowel lining being tightly bound together. If bacteria or yeast do cross the bowel wall, and get into the portal vein carrying blood from the bowel to the liver, the liver takes on important immune functions through the actions of its Kupffer cells and the proteins it produces. All these protective functions are damaged in liver failure. The cells lining the bowel become less tightly bound together (as a result of the toxins present in the blood that are not being cleared by the liver), the Kupffer cells are impaired in their function (or even lost altogether) and the liver cells no longer produce their defensive proteins. Taken together, these effects all significantly increase the risk of bacteria and yeast entering the portal vein and getting past the liver and into the general circulation where they can cause sepsis. One of the effects of sepsis is to reduce blood pressure (it causes the blood vessels to open up, meaning that the blood volume, which is largely fixed, is no longer large enough to fill the circulation effectively) which exacerbates the metabolic effects of liver failure and the risks

to the brain. This exemplifies one of the real challenges of liver failure which is the extent to which all the complications make all the others worse. It really is a series of interlinked vicious cycles.

Regeneration is a property which is almost unique to the liver amongst solid organs, and one which is quite dramatically effective. If half the liver is removed to treat a cancer, then within 3-6 months the liver will have regrown to an identical size to that seen before the operation. It is because of the potential to regenerate that the key first part of treating someone with acute liver failure is to support them by reducing the impact of injury, in order to buy enough time to let the liver recover. Time really is everything. The problem arises if the injury is ongoing and, particularly, if necrosis is a prominent component. Where injury is ongoing the "clean-up" process becomes overwhelmed, and the body is continually exposed to injured or dying cells. In all organs, chronic injury ultimately results in the formation of scar tissue (or fibrosis as it is known technically). This represents the body's attempt to "wall off" injured or infected tissues that it can't control or replace. Scar formation ranges in its impact. In the skin it is unsightly and in a joint it can reduce mobility. Important but not life-threatening. In organs, however, it can significantly reduce function. In lung fibrosis oxygen transport into the blood is reduced and in kidney fibrosis the kidneys malfunction. What about liver fibrosis?

The issues that arise with liver fibrosis depend entirely on the degree, or stage, of the fibrosis. In mild or early fibrosis the impact can be minimal or even non-existent. The reason for this is the simple structure of the liver compared to other organs. As we have discussed, to function the kidney needs to have a complex structure with all aspects of that structure functioning. The basic functional unit of the kidney is called the nephron. This includes a complex structure of cells that first filters fluid out of the blood. That fluid is then concentrated by kidney tubules before collecting into the ureter. The key thing is that each nephron is formed of thousands of cells and the whole structure needs to be intact for the nephron to work. The liver is very different. The basic unit is a single hepatocyte. Each one can do all the functions of the liver. Provided the liver has enough hepatocytes, they are individually healthy, have an adequate blood supply and can drain bile, then the liver will function. Fibrosis in the liver can, depending on the nature and severity of the liver injury, surround the portal tracts, surround the hepatic vein branches or link (bridge) between the portal tracts. Initially, there is no disruption to hepatocyte numbers, blood flow or bile outflow, meaning that in early fibrosis, liver function is normal. The issues arise when the architecture around blood supply and bile flow becomes distorted, typically by bridging fibrosis. As hepatocytes become replaced by scar tissue, so the numbers fall to the point where the normal level of reserve function is lost.

The tipping point is usually when the bridging becomes complete, resulting in areas of hepatocytes becoming walled off by fibrotic tissue. As outlined above, the liver has the capacity to regenerate when hepatocyte numbers are sensed to be insufficient. Where bridging fibrosis is present, the proliferation takes place within a rigid sphere which puts pressure on the cells and the blood supply. This combination of advanced linking fibrosis and proliferation is known as cirrhosis.

At present, there are no therapies that are able to remove fibrosis once it is established (although research and trials are ongoing). The management of cirrhosis, therefore, falls into three phases. The first is to attempt to prevent it from developing in the first place by preventing the chronic liver damage that predisposes to fibrosis. This requires effective, and timely, use of therapy (which in the case of MASLD includes lifestyle changes such as diet and exercise and the emerging drug therapies) to slow, stop and reverse the underlying disease process. There have been major advances in this aspect in a number of liver disease in recent years, most notably viral hepatitis and autoimmune liver disease (although the picture with relation to therapy in MASLD is much more complex). The second phase is, if prevention has not been possible, to manage the complications of cirrhosis that can place the patient at risk. These are outlined in the next section. The third is to consider liver transplantation. Complication management and transplantation have major limitations to them. This means that, for the future, our efforts must be directed at better therapies for underlying disease. If, however, these treatments don't work, or people only present once cirrhosis is present (something that happens more frequently than you might imagine) then effective cirrhosis management becomes essential.

## *CIRRHOSIS AND ITS COMPLICATIONS*

Much of the speciality of hepatology used to be focused on identifying and managing the complications of cirrhosis. The focus is now shifting to identifying liver disease earlier in its course, and treating the underlying processes to prevent fibrosis and cirrhosis from developing in the first place. There will always, however, be people who have one of the forms of liver disease for which disease modification is not yet available, people who don't respond to treatment and people who present late in the disease when cirrhosis is already established. For this reason understanding cirrhosis and how to manage it remains of the utmost importance in hepatology

The clinical complications of cirrhosis reflect a variable combination of two processes. The first of these is impaired liver function; an inadequate amount of liver functional capacity to perform the normal liver roles because of hepatocyte loss through their replacement by fibrotic tissue, and the adverse environment within the cirrhotic nodules. The second is portal hypertension, an elevation in the blood pressure within the portal vein because of the impaired flow through the cirrhotic nodules. The specific complications of cirrhosis that we manage in practice are as follows.

**Porto-systemic varices:** This is the complication of cirrhosis that worries patients and clinicians the most. This is because of the risk of bleeding. Varices arise when the pressure builds up in the portal vein as a result of the obstruction to free flow of portal venous blood through the disrupted structure of a cirrhotic liver; this is called portal hypertension. This must be distinguished from the completely different arterial hypertension which often gets shortened to just "hypertension", which is very common indeed in the population (especially, confusingly, in the MASLD population where metabolic syndrome is such an issue) and which has nothing to do with the liver! Increased pressure in the portal vein leads to opening of alternative ways for the blood to flow; typically blood vessels that were open pre-birth (when blood flow patterns are very different) but which normally close soon after birth. They never, however, completely disappear. When they open up as a result of the increase in portal vein pressure they do so with quite thin walls. This, combined with the high pressure in the portal vein, makes them prone to bleeding. They can be found anywhere in the abdominal cavity and bowel wall, but are classically seen at the base of the oesophagus (the gullet) where it meets the stomach. Bleeding from these oesophageal varices is perhaps the archetypal complication of cirrhosis of all aetiologies. Although varices are predominantly a manifestation of portal hypertension, liver failure can complicate the process through reduced production of the clotting factors that the body needs to form clot and stop bleeding. Although in the vast majority of cases portal hypertension arises in cirrhosis because of the issues around flow through cirrhotic nodules, it can, in some forms of liver disease, arise in non-cirrhotic disease. This means that the presence of varices does not automatically mean liver disease has progressed to cirrhosis (although this is, in practice, usually the case). When varices bleed, the flow rate can be very high. This is an out and out medical emergency. The techniques to prevent bleeding in the first place, and to control it when it occurs are, however, very effective and will be discussed in **Chapter 9.**

**Ascites:** Ascites is the name given for collection of fluid within the peritoneal cavity (the abdominal space). This is another feature of portal hypertension, although, as with varices, liver failure can contribute to the process through reduced protein synthesis. Ascites is made worse if the blood levels of albumin are low, as these proteins play a key role in keeping the fluid in the vessels rather than it leaking out into the abdominal space. Lowered albumin levels are a feature of liver disease of all types, and the reason why albumin forms part of the liver function blood test panel. Ascites causes two problems for patients. The first is that it can be uncomfortable (as well as unsightly) and can hinder breathing when people lie flat (it wedges the diaphragm, which is key for breathing when lying flat, preventing it from moving normally and ventilating the lungs). It can also hinder mobility because of the sheer weight of the fluid. The second problem comes from the complication of ascites becoming infected (spontaneous bacterial peritonitis or SBP). This is usually as a result of bowel bacteria finding their way across the bowel wall, typically in patients who are malnourished. SBP causes the ascites to grow in volume quickly, and there can be abdominal pain. It is also a cause for sudden deterioration in liver function tests as the infection places a significant additional strain on the liver.

**Hepatocellular carcinoma (HCC):** This is a primary cancer of the hepatocytes. It can complicate chronic liver disease of all types and it is emerging to be a really significant issue in some forms of MASLD. A driver for its development is the proliferation of the hepatocytes seen in cirrhosis. When cells of any type proliferate on a continual basis it leaves them open to "going rogue" and escaping from the body's normal control systems. This is a key predisposing step to the development of cancer. HCC is particularly common in viral hepatitis (especially hepatitis B) because of the additional pro-cancerous effects of the virus. HCC is always commoner in men then in women. HCC is unusual amongst cancers in that we largely know who is at risk of getting it (patients with cirrhosis). This allows us to watch for it, allowing early treatment. If it is left unchecked it will progress, growing and metastasising as most cancers do.

**Organ failure:** Over time, the functional capacity of cirrhotic livers usually deteriorates to the point where there is insufficient function for the needs of the body. This is the clinical state of liver failure. There can, on top of this underlying trend of decline in function over time, be acute deteriorations in liver function as a result of episodes of complication such as a variceal bleed or SBP, as well as with intercurrent illnesses unrelated to the liver; all processes which place additional stress on an already struggling liver. The state of liver failure is indicated by rising bilirubin, the onset of encephalopathy (see the next section), falling blood glucose (the liver can no longer buffer sugar) and clotting problems (the liver no longer makes enough clotting factors).

**Hepatic encephalopathy:** Hepatic encephalopathy, as introduced above, is a toxic brain state caused by retention of chemicals by the poorly functioning liver that collect and then impair brain function. It is, perhaps, the archetypal feature of cirrhosis caused by hepatocellular disease. Where it occurs, it is normally as part of a liver failure picture with other features dominating. It is characterised by cloudy thinking and difficulty in concentrating, sleep disturbance and, eventually, coma.

# CHAPTER 2: **INTRODUCTION TO MASLD**

### *The 2-Minute Version*

- The population frequency of metabolic dysfunction-associated steatotic liver disease (MASLD, previously known as non-alcoholic fatty liver disease (NAFLD)) is rising rapidly in most countries of the world, with the highest rates seen in the most affluent countries.
- It represents a spectrum of disease, ranging from the simple, and probably relatively harmless, deposition of fat within the liver cells in the absence of other processes (called simple steatosis), through to fat deposition with inflammation (called steatohepatitis) and, eventually, scarring (fibrosis) and the development of cirrhosis with its complications. The progression of disease can be summarised as: healthy cells ↔ steatosis ↔ steatohepatitis ↔ fibrosis → cirrhosis
- The earlier stages in the process can be reversed with lifestyle change, which can reduce or remove the fat from liver cells.
- MASLD is strongly linked to conditions such as obesity, type 2 diabetes mellitus, hypertension, hypercholesterolaemia and hypertension. There is a strong link to ischaemic heart disease through the latter disease associations. The combination of MASLD with these other conditions is called the metabolic syndrome. The complexity of the condition associations means that the risks to health in MASLD patients go well beyond just liver disease.
- Resistance to the actions of insulin lies at the heart of the metabolic syndrome. MASLD is, therefore, best thought of as arising as a consequence of a failure of normal metabolic pathways. Glucose taken up in the diet, and which would normally be converted into the storage form glycogen under the control of insulin is, instead, converted into fat droplets in the liver cells.
- Fat, both in the liver and elsewhere in the body, is pro-inflammatory, causing the release of chemicals such as cytokines and free radicals that can damage the liver cells. It is the combination of fat deposition and inflammation that drives the cycle of inflammation and tissue repair that lies at the heart of MASLD.
- MASLD has its impact on the lives of patients in two distinct ways. These are progressive liver damage leading, eventually, to the development of cirrhosis and chronic liver failure, and systemic symptoms such as fatigue which can develop at any point in the

disease course. Quality of life can be a major issue for MASLD patients, and one that is often neglected by clinicians.
- MASLD can develop at any point in life and is increasingly being seen in children and young adults. This is a reflection of the rapid rise in childhood obesity which is being seen in many populations. Significant MASLD can have a major impact on the life chances of children.

More than is the case for any other liver disease, it is really important to "set the scene" in MASLD before diving into the detail of causes, diagnosis and treatment. There are several reasons for this. The first and most important is that in terms of the history of medicine, and our understanding of disease, MASLD is a real newcomer. One of us remembers giving a lecture to GPs around 25 years ago on the topic of "what GPs need to know about liver disease". This focused on alcohol, viral hepatitis and the other forms of liver disease that we have known about for a long time. Fatty liver disease (MASLD as we know it today) was included in a slide of "things that you will hear about but don't need to worry about". How wrong that was in retrospect.

MASLD has, in fact, emerged as a major, if not *the* major, form of chronic liver disease in western populations. How do we explain such a rapid and dramatic change in disease patterns over the last quarter century? There are two potential explanations. The first is that it was always there, its just that we didn't recognise it for the problem it is. The presence of fat in the liver on ultrasound scans has been reported since ultrasound first became available, but for many years it was thought just to be an obesity feature unrelated to actual liver injury. We now know that this isn't the case. We have also, for many years, known that there is a group of patients developing chronic liver disease for reasons that were not understood. This group were labelled as having "cryptogenic liver disease" (a name which in essence says it is a liver disease where we don't know the cause!). In retrospect, it is likely that many of these people had one of the more severe forms of what we now know to be MASLD. The second explanation is, of course, that this is genuinely becoming a much commoner problem. It is likely that both factors come into play.

If MASLD is becoming much commoner, why might this be the case? The obvious answer is the increase in obesity in our population (and the nutritional factors that lie behind it). In simple terms, we are, as a society, becoming more overweight. Data from the USA show that the increase in obesity rates is followed, entirely predictably in terms of timing, by an increase in MASLD. This was initially seen in adults, but the same trend is now, worryingly, also being seen in children. This is really storing up problems for the future. The increase in obesity has reasonably predictable causes; we eat more than we used to, and we do less exercise. There is also, as we will explore in later chapters, another, more subtle influence, which is the nature of what we eat and drink. It is likely that there are specific elements in our diet that particularly drive the development of MASLD. Understanding and modifying diet and exercise is a really critical aspect of living with, and beating, MASLD.

The link between MASLD and obesity (and it is a link rather than a direct connection; many people who are overweight don't develop significant

MASLD and there are certainly people with MASLD who are not overweight) lies at the very heart of one of the really critical aspects to MASLD, which is that it almost never exists in isolation. Instead, it is part of a complex series of linked clinical problems which frequently co-exist, and which need to be thought about, and treated as, a whole, rather than in isolation. This is the metabolic syndrome.

## *THE METABOLIC SYNDROME AND MASLD*

"The Metabolic Syndrome" is a term in common usage to describe the presence, in combination, of some or all of MASLD, type 2 diabetes mellitus (the adult-onset form of diabetes rather than the form that develops typically in childhood), obesity, ischaemic heart disease, hypertension and raised blood cholesterol. The nature of the inter-relationship of the components is complex, with an element of cause and effect. At the heart of the syndrome is the combination of type 2 diabetes and MASLD, which do appear to be closely linked in terms of risk factors and mechanism (ischaemic heart disease may be, in contrast, a consequence of the presence of other "syndrome" components).

The concept of the metabolic syndrome is important in practice for three reasons. The first is that it tells us important things about why people develop MASLD in the first place, which will increasingly guide us in relation to how to treat MASLD better. We will expand on this in the next paragraph, and in the next chapter. The second is that it potentially gives us an "early warning" about the development of MASLD. In simple terms, we know who is at risk of it and therefore where to look for the problem in practice. Earlier diagnosis will, in all probability, lie at the heart of better treatment in the future, and knowing which people are at risk is a major opportunity. The third important reason why metabolic syndrome really matters is, in many ways, the most challenging. It is the fact that people with MASLD almost never have that condition in isolation. It is accompanied by one or more other related metabolic conditions. This means that the clinical problem set in MASLD patients is almost always complex. Several problems coming together to cause risk to life and, importantly, symptoms. This matters because a treatment for one component of the metabolic syndrome may well be compromised by another component, limiting treatment options. For example, liver transplant (an approach to the treatment of advanced MASLD) can be made significantly more risky by significant obesity and may be precluded altogether by ischaemic heart disease. There have also been major issues with cardiac risk with some of the drugs which have been tried for both type 2 diabetes and fatty liver. What this all means in practice is that we can never look at, and think about, MASLD in isolation. It needs to be thought of in the round.

The two cardinal processes in the metabolic syndrome, MASLD and type 2 diabetes, share an important underlying process which is probably at the heart of the syndrome. They are both characterised by abnormal handling of the nutrients that are taken up in the diet. To understand the issues that might be arising it is helpful to think of the "life" of a sugary drink that someone might drink on a hot day.

The sucrose in the drink (sucrose is the technical name for the type of sugar which is present in food and drink) is rapidly split into two smaller sugar molecules (one glucose and one fructose molecule) through the actions of an enzyme called sucrase which is released by the cells lining the small bowel wall. The glucose and fructose are then taken up across the small bowel wall and enter the portal vein. The uptake happens very rapidly, leading to a "spike" in the level of glucose in the portal vein which delivers blood to the liver. This glucose spike stimulates specialised cells in the pancreas to release the hormone insulin. Insulin plays a critical role in how the body handles glucose (amongst other things). In simple terms, it controls the "smoothing out" of the glucose levels, lowering the very high levels seen immediately after you have drunk that sugary drink by stimulating storage of glucose in cells; glucose that can then be released between drinks when the glucose level plummets to ensure that the glucose level isn't too low (something that the brain doesn't like!). The main store for glucose is a complex carbohydrate molecule called glycogen which is found in the liver (and skeletal muscle). In type 1 diabetes (the type that typically develops in children and young adults) the specialised insulin-producing cells are damaged by the immune system, meaning that insulin production is reduced, and then stops altogether. The immediate short-term effect of that is for glucose levels to increase rapidly as the lack of insulin precludes the uptake of glucose into liver and muscle cells and conversion into glycogen. Insulin injections restore the capacity to convert glucose into glycogen.

How does this life cycle of a sugary drink change in people with MASLD? At the heart of the problem is a process called insulin resistance. This is a state where the insulin response to a glucose spike is normal, but there is a failure of the body to respond appropriately. The lack of an effective insulin signal then causes glucose to continue to rise. The body responds to this by triggering an alternative energy storage pathway to replace glycogen synthesis, which can't take place because the insulin signal isn't getting through. This is the formation of fat in the cells of the liver. High levels of fat synthesis in the liver because of prolonged insulin resistance gives rise to MASLD in the form (initially at least) of simple steatosis (the deposition of fat in liver cells without any additional complicating processes).

Initially, in an insulin resistance state, the liver has the capacity to "soak up" the glucose that can't be converted to glycogen though fat formation. This means that, initially at least, glucose levels in the general circulation remain largely normal. There comes a point, however, where the liver's capacity to soak up glucose is saturated, and glucose is then released into the general circulation. A good analogy for this is a tap dripping into a sink with a plug in it. For a long time, there is no water spilling onto the floor. This isn't because the tap isn't dripping, it is because the sink can hold the water. This is the capacity of the liver to soak up excess glucose in the form of fat. Eventually, the sink (or liver) is full and the water (or glucose) spills over. This is type 2 diabetes, a form of diabetes resulting almost entirely from insulin resistance. This pathway, of course, instantly explains why MASLD and type 2 diabetes go together in the metabolic syndrome. They share the same underlying issue of insulin resistance.

## *LIVER INJURY IN MASLD*

Although part of a much larger complex of clinical issues, MASLD is, fundamentally, a disease of injury to the liver cells or hepatocytes, with clinical features of the disease arising as a consequence of that injury and/or the body's response to it.

There are two main drivers of liver cell injury in MASLD, steatosis (fat deposition) itself, and steatosis with inflammation, which combine in the more aggressive forms of the disease, as steatohepatitis. Liver injury can then be followed by scar formation in the form of fibrosis and, ultimately, cirrhosis. The progression of disease can be summarised as:

**healthy cells ↔ steatosis ↔ steatohepatitis ↔ fibrosis → cirrhosis**

The clinical features of the disease reflect the balance of these processes at any one time, and each presents a potential target for treatment; something that we will describe in detail in later chapters. One thing that will emerge as a really important issue is the need to get the sequencing of treatment right. In simple terms, steatosis needs treatment for steatosis, steatohepatitis inflammation needs treatment for inflammation and fibrosis needs treatment for fibrosis. As we discussed in the previous chapter, hepatologists have, historically, tended to focus on identifying people with advanced fibrosis and cirrhosis and managing that (largely through screening for and mitigating the complications of cirrhosis). The direction of travel in modern hepatology is, however, earlier diagnosis and appropriate treatment to stop the stages progressing, and ideally to reverse them, with the goal of never needing to manage cirrhosis. This will clearly benefit patients in the long term, but it does need a different approach in the here and now.

**Steatosis:** Fat deposition in the cells of the liver is the starting point for injury in MASLD (and therefore, logically, the first target for treatment; if there is no more fat in the liver in someone with early MASLD, and no additional features such as inflammation, there is no disease). It is important to say that fat deposition in hepatocytes does not cause significant injury per se. Many people have fat in their liver cells. This used to be called "simple steatosis" with the word simple being in the medical sense of "with nothing else" (i.e. inflammation). There can be some metabolic dysfunction in cells (they aren't being fuelled correctly) and certainly physical distortion can alter the way cells and the whole liver functions (in essence the fat droplets that form in the cells alter the shape of both the cell and the whole organ). This can lead to abnormality in liver blood tests (related, as we will outline in **Chapter 4,** to low grade liver damage rather than a failure of liver function) and abdominal discomfort as the liver capsule is stretched by an expanding liver (often the first sign of the presence of the condition) but rarely more than that. What is critical to the conversion of an abnormal, but tolerable, state into a high risk one is the development of inflammation.

**Steatohepatitis:** Inflammation is the natural body response to any form of injury and is part of the recovery process. Injured cells are cleared so they can be replaced, and the tissue returned to normal. The state of inflammation (which is a non-specific one, responding to the presence of injury in the tissue whatever its cause) also triggers the development of the specific immune response (the response that fights particular infections and which gives rise to the long-term immunological memory that underpins vaccination). In the case of MASLD the key thing is that **fatty tissue can activate inflammation**, resulting in the fat containing liver cells being inappropriately targeted by the immune system.

People often assume that the body responds to injury in a "smart" way, tailoring what it does to the nature of the challenge. This assumption is based on our experience of situations such as vaccination where just such a bespoke, targeted response of the body is seen. In fact, the body responds in pre-programmed ways. We have evolved to have a system that protects us from the threats that our ancestors faced as the major challenge to their survival (genes that allowed them to survive something meant that they lived to pass those genes on, genes that didn't allow survival died off with their host). For the vast majority of human evolution there have been two primary threats. The first was from infection. In essence, the inflammatory and subsequent immune response treat every threat as an infection because infection was what drove the evolution of the inflammation response in the first place. Inflammation developing in MASLD is therefore, in the "eyes" of the immune system, a response to infection which has arisen to an infection that isn't there. Because there is no infection there, it can't be cleared, and this risks the development of an endless loop of injury. The other long-term threat, throughout human existence, has been starvation, meaning that genetic adaptations that helped with food "hoarding", so that no nutrition was wasted, assisted with survival and thus were progressively enriched in the population......the adaptations that might today give rise to fatty liver, in an era where food is plentiful and more calorific.

The critical issue with MASLD, and many other chronic or long-term conditions driven by inflammation, is that the response that has evolved to clear infection through its sequential steps is far from optimal for non-infection. Ultimately, what stops inflammation completely, and the immune response, is the clearance of the infection. The body's inflammation and immune responses have a type of automatic shut-off built into them. They will naturally switch themselves off if they aren't being actively switched on (think of your TV defaulting to standby mode). If an infection has been cleared, the "on switch" is no longer being pressed, which means that the automatic "off switch" kicks in and the response is switched off. Without inflammation being activated, the natural clean-up process dominates and tissue returns to normal. In MASLD, in simple terms, the fat drives inflammation but isn't cleared by the inflammatory response (as it isn't an infection, there is nothing for a specific immune response to be mounted to). This means that the "on switch" remains pressed continually and the "off switch" never has the chance to be pressed. This means ongoing inflammation and damage to the liver.

The pro-inflammatory actions of fat have two aspects to them in MASLD. The first is the general pro-inflammatory action of fatty tissue around the body. Although not all patients with fatty liver tissue are overweight, with enlarged stores of fat, the majority are, and that fatty tissue produces high levels of the chemicals (called cytokines) that drive inflammation. This is presumably a consequence of a constant low level of irritation to the body's protective inflammatory system caused by the presence of fat droplets in cells and the low-grade harm caused to those cells. The presence of these inflammatory chemicals at enhanced level in people with a lot of adipose tissue (the technical name for tissue fat stores) probably underpins many of the clinical problems that are associated with obesity (including, as we will discuss later, symptoms such as fatigue). It certainly contributes to injury in the liver. It appears very likely that the distribution of fat in the body plays an important role in determining the degree of risk it poses. It seems that visceral fat, that form of fat that is deposited in the abdomen around the gut and which contributes to the classic "beer belly", is a particularly high-risk pattern of deposition.

The second aspect to fat and inflammation is the role that fat stores within hepatocyte play in actual liver cell damage. Fat increases the levels of oxidant stress (i.e., the chemical action of fat is to increase the release of free radicals within and around the liver cell, which damage and ultimately kill the cell). In simple terms, therefore, the cause of liver injury in MASLD is fat. There is a further aspect to inflammation and obesity that place a critical additional role in the origins of MASLD. Inflammation alters the way cells generate and use energy and thus makes insulin resistance worse. Given that insulin resistance lies at the very heart of both type 2 diabetes and MASLD this helps to explain how obesity can contribute so much to the development of the metabolic syndrome.

One question which we will return to later in this book is a paradoxical one. It is not why do people with fat in their liver go on to develop liver injury, but why do many people not do so, given the presence of fat in their liver cells and the general pro-inflammatory effect of obesity? This is, of course, of more than just academic interest as if we can understand what controls the transition from a safe (or probably more accurately a safer) form of fat deposition (steatosis) to an unsafe form (steatohepatitis) it may give us insights into how to reduce disease risk.

**Fibrosis:** Where fat deposition and inflammation combine, in a setting where there is no natural "off switch", a pattern of chronic liver injury will arise. This ongoing injury to the hepatocytes then gives rise to the next part of the cycle, fibrosis or scarring. Our bodies are designed with a "failsafe" second process to survive infection if that infection can't be cleared completely by the immune system. The body, in simple terms, tries to wall it off. When we started as junior doctors, we used to see lots of people born in the era before antibiotics, with areas of scarring in their lungs. These were walled off areas of TB infection. Without ever knowing it they had been infected with TB, but the immune system had not been able to get rid of it (the TB bacterium is a tricky one for the immune system to handle). If the TB bacterium spreads throughout the body it is fatal, so to avoid that the next best thing, if clearing it is not possible, is to wall it off. Hence, the scarred areas which people didn't even know they had. The same process is activated in the liver in any situation when the body's systems can't effectively clear or resolve damaged and dying cells. In the severe forms of MASLD, typically where inflammation accompanies fat deposition in the hepatocytes, this means scar formation, initially around the portal tracts, and eventually between portal tracts. At first this doesn't really have an impact, and most people developing liver fibrosis with MASLD don't even know it. The problem is that, as it grows more extensive, it begins to replace hepatocytes to a significant degree (whereas in the early response to an infection that is cleared a dead hepatocyte is replaced by another hepatocyte, where the injury is ongoing the dead hepatocyte is replaced by scar). The scars also disrupt the architecture of the liver, meaning that it just doesn't work as well as a normal liver.

**Cirrhosis:** The final part of the cycle is the development of cirrhosis. Cirrhosis arises in the liver when scarring becomes extensive, with complete cross-linking of the portal tracts. This means that there is a network of capsules of scar tissue with the hepatocytes walled off within them (think bubble wrap, with the plastic being the scar tissue and the air pockets the hepatocytes). This has two effects. One is that by this point the amount of lost liver tissue is extensive, meaning that the liver capacity to function is substantially reduced. The other is that, as they have throughout the disease, the hepatocytes try to respond normally by dividing to create more hepatocytes. They are, however, doing so within a rigid structure of scar tissue. What this does is to increase the pressure within the "bubbles" of the bubble wrap. This squeezes the blood vessels, with the main effect of increasing the pressure in the portal vein. This leads to all the complications of portal hypertension outlined in the previous chapter. If there is active inflammation of the liver as well, the swelling that this causes further increases the pressure.

So, to summarise, the progression of disease can be shown as:
**healthy cells ↔ steatosis ↔ steatohepatitis ↔ fibrosis → cirrhosis**
Note that the first three stages can be improved and reversed with treatment (essentially lifestyle change for the early stages, possibly drugs for the later stages), but that the damage is effectively irreversible once cirrhosis develops.

The fundamental issue with severe MASLD forms, therefore, is not the degree of disease activity at any one time, it is the failure to control the disease over a period of time. It is the "drip drip drip" of long-term injury driving inflammation on to fibrosis, then on to cirrhosis, that we need to actively prevent. The message is therefore simple. Control the disease completely as soon as possible and after that keep it controlled!

## *THE IMPACT OF MASLD ON PATIENTS*

There are two broad ways in which MASLD in its different forms impacts on patients, and understanding and approaching these is the focus of much of this book. There is a significant degree of misunderstanding about disease impact, however, amongst both patients and clinicians and it is helpful to take an overview before exploring the detail later in the book. It is important, always, to remember that MASLD rarely exists in isolation and the problems it causes directly will be complicated and added to by the clinical features of the other clinical manifestations of the metabolic syndrome.

**Impact through chronic disease and risk to life:** Historically, the main (indeed essentially only) focus of management in all liver diseases was to reduce the rate of progression of liver injury to avoid the development of the complications of cirrhosis, with their risk to life. These included, as we have discussed, varices, ascites, hepatocellular carcinoma, and hepatic encephalopathy as well, of course, as liver failure. This remains the main focus of what we do in MASLD but needs to be seen in the context of the broader impacts of the disease and its treatment.

**Impact through symptoms and impaired quality of life:** Whereas the problems associated with cirrhosis development impact on a minority of patients at any one time (only those with advanced disease) the majority of patients at any one time will experience one or more of the symptoms of the disease. One of the mistakes that clinicians make in the management of MASLD is the failure to appreciate that some of the symptoms occur throughout the disease course and are not just a feature of advanced disease. For many people with non-cirrhotic disease, they can, in fact, be the biggest source of clinical problems. They can also contribute to disease risk because they can interfere with lifestyle modification as a therapy. The classic example of this is the impact that fatigue, a common and rather under-recognised symptom in MASLD, has on perceived and actual ability to do exercise; a critical aspect of effective lifestyle modification in MASLD. The causes and treatments of MASLD symptoms are discussed in detail in **Chapter 11**. An important concept in understanding the impact of symptoms on patients with MASLD, as with any disease, is that of Health-Related Quality of Life (HRQoL); the extent to which health states impact on that aspect of life quality determined by health. In simple terms, this is a case of understanding the nature of the problem in order to attempt to find a solution. It is important, in the setting of symptoms, to think in terms of the cumulative impact of all symptoms on quality of life, rather than to focus on a single symptom, no matter how seemingly important that individual symptom is. Improvement in a single symptom will not typically improve life for patients if others are left untreated. Even worse, over-focus on a single symptom can lead to the use of treatments that improve that symptom whilst making others worse.

**MASLD across the age spectrum:** MASLD can, and does, arise at any age. Originally described in people in the later middle years of life (the demographic group most impacted by type 2 diabetes and the other manifestations of the metabolic syndrome), it is increasingly clear that the condition can develop in childhood, with increasing numbers of children and young adults presenting with cirrhosis. This is a, perhaps unsurprising, consequence of the rapid rise in childhood obesity in affluent societies. It may also be that some of the dietary drivers for childhood obesity in western societies may play a particular role in driving the disease process.

In terms of the clinical impact of MASLD in childhood, the simple way of thinking about it is that children face all the issues that adults face, but with added problems unique to childhood. The additional issues are the impact of ill health on education (and thus life chances), the obvious need for more years of "liver life" for people developing a liver disease in early life and the impacts on self-esteem and social development that come from childhood obesity. Children really can be very cruel to other children. This all-encompassing impact means that it is of the greatest possible importance that we take all possible steps as a society, as parents and as clinicians to tackle childhood obesity/MASLD.

## ***MASLD: WHAT'S IN A NAME?***

In the "how to use this guide" section we introduced some of the challenges and complexities around terminology in MASLD. What was already a complex area has, with the name change, become even more challenging. The large number of different terms used can, and does, cause confusion amongst patients and doctors. In the first edition of this book we said that "if we could go back to the beginning, it would be really useful to have a more descriptive approach to what we think is happening". To an extent this is what is happening with the new terminology; the challenge will be the time lag before it becomes fully accepted and used in practice. Using the thought process behind the new name we have "fat in the liver" (***steatotic liver disease***), "fat in the liver as a result of abnormality in the body's metabolism" (***metabolic dysfunction-associated steatotic liver disease (MASLD)***) and "fat in the liver as a result of abnormality in the body's metabolism accompanied by inflammation and, potentially fibrosis or cirrhosis" (***metabolic dysfunction-associated steatohepatitis (MASH)***).

Why was the name changed? In simple terms, words can be very powerful indeed and we all need to be careful in how we use them. There are, in particular, certain words that trigger specific anxieties in people, to the extent that once they are used people can end up switching off and not hearing anything else that is being said to them. In the case of NAFLD in all its forms there were, unfortunately, three such words. The first, for patients with NASH was "alcoholic". Although the full expression is "non-alcoholic" it is amazing how often the "non" element was ignored. NASH had nothing to do with alcohol (in fact significant alcohol consumption de facto ruled the diagnosis out). It did, however, still cause problems.

The second problem word in the context of NASH was "hepatitis" and this issue remains in the revised term MASH. It actually simply means inflammation in the liver and has no implications as to the cause. In the lay world, however, it is often taken to mean viral hepatitis, which may be incorrectly interpreted as implying certain lifestyles, or that people are infectious.

The other problem word is "cirrhosis" when used to describe advanced MASLD. In the eyes of the public and media this is synonymous with alcoholic liver disease. This absolutely isn't the case. Cirrhosis is a pathological term to describe the combined process of liver regeneration and scarring and has no implications whatsoever with regard to the cause of the liver disease. Many people with alcoholic liver disease don't have cirrhosis and most cirrhosis is not caused by alcohol.

# CHAPTER 3: **THE CAUSES OF MASLD**

## *The 2-Minute Version*

- There are two aspects to the question of "what causes MASLD?" These are **aetiology** and **pathogenesis**. The question of the aetiology of any disease is about why you got it rather than someone else, and why it developed at the time that it did. Pathogenesis is the process by which the disease caused injury to your body and caused the symptoms and complications you experience. Understanding aetiology can help prevent a disease. Understanding pathogenesis can help treat it once it is established.
- The aetiology of MASLD is an interaction of genetic risk factors and environmental factors. In this sense, it is typical of most chronic diseases.
- The genetic factors in the aetiology of MASLD are predominantly related to the regulation of metabolism and, in particular, control of energy storage and use. There is a strong association between MASLD and type 2 diabetes and, unsurprisingly, genetic overlap.
- The environmental factors in the aetiology of MASLD are largely dietary, relating to the volume and nature of food in the diet. Perhaps counter-intuitively, the fat that is deposited in the liver in MASLD is largely not dietary fat that is taken up and stored, instead it is de novo fat which is made from other dietary components and stored in the liver. The chief culprit is carbohydrate.
- When glucose is taken up in the diet (either directly through glucose that has been consumed or, more commonly, from more complex carbohydrates that are broken down into glucose) the majority is incorporated, by the liver, and under the control of insulin, into a storage form called glycogen. This is then broken back down again into glucose and released into the blood to keep the glucose level up. If too much glucose is taken up in the diet, or insulin is not produced in sufficient levels (or the body stops responding to it), glucose can't be incorporated into glycogen and it is, instead, turned into fat.
- Fructose is another form of sugar which is increasingly used as a "low sugar" sweetener. Its chemical properties mean that it doesn't lead to an increase in blood sugar level. The body can't handle it, however, in any other way than to convert it into fat. It is therefore probably a major factor in the development of MASLD.

- Whereas fat deposition in the liver or elsewhere in the body is largely not, in and of itself, harmful, the fatty tissue can increase the levels of inflammation. The combination of fat and inflammation in the liver is harmful and gives rise to hepatocyte injury (through the processes of apoptosis and senescence). This reduces the number of functioning hepatocytes, although the body copes to a degree by making replacement cells.
- A key response of the body to ongoing injury is through scar tissue formation. The combination of scarring (or fibrosis as it is termed by pathologists), and regeneration of the hepatocytes gives rise to cirrhosis

The question as to why people get MASLD is, at the same time, both a simple and a complex one to answer. At a simplistic level, fat gets deposited in the hepatocytes in a way that shouldn't normally happen. In some people this is harmless, whilst in others it causes irritation in the form of inflammation. This leads to liver injury, and the response of the body to that injury in the form of scar formation. Progressive scarring liver injury leads eventually to the development of cirrhosis. There are, as a result, two fundamental questions to answer if we are to understand the causes of MASLD. The first is why does fat get deposited in the liver in some people (but not in others) in the first place? The second is why, in some people, the fat has the irritant effect that leads to liver injury. Answer these two questions and we are well on the way to being able to treat the disease better.

When doctors and scientists think about the causes of any disease, they split them into two aspects. Aetiology and pathogenesis. You will hear these terms used frequently (and often incorrectly). **Aetiology** refers to the true cause of the disease. Why did it develop in you as opposed to someone else, and why did it develop at the time that it did rather than at some other time? **Pathogenesis** refers to the pathways by which the aetiology of disease results in tissue damage and the clinical features of the disease. The "how" as opposed to the "why". Patients frequently ask in the clinic what causes their disease. We strongly suspect that this question is actually a combination of two, rather more focused, questions:

1) "How can you treat the disease?" This requires understanding of disease **pathogenesis.**

2) "Will my daughter or son get it, and can you prevent it?" This requires understanding of **aetiology**. This question also becomes highly relevant when thinking about how to prevent the recurrence of MASLD after liver transplantation.

We suspect there is often a third question set that is in the background. This is "did I cause it by something that I did, and will I be the cause of it in my daughter or son". These questions reflect an element of guilt that patients all too often feel.

## *THE AETIOLOGY OF MASLD*

MASLD is, as is the case with essentially all inflammatory disease, thought to arise through the interaction of a combination of genetic and environmental factors. This combination of factors is conventionally known as "complex disease" to distinguish it from purely genetic disease (which is thus implied to be "simple"; something that I am not sure all clinicians would agree about!). Complex disease has traditionally always been explained as the "ploughed field and the seed". The genetic aspect is the underpinning risk environment, the way in which a person is "built", without which you will never get the diseases. The "seed" is the trigger that converts one of the many people in the population who are in theory genetically susceptible into the smaller number who actually develop the disease. The way we explain this to patients in the clinic is about the risk of banging your head on the door frame! Only the very tallest people will bang their head on the doorframe as they pass through it. Height is largely genetically determined and is predictable from the height of a person's parents. The height of the door frame clearly plays a role, though, and equally clearly has nothing to do with an individual or their genetic make-up. The genetics of height, and the environment of the door frame, therefore combine to put a small proportion of the population at risk of developing a bruise on their forehead!

**The Genetic Basis of MASLD:** The study of the genetic basis of disease has increased exponentially in recent years, with the advent of new genotyping technologies following on from the Human Genome Project. This will undergo a further expansion in the next few years as whole genome sequencing becomes an easily accessible tool, potentially reaching into routine clinical practice. Sequencing a whole genome, which took years and millions of dollars in the Human Genome Project, is now available for $1000 and can now be done literally overnight (although the analysis of the large amount of resulting data can take a lot longer!). The easy availability of genetic data in some diseases can lead to the perception that genetic factors play a dominant role in aetiology. This is, in fact, probably not the case in MASLD, with environmental factors related to nutrition level and type playing an equal, if not dominant role (although food consumption itself is thought to have a genetic component; we did say that this was complex!)

There are several strands of evidence pointing to a genetic component to MASLD aetiology. The traditional starting point for studying genetic basis of any disease is what are called twin studies. This is the concordance rate in monozygotic (identical) and dizygotic (non-identical) twins (i.e. the rate with which the disease being studied develops in both of a twin pair). Identical twins are, as the name suggests, identical in terms of their inherited gene set. They also, typically, share the same environment (they usually live together throughout childhood when a lot of key disease risk factor exposure occurs). Non-identical twins share the same environment, and a proportion of their genetic make-up, but this is only to the same degree as would be the case for non-twin brothers and sisters. If the disease rate is the same in both identical and non-identical twins, and that rate is higher than in the normal population, it points to an environmental factor in disease aetiology. In contrast, if the disease rate is higher in identical twins than non-identical it suggests that the shared genetic make-up is the predominant factor. As with much research in MASLD, the twin studies give a slightly mixed and contradictory picture. This probably reflects, in part, the aspect of the disease pathway that is being considered. It is likely that the further down the pathway to high-risk disease, the more the twin studies suggest concordance in monozygotic twins. In simple terms, there appears to be a greater genetic component to aggressive disease than there is to simple obesity related fat deposition. This effect is seen in its most extreme form with type 2 diabetes, a key part of the metabolic syndrome and a condition very strongly associated with MASLD. In type 2 diabetes the concordance rate in monozygotic twins is close to 100%, with environmental factors (such as diet) seemingly only impacting on when the disease develops, with the issue of whether it develops being pretty much totally genetic. The limitations of twin studies are obvious. Although the notion of environment being shared in all twins, with genetics only being shared if monozygotic is appealingly clear cut, reality is more complex than that. Monozygotic twins are much more closely aligned than dizygotic when it comes to behaviour patterns (a good example being retention of a similar appearance with factors around body image and body weight). This is a factor even before we consider the obvious fact that dizygotic twins can be different sexes (unlike monozygotic); an important factor when we consider that MASLD is commoner in general terms in males than in females.

In recent years, the precise nature of the genetic risk of MASLD has begun to be understood in detail. This has occurred with the advent of modern genetics tools. MASLD has been studied extensively using genome wide association study (GWAS) methodology in large cohorts of patients across the world, indeed some of the people reading this book may well have taken part in these studies. The basis of the GWAS approach is that throughout the genome (the name for the whole genetic sequence that we all have, divided into 23 pairs of chromosomes) there are areas where there is predictable variation. This acts as a map of "coordinates" throughout the genome. These coordinates link to variations in the genes, the parts of the genome that are translated into the proteins that go to make up the body. Mapping the coordinates therefore allows us to build up a picture of the gene variations that each of us have. It is important to realise that what is mapped in these studies is not abnormal gene variants (the single disordered genes that give rise to conditions such as cystic fibrosis) but variations in normal that, combined together for all genes, make us all different (unless we have an identical twin). There isn't, therefore, a genetic "cause" for MASLD as such. Rather there is a genetic "explanation". This is a subtle but important distinction.

The GWAS studies in MASLD have given rise to three broad conclusions that increase our understanding of the disease. The first is that it is not the case that one or even a small number of genes make a significant contribution to MASLD. Rather, the risk appears to be because of the cumulative impact of a large number of small effects. This finding is in keeping with many of, if not all, the complex diseases studied to date, and mirrors personal traits such as height. As we have discovered earlier (remember the door frame?) height is, to a significant degree, genetically determined (nutrition also plays a role). There is not, however, a "height gene". Instead, multiple variations in normal genes combine to have the effect. The second is that the genes shown to be associated with MASLD to date relate to a wide range of biological processes; something that is in keeping with a multi-step, multi-factorial element to disease aetiology. The third conclusion is that, even despite the large amount of work carried out to date, we probably understand less than 30% of the genetic influence on the disease. Presumably the genetic factors that we don't yet understand represent an even larger number of even weaker disease association effects. We would hazard a guess that the ongoing genetic research in MASLD will provide additional "information infill" about disease processes but will not provide fundamental additional insights into the disease.

Paradoxically, the study of the genetic basis of MASLD does not give rise to the one thing that everyone expects it to, which is a genetic test to determine who is at risk of disease. Patients ask about this very frequently because of the familial risk of disease, and the desire to work out who within a family might be at the greatest risk. The reason why there is not a genetic risk predictor is precisely the same one as to why MASLD is not a genetic disease. Genetic tests require there to be a single gene (or very small number of genes) which are very strongly associated with the disease. As we have seen, in MASLD the genetic component of risk comes from the cumulative impact of a large number of genetic variants, the individual contributions of which are very small. It would be theoretically possible to combine a large number of these variations into a composite genetic score that gave a high degree of certainty of the disease in people that had all of them (this approach is currently very much in vogue and is called "predictive risk score" development). The challenge would be that the vast majority of people who actually went on to develop the disease would not have all of them. The test would therefore be of very limited use clinically.

Where genetic study in MASLD has been informative is in helping us to understand the key pathways that are implicated in the disease process. In simple terms, if a genetic variant associated with over or under activity of a key biological process is seen more or less frequently in MASLD patients than in the normal population, then it strongly suggests that the pathway is in some way implicated in the disease (and may, by extrapolation, be a target for treatment approaches). A number of such genetic associations have been seen in MASLD. What do they tell us about the disease? The strongest and best characterised association is, for example, with a gene called PNPLA3. Genetic variants are associated with histological severity in MASLD. The enzyme encoded by the gene plays a key role in the handling of one of the key types of fat, triglyceride, within the hepatocyte (it acts as a lipase breaking down the fat). The breakdown of triglyceride into its components (glycerol and free fatty acids) is a key part of normal energy generation and consumption. The PNPLA3 genetic association strongly suggests a role for fatty acid metabolism within hepatocytes in the aetiology of MASLD.

**The nutritional basis of MASLD:** Diet is fundamentally important when it comes to MASLD; that much is probably obvious in a disease where energy, and how it is handled by the body, is at its heart. It is important to also understand that, whereas diet is key as a cause of MASLD, it can also play a really important role as a treatment, so much so that when we refer to treatments, we include dietary control, along with exercise, within that term. This is something that we will explore in detail in **Chapter 6**. Whilst the general importance of diet as the cause of MASLD is widely recognised, the nuances are less well appreciated. The common perception is that MASLD is simply caused by excess calorie intake, and that the treatment is to lose weight by reducing calorie intake. The reality is, however, more complex than that. Firstly, because it's not simply a matter of the total amount of all the calories going in, but that some foods are more likely to cause MASLD than others. Secondly, as many people know, losing weight is not as simple as reducing calorie intake, which can be difficult in itself, but may not even lead to weight loss. In this section we will look at the nutrients in the food we eat, what their role is in the body, and how they contribute to MASLD. There are some food groups that are a particular risk for the development of MASLD to be aware of. The good news is that, once you are aware of the way that foods and eating patterns contribute to MASLD, it will give you the means to improve it. This will be covered in more detail in **Chapter 6.**

One of the fascinating things about the liver is how reactive it is to diet, and how quickly it can alter its fat content in response to dietary change. This is demonstrated by giving two (extreme) examples. The first is possibly the ultimate example of a fatty liver, that of pâté de fois gras made from duck or goose liver. This is a traditional delicacy in France, the term actually means "fat liver". The birds are overfed with a highly starchy diet of grain or corn, which is converted into fat by the liver, where it is then stored. This results in an extremely fatty liver which is seen by some as a delicacy. What surprises many people is that it is a starchy carbohydrate rather than fat that is fed to the birds.

The second example is that of a liver-reducing diet. This is a low calorie, and in particular, low carbohydrate and fat, diet that is used for 2 weeks before laparoscopic (keyhole) surgery in people who are thought to have MASLD, and who are having surgery near the liver. This is because MASLD causes the liver to be enlarged and stiff. During surgery near the liver, the liver needs to be retracted out of the way, and the fatty liver is more at risk of injury from this. Just two weeks of following the liver reducing diet is enough to shrink the liver and make surgery safer and easier. These are extreme examples, but they make the very important points that the liver can respond very rapidly indeed to short term changes in the diet (both positively and negatively), and that fat in the liver does not simply result from excess fat in the diet. From these observations alone it should be obvious as to the potential power of diet modification as a treatment in MASLD.

To understand the inter-relationship between diet and MASLD it is essential to understand a little about nutrition. The cells in our bodies need nutrients to function. These split into **micronutrients** and **macronutrients**. As the name suggests, micronutrients are those elements of the diet that we need to take in in very small amounts. These include vitamins and metals; things that are essential for the ways in which cells function and which can't be made by the body. Some micronutrients can be important in MASLD when deficiency arises. They are not, however, the major focus of this section. Macronutrients are, in contrast, the nutrients that your body needs in large amounts to function. The three main macronutrients are **carbohydrate, protein,** and **fat**. Unlike micronutrients, they provide the energy that is needed for the body to function. **Fibre** is often considered a macronutrient, although it is actually part of the carbohydrate group. It provides, however, little, if any, energy supply to the body beyond the gut.

*1) Carbohydrate*

The basic building blocks of carbohydrates are small molecules such as glucose, fructose, or sucrose (sugars, in simple terms). Glucose and fructose are like mirror images of each other. They have the same chemical formula but make up a slightly different shape. This minor difference in shape has hugely significant biological effects, however, in terms of how the liver can process and use fructose. Glucose can be taken up and used for energy by most of the cells in the body. However, fructose can only be used by the liver, where it is converted into glucose or fat. Sucrose (table sugar) is a mixture of glucose and fructose, which is what it is broken down into during digestion. Larger carbohydrates, whatever their origin, are broken down into glucose, which is the carbohydrate molecule of energy used by the body, and which is transported in the blood for use by the cells. Most carbohydrates come from plant sources, with the exception of animal sources that developed to feed their young, i.e., eggs and milk.

Larger carbohydrates consist of chains or groups of these smaller molecules, predominantly glucose. Carbohydrates are often described as simple or complex, but these descriptions can be misleading. This is partly because the description is usually based on the molecule's structure, rather than the way it behaves in the body, and because a food may consist of more than one type of carbohydrate, which may affect how the body can process it. This is relevant because it has implications for the rise in blood glucose which occurs following a meal, which is described later in this chapter.

When we eat larger carbohydrate molecules, they get digested in the stomach and small bowel, and broken down into glucose molecules which are then transported into the liver via the portal vein. Once in the liver, the glucose is processed. Some glucose goes into the blood stream to provide energy around the body, whilst the rest needs to be stored in some way for later use between meals. This is a bit like using cash, having an instant access bank account, and a savings account. Glucose is the cash, and the instant access account is in the form of glycogen, which is a molecule made up of multiple glucose molecules. Glycogen is easily made from, and broken back down into, glucose to provide ready storage and supply as needed. However, there is a limit to how much glycogen the liver can store. Once that limit is reached, glucose must be converted into an alternative storage molecule type; fat (and in particular the triglyceride form of fat). This is stored in the liver or sent elsewhere in the body to be stored as visceral (around the body organs, particularly in the abdomen) or subcutaneous (around the outside of the body under the skin) fat. This is the savings account, which may not be as instant access as we would like it to be. Sometimes it seems like one of those accounts with strict withdrawal restrictions! The hormone insulin has an important regulatory role in these processes. Insulin release is triggered by the blood glucose rise following carbohydrate intake and is essentially designed to push glucose into cells for use or for storage, as glycogen or by converting it to fat. As a result of this process, blood glucose levels will be reduced. Insulin levels fall in between meals, and the reverse process happens, with breakdown of glycogen into glucose, and release of fat from storage to be converted back into glucose, which is regulated by the hormone glucagon. To stretch the bank account analogy a bit further, insulin and glucagon are the logins for the online bank.

Apart from fructose, which will be discussed later, pretty much all carbohydrates end up as glucose. How quickly this process happens depends on the properties of the food – this is where the difficulty with classifying foods as complex carbohydrates based on their structure or function comes in. Some carbohydrates, like white rice, have a complex structure, but behave more like glucose, the 'simple' carbohydrate, by being broken down and digested quickly. This results in a rapid rise in blood glucose and insulin. Other carbohydrates, for example fruits and vegetables, which are structurally 'simple' have slower digestion and absorption, causing a slower rise in blood glucose, and less insulin response. A useful concept for looking at this issue is that of the **glycaemic** index. This measure describes how foods increase the blood glucose with time. A high glycaemic index means that the food causes a rapid increase in blood glucose over the first hour, compared with a low glycaemic index food.

Foods that have a high glycaemic index, resulting in a rapid rise in blood glucose, even faster than that of sugar, include bread, cereals such as cornflakes, shredded wheat and porridge and white rice. It also includes root vegetables like parsnips, potatoes, and carrots. People may choose to follow a low glycaemia index (low GI) diet to reduce their blood glucose levels, and therefore their insulin levels, to prevent or treat type 2 diabetes mellitus (and by extension MASLD). However, glycaemic index is not the whole story. This is where the concept of **glycaemic load** (GL) comes in… The amount which foods raise blood glucose depends on several factors – the type of carbohydrate, the other nutrients in the food (such as protein, fat, fibre) and the amount of carbohydrate in a serving, which is related to the carbohydrate density and the size of a portion.

Examples of food and drink with both a high GI and high GL are – potatoes, soft drinks, white rice. These foods cause a rapid and substantial rise in glucose. However, high GI foods such as carrots, apples, milk, and lentils may cause a rapid rise in blood glucose but have a smaller overall carbohydrate load. The higher the carbohydrate load, which is reflected in a high GL, the more glucose needs to be processed, resulting in a higher blood glucose (leading eventually to type 2 diabetes mellitus) or conversion and storage as fat (in the liver and elsewhere in the body), or most likely both of these.

It should, therefore, be starting to become clear that all carbohydrate, if enough is eaten, will contribute to weight gain, and the metabolic syndrome in all its forms. Whilst people have been encouraged to eat 'complex' carbohydrates in the past, it has become clear that many of these, such as potatoes, have effects on the body that are not much different to eating sugar. A baked potato contains the equivalent amount of glucose as 8 sugar lumps! We suspect that most people would regard a baked potato as being a healthy eating option (and 8 sugar lumps a most definitely unhealthy option) and yet in terms of the metabolic syndrome and MASLD risk they are, in essence, identical.

Comparing the carbohydrate content of foods to an easy to visualize equivalent amount of sugar is, we think, a useful thing to do. One teaspoon of sugar contains just over 4 grams of glucose. The equivalent number of teaspoons of sugar to a serving of food is shown in the table below. This is divided up into food categories, listing foods with the highest carbohydrate content first in each group. Be aware that throughout this section, the term carbohydrate is used with the UK meaning, which is not including fibre. This would be termed as net carbohydrate in some countries.

| Food | Portion size | Carbohydrate (grams) | Equivalent Teaspoons of sugar |
|---|---|---|---|
| *Vegetables and Fruit* | | | |
| Baked potato with skin | 1 medium | 33 | 8 |
| Sweet potato | 1 medium | 26 | 6.5 |
| Banana | 1 medium | 24 | 6 |
| Mango | ½ medium | 22 | 5.5 |
| Apple | 1 medium | 19 | 5 |
| Blueberries | 1 cup | 18 | 4.5 |
| Sweetcorn | ½ cup | 14 | 3.5 |
| Orange | 1 medium | 12 | 3 |
| Kiwi fruit | 1 medium | 8 | 2 |
| Strawberries | 1 cup | 4 | 1 |
| Carrots | ½ cup | 4 | 1 |
| Rhubarb | 1 cup | 3 | 1 |
| Broccoli | ½ cup | 3 | 1 |
| Tomato | ½ cup | 3 | 1 |
| Red pepper (raw) | ½ cup | 3 | 1 |
| Cauliflower | ½ cup | 1 | 0.5 |
| Avocado | ½ medium | 1 | 0.5 |
| Leafy green vegetables | 1 cup | 1 or less | 0 |
| Olives | 5 | 0 | 0 |
| *Grains and cereals* | | | |
| Brown rice | 1 cup when cooked | 48 | 12 |
| White rice | 1 cup when cooked | 44 | 11 |
| Quinoa | 1 cup when cooked | 35 | 9 |
| Bulgar wheat | 1 cup when cooked | 32 | 8 |
| Whole rolled oats | ½ cup before cooking | 23 | 6 |
| Pearl barley | ½ cup when cooked | 22 | 5.5 |
| *Beans and legumes* | | | |
| Kidney beans | ½ cup | 14 | 3.5 |

| | | | |
|---|---|---|---|
| Lentils | ½ cup | 14 | 3.5 |
| Chickpeas | ½ cup | 13 | 3 |
| Green beans | ½ cup | 2 | 0.5 |
| | | | |
| **Nuts and seeds** | | | |
| Cashews | ¼ cup | 10 | 2.5 |
| Peanuts | ¼ cup plain | 5 | 1 |
| Sunflower seeds | ¼ cup | 5 | 1 |
| Chia seeds | ¼ cup | 3 | 1 |
| Walnuts | ¼ cup | 2 | 0.5 |
| Pecan | ¼ cup | 1 | 0.5 |
| | | | |
| **Dairy** | | | |
| Skimmed milk | 1 cup | 12 | 3 |
| Full fat milk | 1 cup | 12 | 3 |
| Cheddar | ½ cup grated | 2 | 0.5 |
| | | | |
| **Processed food** | | | |
| Spaghetti (white) | 1 cup | 41 | 10 |
| Couscous | 1 cup | 34 | 8.5 |
| Spaghetti (wholemeal) | 1 cup | 26 | 6.5 |
| White bread | 2 medium slices | 26 | 6.5 |
| Wholemeal bread | 2 medium slices | 24 | 6 |
| | | | |
| Macaroni cheese frozen meal | 1 portion | 72 | 18 |
| Chicken curry frozen meal | 1 portion | 60 | 15 |
| Pepperoni pizza | ½ pizza | 44 | 11 |
| Baked beans 415g tin | ½ tin | 26 | 6.5 |
| Vegan 'meat' burger | 1 burger | 7 | 2 |
| | | | |
| Granola | 1 cup | 45 | 11 |
| Wheat biscuit cereal | 2 biscuits | 25 | 6 |
| Corn flake cereal | 1 cup | 23 | 6 |
| Rice pop cereal | 1 cup | 23 | 6 |

|  |  |  |  |
|---|---|---|---|
| Fruit jam | 1 tablespoon | 13 | 3 |
| Honey | 1 tablespoon | 11 | 3 |
| Chocolate hazelnut spread | 1 tablespoon | 8 | 2 |
| Peanut butter (sweetened) | 1 tablespoon | 2 | 0.5 |
| Peanut butter (unsweetened) | 1 tablespoon | 1 | 0 |
|  |  |  |  |
| Fruit smoothie (shop bought) | 1 cup | 30 | 7.5 |
| Apple juice | 1 cup | 27 | 7 |
| Banana corner yoghurt | 1 yoghurt | 24 | 6 |
| Fruit corner yoghurt | 1 yoghurt | 16 | 4 |
| Plain yoghurt | 1 cup | 15 | 4 |
| Low fat fruit yoghurt | 1 pot | 14 | 3.5 |
|  |  |  |  |
| 'Diabetic' ice cream made with fructose | ½ cup | 30 | 7.5 |
| Toffee chocolate ice cream bar | 51 ml bar | 17 | 4 |
| Vanilla ice cream | ½ cup | 17 | 4 |
| Frozen fruit lolly | 80 g lolly | 12 | 3 |
|  |  |  |  |
| Lemon slice | 1 slice | 22 | 5.5 |
| Chocolate biscuit | 2 biscuits | 20 | 5 |
| Oat biscuits / digestive | 2 biscuits | 18 | 4.5 |
|  |  |  |  |

*Meat, eggs, fish, butter, margarine, oils all contain minimal or no carbohydrate.*

Once we recognise that all carbohydrates are turned into either glucose or fat, there are several things that are striking about this table. The first is that many of the foods that we have been led to believe are healthy for us, such as the starchy rice, pasta and potatoes, and breakfast cereals, are in fact filling us up with glucose. Excessive intake of these foods can result, in time, in a rise in blood glucose, leading to type 2 diabetes mellitus, and an increase in fat deposition, leading to MASLD and obesity. The second is that not all fruit and vegetables are the same. There is a great deal of variation in the carbohydrate content between some of them. If banana, apple, and mango make up your 5-a-day, this will result in a lot more sugar equivalent that leafy vegetables, tomatoes and strawberries. Shop bought fruit smoothies are not the same as homemade smoothies using whole fruit either. Thirdly, even if you are looking at nutritional information on the packets of the food you buy, it isn't always easy to compare foods due to variation in the quoted portion size. This table uses measures that are visible, realistic, and relatable. Often the quoted portion size is less than what is commonly eaten, for example with breakfast cereals. The fourth thing to note is that the carbohydrate content is not related to sweetness of taste. One cup of strawberries would be a sweet and tasty dish but has around 1/8$^{th}$ the total carbohydrate of a baked potato, and a quarter of the carbohydrate of a fruit yoghurt. The fifth point is that wholemeal or wholegrain foods do not necessarily have lower carbohydrate content than the white alternatives. All, if you will pardon the pun, food for thought!

Although most carbohydrates that we eat get digested and broken down into glucose, there is a particular problem that comes from eating, or drinking, fructose. As mentioned earlier in this chapter, fructose is a mirror image of glucose, that can't be used anywhere in the body (it doesn't "fit"). It must, therefore, be metabolised in the liver. A small amount of fructose occurs naturally in fruit and vegetables. At the amounts that occur in fruit, when eaten whole, along with the fibre that makes up the pulp of fruit, this is not usually a problem and the relatively small, and smoothly absorbed, fructose load can be handled by the liver. However, if a large amount of fructose is delivered to the liver, such as when large quantities of fruit juice are drunk, this gets converted into fat, and stored in the liver. Because fructose is metabolised in the liver, it doesn't get into the blood stream, so doesn't cause a rise in blood glucose. This can be perceived as being a good thing for people with diabetes, and there are foods marketed as being good for diabetics based entirely on the fact that they use fructose rather than glucose. The reality is that these foods are loaded with calories, which can only be used by the liver, and are a very rapid route to developing MASLD. Fructose is also present in sucrose, table sugar, where it is present in equal amounts with glucose. A sugar load therefore will also deliver a significant amount of fructose to the liver. High fructose corn syrups are a highly processed form of sweetener used predominantly in the USA, and there has been much discussion in the media and literature as to whether this is, quite literally, fuelling the American MASLD epidemic.

This all sounds very grim and rather begs the questions, do we need to eat carbohydrates and what would happen if we didn't eat them? We have all been led to believe that carbohydrates are essential to provide us with energy. This is not actually true. While some of our cells need a continuous supply of glucose, this can be provided by the liver breaking down stored energy in the form of fat and protein (a process called gluconeogenesis which means, literally, "making new glucose"). Some of our cells are even able to run off energy provided directly by fat, as happens with a ketogenic 'keto' diet, which many marathon runners have trained their body to do. However, foods are not usually just one type of molecule, and unprocessed carbohydrates provide valuable micronutrients, which are essential for the body to function, along with fibre, which helps keep the bowel healthy. It's important to differentiate which foods contain 'empty calories'; a large amount of carbohydrate without any of the beneficial micronutrients and fibre. These are often referred to as energy dense 'beige carbs', and include rice, pasta, flour and potatoes. We are advised to eat wholemeal products or whole grains, as these contain the outer layer of the cereal seed, which contains valuable micronutrients and fibre, but even with this extra nutrition, the carbohydrate load may outweigh the benefit for some of these foods in some people.

Food processing removes many of the micronutrients in food. Nutrient dense foods are those which have more beneficial micronutrients (vitamins and minerals) compared with their energy provision. Fruit and vegetables are great sources of micronutrients, so in answer to the question, should carbohydrates be removed from one's diet, the answer is to pick them wisely. A diet where the predominant carbohydrates come from whole vegetables and fruit, rather than starchy or sugary foods, is the best option for those with MASLD in terms of providing essential nutrients without delivering as much glucose which will be stored as fat. This is also beneficial for the prevention and management of type 2 diabetes, as high intake of carbohydrate leads to high blood glucose, leading to higher insulin levels, then insulin resistance and the vicious cycle of further high blood glucose.

So what is the "bottom line" with regard to carbohydrates and MASLD? It is probably quite simple. Starchy and sugary carbohydrates can cause MASLD and offer little benefit to you in return for this risk. Less processed carbohydrates provide useful nutrition as they include fibre and micronutrients. Foods with added fructose should be avoided completely.

*2) Protein*

Whereas most carbohydrates come from plants, protein can be obtained from both plant and animal sources. Proteins are the main building blocks of the body and are essential for many roles, including making muscle. Protein can be used as an energy supply, but this is to the detriment of its other roles such as maintaining strength and renewing and rebuilding cells. It would only be used as an energy source in the event of starvation and energy deficiency; fat and carbohydrate are the main sources of energy.

The amount of protein we need in our diet varies depending on our age, activity level and other factors, but as a minimum we need around 0.75 grams per kilogram of body weight a day. For a 100kg person, this is the equivalent of around 4 cans of tuna a day. Animal sources provide more protein dense foods than plant sources. The evidence for any effect of high protein intake causing MASLD is mixed, but what are well recognised are the risks of protein deficiency. It is important, therefore, to ensure that protein intake is adequate, whatever source it comes from. High protein level sources include meat, fish, eggs, and dairy. Plant products provide less protein, but good sources are seitan, soybean, lentils and some beans. Many people in the UK do not consume an adequate daily amount of protein. Protein also has a beneficial effect in reducing appetite, and giving a feeling of fullness, which can be helpful when trying to lose weight. This can indirectly improve MASLD. It has much less of an effect on blood glucose than carbohydrates, so eating protein helps with control of type 2 diabetes.

The bottom line for proteins and MASLD is probably that protein intake is not linked to MASLD, but low protein intake is detrimental to health.

*3 Fat*

It feels perhaps a little counter-intuitive that only now do we talk about fat in the diet, despite fat deposition in the liver being the very essence of MASLD. As we outlined earlier, however, the key thing here is that the fat present in the liver in MASLD is typically made from other nutrients (in essence carbohydrate) rather than being dietary fat per se. The relative lack of focus on dietary fat is, therefore, not as paradoxical as it perhaps originally seemed. There are, however, important questions about dietary fat, and it is an area where there has been a huge amount of change in advice and opinion over the last few years. For several decades fats were demonised as the cause of heart disease, amongst other things. There is now a more nuanced approach to dietary advice. Some fats are good, some are bad, and there are many grey areas. To start with, let's look at some facts.

- Some fats are essential in the diet as the body needs them for healthy function and cannot make them.
- Intake of fats in the diet is necessary to absorb the fat soluble vitamins (A,D,E and K).
- Fats provide energy and precursor molecules for some essential hormones (steroid hormones for example) and chemicals.
- Naturally occurring fats can be divided by their structure into saturated, mono-unsaturated and poly-unsaturated (the term "saturated" in this setting refers to the nature of the chemical structure of the constituent molecules).

- Industrially produced trans-fats (iTFAs) are used by the food industry, and cause a big increase in risk for heart disease, strokes, diabetes. They are also perhaps the only fats to directly drive MASLD development.
- Our bodies are designed to safely store fat to allow an energy reservoir for times of fasting or famine.
- Excess energy from consumed fat is stored in the adipose (fat) tissue around the body (although trans-fats lead to accumulation in the liver specifically).
- Cholesterol in the blood is predominantly made by the body, and is not directly linked to the amount that is eaten. Cholesterol is also essential for the cells to function.

Fat comes from animal and plant sources, although the cholesterol form of fat is found exclusively in animal sources. There are multiple different fatty acids, one of the molecule types that make up the group of fats. One source may contain several types of fatty acids. Some fatty acids are good, some are harmful. Food processing can have an effect on the structure of the fatty acids, which may mean that a product of a food no longer has the healthy benefits of the original food. This is particularly the case for seed oils, where the seeds contain beneficial fats, but undergo considerable processing to make the oil.

Saturated fats come from animal and plant sources, and are usually solid at room temperature. This includes the fat from meats, dairy products and tropical oils (coconut and palm oil, and cocoa butter). In the past they have been thought to cause heart disease, although this link has now been questioned. Eaten in moderation they are unlikely to cause health problems, although excessive intake will contribute to obesity due to excess energy intake.

Mono-unsaturated fats come from nuts, vegetable oil (olive oil, peanut oil), nut butters and avocado. These can improve cholesterol levels and reduce heart disease.

Poly-unsaturated fats include omega-3 fatty acids, which have heart benefits. Poly-unsaturated fats sources that have omega-3 fatty acids include oily fish such as salmon, herring, sardines, and trout, and nuts and seeds such as walnuts, flaxseed (linseed), chia seed and canola oil. Whilst there is much evidence to show benefits from eating omega-3 fatty acids, there is a much higher intake in the Western diet of omega-6 fatty acids, which come from sources such as tofu, soybeans, seeds, corn and seed oils and margarine. Omega-6 fatty acids may promote harmful inflammatory processes, although they are essential fatty acids (ones that the body needs but can't itself produce) meaning that we need at least some in our diet. The process for making oils such as corn oil from maize, or the seed oils such as canola/rapeseed, sunflower and safflower oil is heavily industrialised, the end products are high in omega-6 fatty acids and can create unnatural and harmful molecules. It is likely that we need a ratio of 1:1 between omega-3 fatty acids and omega-6 fatty acids, whereas the ratio in the Western world has been around 1:20 for the last few decades. A high ratio of omega-6 fatty acids compared to omega-3 fatty acids has been shown to cause fatty liver changes. The high intake of seed oils and margarine has been a major contributor to the high intake of omega-6 fatty acids over the last few decades. Many Asian countries have followed the move to using more seed oil over the last few years too.

Industrially produced trans-fats were developed by the food industry as they can prolong the shelf life of processed food. They have now been identified as causing a substantial increase in overall risk of death, specially from cardiac causes. They have also been identified as causing MASLD. To identify if a food contains trans-fats, look on the label for partially hydrogenated or hydrogenated vegetable oil. Try and avoid all foods containing trans-fats if you have MASLD.

There are benefits of fat in terms of adding taste to food. One of the consequences of the demonising of fat over the last few decades has been that sugar, salt, or both, have been used to replace the satisfaction of taste that was lost with removing fat. Fat also delays the emptying of food from the stomach, which gives a feeling of fullness, thereby reducing further food intake.

To conclude, although fats have been categorised as saturated and unsaturated, this is unhelpful as the benefits and harm caused by different fats does not fit well within this simple categorisation. It is more useful to consider them by source. Animal sources of fat can be enjoyed in moderation. Fish sources provide valuable omega-3 fatty acid. Vegetables and vegetable oils that are obtained by simple pressing processes, such as olive oil or coconut oil, have some health benefits. Nuts and seeds provide essential omega-6 fatty acids, but seed oils and margarine provide a level of omega-6 fatty acids that may be causing or worsening MASLD. Trans-fats are a significant cause of MASLD, and foods containing them should be avoided completely if possible. Eating fat does not increase the blood glucose level.

The "bottom line" in relation to dietary fat in MASLD is to avoid trans-fats completely, and to limit intake of seed oils and margarine.

### *4) Fibre*

Fibre is indigestible plant material that doesn't contribute to our energy intake. However, it is an important part of our diet. In some countries fibre is included in the nutrition information of food products within total carbohydrates, with the non-fibre carbohydrates described as net carbohydrates. It has traditionally been categorised into soluble fibre and insoluble fibre.

Soluble fibre dissolves in water. It delays the absorption of glucose and fatty acids, therefore reducing the rise in blood glucose after a meal, and thus the level of the insulin response. It has beneficial effects on blood lipids and cholesterol. Porridge oats are an example of soluble fibre. Insoluble fibre, as its name suggests, doesn't dissolve in water, and helps bulk up the bowel contents; a property which increases the movement of waste through the bowels.

There has been an increasing awareness recently of the importance of the trillions of bacteria that live in our large bowel or colon, that work in a symbiotic way with our bodies. This is known as the gut microbiome, and evidence suggests that these bacteria may have an important role to play in weight management, blood glucose control, immunity, brain function, mental health and MASLD. They use dietary fibre for their nutrition. What we eat, and the quantity and type of fibre we eat determines the gut microbiome constituency. The types of fibre that the bacteria can digest are known as fermentable fibres or prebiotics. Common sources of fermentable fibre include oats, beans and legumes. A by-product of the fermentation of the fibre by bacteria is gas production, causing the well-known side effects of flatulence and abdominal cramps, which usually reduces if these foods are eaten regularly. Some people also like to take probiotics, which are foods or food supplements containing cultures of healthy bacteria. This includes some foods which are produced naturally using fermentation, such as live yoghurt, kefir, sauerkraut, tempeh, kombucha tea and kimchi. It's uncertain how much of the live bacteria fraction in fermented foods or probiotic supplements reaches the colon alive as the acid production in the stomach has evolved specifically to protect the upper GI tract from bacterial colonization! There is a recognition that a healthy gut microbiome is important for our health, and changes in it are associated with MASLD. It is, however, very difficult to separate cause and effect. The best advice is to ensure that diet includes plenty of fibre from a variety of sources, to optimise the gut microbiome nutrition.

Good sources of healthy fibre include vegetables, fruit, nuts, seeds, some whole grains like oats, legumes and, happily, cocoa and thus dark chocolate. However, some people get significant gastrointestinal side effects, causing irritable bowel syndrome (IBS) or symptoms similar to those of coeliac disease, with some of the fibres, which come under the umbrella term FODMAPs (Fermentable oligo- di-monosaccharides and polyols). Common culprits include fructose, lactose (lactose intolerance), some grains, legumes and sweeteners like xylitol, sorbitol and mannitol.

Fibre increases the sensation of fullness, and reduces hunger, which is a valuable aid when trying to lose weight.

The bottom line for dietary fibre in MASLD is that it is important for the health of the gut microbiome and poor microbiome health is associated with MASLD. A diet containing a mixture of dietary fibre sources is, therefore, likely to be beneficial.

**Alcohol:** It is important to discuss alcohol in a section on nutrition in MASLD because of the role it can play in dietary energy intake for too many people in our population. It is very easy to slip into thinking about alcohol having specific properties that lead to it causing liver disease. This is, to an extent, true as it can modify natural body proteins leading to their recognition by the immune system, triggering a harmful immune response. There is, however, a significant additional issue relating to the nutritional load associated with alcohol consumption. Ethanol, the main ingredient of alcohol, is in its own nutrition category, as it is not actually a carbohydrate, although it is derived from carbohydrates. There is some benefit for heart disease, and for type 2 diabetes, when used in small to moderate amounts. The benefits are mainly seen with red wine, which may be because of the antioxidants in the grape skin, rather than from the alcohol itself. To counterbalance these benefits there are the well-known harms, not just liver disease, but also cancer.

The key issue is that ethanol is more calorific than carbohydrate and drinking alcohol results in fat accumulation in the liver as a result of its nutritional load. In addition to this effect from the ethanol, many alcoholic drinks also include a large amount of conventional carbohydrate, which also, as we have discussed, drives accumulation of fat. Cocktails containing sugar and beers containing starch are particular culprits. There is also a tendency to drink significant amounts of alcohol at one go.

The "bottom line" with alcohol is that alcoholic drinks can contribute to MASLD, and intake should be limited. The co-existence of both an alcohol and metabolic aetiology in steatotic liver disease was formally recognised during the re-naming exercise for steatotic liver disease with the inclusion of the category of "MASLD and increased alcohol intake" (MetALD). Within this category of steatotic liver disease there are MASLD and ALD (alcohol-associated liver disease) variants. This does rather end up complicating the picture and it is perhaps sensible to regard metabolic liver disease as a single spectrum with the calorie load from alcohol playing an important, if variable, role.

**Micronutrients:** Unlike macronutrients, where excess intake of certain forms is common in MASLD and is, indeed, a key part of the disease process, shortage in MASLD is common for many micronutrients. Micronutrients are electrolytes, vitamins, minerals and carotenoids (the brightly coloured red, yellow and orange pigments in plants). They are required in small amounts by the body, usually milligram or microgram quantities, and do not provide a source of energy. Instead, they fulfil essential roles in many metabolic functions throughout the body. Many people with MASLD have micronutrient deficiencies, but separating out whether this is a cause of the MASLD, just coincidental due to lack of dietary intake, or an effect of MASLD is difficult.

There is some evidence to suggest that the following micronutrient deficiencies may contribute to development of MASLD:

- *Zinc* (found in shellfish, red meat, legumes, nuts)
- *Copper* (found in shellfish, legumes, nuts, seeds, absorption may be reduced by zinc supplements)
- *Vitamin A* (found in dairy, coloured vegetables, and fruit)
- *Vitamin D* (found in oily fish, red meats, egg yolks)
- *Vitamin E* (found in nuts, seeds, and whole grains)
- *Carotenoids* (found in coloured vegetables and fruit)

Many people choose to take vitamin and mineral supplements and there are certainly many different forms on the market. Many in the scientific community believe, however, that these supplements are less beneficial, and potentially more harmful, than getting these essential micronutrients as part of a balanced diet. Food supplements do not act the same as when the nutrient is taken in food. For example, iron tablets given in a high dose to treat anaemia cause black stool and diarrhoea, but when eaten in food it has better absorption at a lower concentration. A reasonable conclusion is that adequate intake of micronutrients in a healthy and balanced diet is probably ideal. Supplements are not as good, but still better than ongoing deficiency.

See **Appendix 3** for a more detailed description of the many micronutrients, sources, and biological functions.

**Effects of Food Processing:** "Processed food" is frequently mentioned as a cause of obesity and MASLD. However, there are different degrees of processing, and many processed foods are useful parts of our diet. Indeed, it would be very difficult to live without the benefits of some processed foods. The NOVA classification breaks it down into four levels of processing.

*Group 1:* Unprocessed or Minimally Processed:
**These are the foods that should be eaten the most**. This group includes fruits, vegetables, legumes, meats (unprocessed), nuts, seeds, milk, eggs, whole grains (oats, brown rice). It can include frozen or vacuum-packed food provided it isn't processed.

*Group 2*: Processed Culinary Ingredients:

This includes sugar, honey, canned coconut milk, oils from nuts or fruits such as olive oil, butter, white flour or rice, salt, live plain yoghurt. They may contain additives to preserve freshness.

*Group 3*: Processed Foods:
This group includes processed food containing just 2 or 3 ingredients, such as canned fish, legumes, fruit or vegetables, salted nuts, cured meats, beer, wine, cider, freshly baked bread, simple cheeses, pasta.

*Group 4:* Ultra-Processed Foods
**These are the foods that should be eaten the least.** They often include artificial colours, dyes, additives, sweeteners. Examples include many cereals, packaged bread, ready meals, cakes, biscuits, deserts including flavoured yoghurt, carbonated soft drinks, margarine, seed vegetable oils, sausages, pizza.

This list is not exhaustive but should give you some idea of the issues. An easy way to tell if something is ultra-processed is to look at the ingredients list. If it contains ingredients that you wouldn't reasonably expect to come across in a home kitchen, then it is likely to be ultra-processed. There is a difference between items you may make at home from unprocessed or processed ingredients, such as homemade burgers, and shop bought packaged burgers, which may be either processed or ultra-processed. They may look similar, but packaged prepared shop-bought food is likely to have less in the way of the nutrients that we need, in particular fibre and micronutrients, and more nutrients that are harmful, such as unhealthy fats, added sugar, artificial sweeteners and other additives, and to be more calorific. The addition of sugar to many savoury foods also has the effect of altering our sense of taste. Many people who cut back on their sugar and carbohydrate intake comment on how much their sense of taste and sweetness improves, and that they can then appreciate flavours other than sugar!

Does all this matter? **The answer is a clear yes!** Regular intake of ultra-processed food is strongly associated with MASLD, type 2 diabetes, obesity and other aspects of the metabolic syndrome. Effective control of MASLD needs these foods to be avoided as much as is possible.

**Artificial and natural sweeteners:** Artificial sweeteners are chemicals added to food to replace the sweetness of sugar. Commonly used ones include aspartame, sucralose, saccharin, neotame and acesulfame potassium. They provide minimal or no energy, therefore the food consumed has a lower calorie content than if sugar was used to provide the same level of sweetness. Despite this, the evidence is mixed as to whether they actually aid weight loss.

There is increasing evidence that they cause disruption to the gut microbiome, which may be associated with causing or worsening MASLD. Intake of foods containing artificial sweeteners is, therefore, probably best avoided in people with MASLD.

Natural sweeteners are, as the name suggests, chemicals that occur naturally. It is important to remember, however, that the product that you buy may be an industrially produced copy of the natural substance. This class of sweetener includes stevia, erythritol, xylitol, monk fruit sweetener and trehalose. There is no evidence they worsen MASLD (indeed there is actually some positive evidence that stevia and trehalose may improve MASLD) but be aware that trehalose has been associated with an increase in a severe form of infective bowel disease, clostridium difficile infection. The conclusion is that artificial sweeteners are best avoided in MASLD. If natural sweeteners can help you reduce calorie intake, then this is a positive. They should still, however, be used with a degree of caution.

**Eating patterns and timing of dietary intake:** The last topic in this section is not about what we eat, but when we eat it. The starting point to thinking about this is actually the endpoint, which is that we need to have a continuous supply of glucose in our blood at all times to provide energy to our cells. The liver is a very effective organ and is able to provide this continuous supply of glucose, within the safe limits that the body needs, regardless of whether we have consumed glucose or not. After a carbohydrate containing meal, when glucose is entering the liver from the bowel, this will be the source of blood glucose that is delivered around the body. Within a couple of hours, though, the supply of glucose from the meal will have been used up. The liver seamlessly kicks into its second mode, which is to break down the stored glycogen in the liver into glucose and release it into the blood stream. After around 4 hours, assuming no more food is eaten, the liver starts to engage its third glucose providing mode, which is called gluconeogenesis. This means making new glucose, which it does from fat obtained from both within the liver and elsewhere in the body. Around 16 hours after a meal, the gluconeogenesis process is providing more glucose than the remaining glycogen. This means it is using up the fat stored in the liver, the same fat that makes it MASLD, for providing glucose. After around 2 days, the glycogen is used up, but the fat burning gluconeogenesis process can continue to provide a steady supply of glucose almost indefinitely, until all the body fat is used up. That is not to say that continuous fasting is recommended, but it has been done effectively and safely. There are many marathon runners who choose to run having fasted, as it trains their bodies not to rely on glycogen, the supply of which can be exhausted during long distance running.

How does all this relate to MASLD? If we eat something every four hours, for example a snack or calorie containing drink between meals, the liver never needs to switch to the fat burning gluconeogenesis mode. The longer the gaps between intake, the more the process of burning fat happens. We have been told how important it is to eat 3 meals a day, that breakfast is the most important meal of the day, and that snacks help keep our blood sugar up. These traditional views are not, however, backed up by the physiology. A normal functioning liver (in the absence of type 1 diabetes or diabetes medication) can safely provide a supply of blood glucose for many days even in the absence of any dietary input. The "bottom line" is that frequent meals or snacks worsen fat accumulation in the liver, longer gaps between meals means fat gets used for energy.

**Diet as the "cause" of MASLD: a summary:** There are some things about what we eat, and when we eat, that predispose people to MASLD. The biggest culprits are high total carbohydrate intake, and especially fructose, highly processed fats such as trans-fats and some seed-based oils and margarines, lack of fibre and micronutrients, highly processed foods, and frequent snacking or meals. In **Chapter 6** we will discuss strategies to change this.

## *THE PATHOGENESIS OF MASLD*

Ultimately, treatment of existing MASLD requires us to understand what the processes are that are resulting in liver injury so that we can control and, ideally, then reverse them. This is where the concept of pathogenesis is so important. In understanding the pathogenesis of MASLD, we need to explain and link five cardinal disease processes:

1) Fat deposition within the liver (and elsewhere in the body).
2) Inflammation in the liver which impacts both on the liver and the body generally
3) Insulin resistance
4) Hepatocyte injury
5) Development of fibrosis and, eventually, cirrhosis.

What is challenging in MASLD is that although the progression of hepatocyte injury through to fibrosis is well understood, how the first three processes interlink is far from clear. In this section we will explore some of the current thinking about the pathway to liver injury, and then reach some common-sense conclusions about the implications for disease treatment.

**The original model:** *The "2-hit hypothesis":* One of the early key discoveries in MASLD was that, whereas fat deposition in the liver was very common in the population, the development of overt liver injury (inflammation, hepatocyte damage and fibrosis) was less common (although the frequency is now growing). It was this observation that led directly to some of the terminology that is still in use today (and which gives rise to a lot of the confusion in MASLD). The "2-hit hypothesis" was a model which set out to explain this. In this model the first "hit" was the deposition of fat in the liver. This was, in isolation, not harmful. Hepatocyte injury only occurred when a second, independent "hit" occurred which triggered inflammation. Think of a petrol cigarette lighter. A flame needs 2 elements. The first is a flow of fuel. The second is a spark to ignite that flame. In the 2-hit hypothesis model the fat deposition in the liver was the fuel and the inflammation provoking event (perhaps an infection of some sort) was the spark. One element without the other would not lead to hepatocyte injury and its sequelae. In this model, the driver for fat deposition in the liver would be insulin resistance. This would explain the link between MASLD and type 2 diabetes; insulin resistance is a key part of the disease process in both settings. As we have discussed earlier in the chapter, the risk of type 2 diabetes has a very significant genetic element to it.

**The problem with the "2-hit" model:** The 2-hit hypothesis is a very attractive one, and it certainly fits with cross-sectional cohort observations (the mixture of disease components seen across a large group of patients at a single "snapshot" point in time). This approach lacks one element, however. This is the impact of time and thus the sequence in which events occur. When this more rounded approach is taken, some problems with the 2-hit model emerge.

- The difference between low-risk patients (simple steatosis) and high risk patients (MASH) is much less black and white than was originally thought to be case. The difference in risk profile is much more one of rate of progression from one state to another rather than one of an absolute dichotomy between the two states. This makes the role of any "second hit" much less clear cut.
- A cardinal feature of the 2-hit model is that the first hit of steatosis predates the second hit that triggers inflammation. The onset of insulin resistance, which in the model is upstream of fat deposition, must logically occur first if this is the case. However, it is now clear that inflammation promotes insulin resistance. People with type 2 diabetes will be very familiar with a worsening in their diabetic control when they get infections. This is through a direct effect of both infectious organism components such as endotoxin and cytokines, the chemicals that the immune and inflammatory systems use to communicate, altering the way in which key enzymes that regulate metabolism function. What this means is that inflammation probably occurs at least in parallel with insulin resistance and fat deposition, as a linked process, rather than being

an independent second process that occurs once fat deposition is established.

From this it will be very clear that, rather than a simple sequential step process, where one change begats another, there is a complex web of inter-relationships of the components of the disease process that we see across MASLD patients.

**An alternative model for pathogenesis:** An alternative way of thinking about disease pathogenesis in MASLD is that it is all driven by fat deposition in the liver and adipose tissue (at the end of the day, the one thing that everyone with MASLD has is a fatty liver). This fat is inherently pro-inflammatory (it is what fat does). The degree of inflammation presumably has several factors controlling it, including genetic factors (the genetic factors that influence the degree of any inflammatory process). For a given amount of fat in the liver, and elsewhere in the body, different people will have different levels of inflammation. This inflammation will lead to hepatocyte injury which, if sufficient in degree, and present for long enough, will give liver damage and activation of the fibrosis pathway. The combination of ongoing liver injury and fibrosis will lead, ultimately, to cirrhosis. In this model, insulin resistance is probably there at the outset of the disease to some degree and contributing to fat deposition in the first place. This is likely to be, again, a genetic effect (remember the strong genetic contribution to type 2 diabetes; the defining example of insulin resistance and its effects). When fat-related inflammation develops, this is likely to exacerbate insulin resistance, leading to even more fat deposition. The key aspect to this model is that the older 2 hit hypothesis concept, that fat in the liver is fine unless a second hit happens, is almost certainly wrong. There is a continuous spectrum of risk once fat deposition has begun, with the onset of inflammation and worsening insulin resistance acting as a "booster" for the disease process.

**Hepatocyte injury in MASLD:** The "why" of the pathogenesis of MASLD is, as we have discussed in the previous section, a complex and not yet resolved question. In contrast, the "how" of pathogenesis is relatively straight-forward. The localised inflammatory response in the liver damages hepatocytes, and the body then reacts to clear them in the same way it would do infected cells. As we outlined in **Chapter 2**, two processes predominate in terms of the actual process of hepatocyte "death". The first is apoptosis or programmed cell death, and the other in senescence.

To recap, apoptosis is a process by which a cell is given a signal to die by an external or internal process. A classic example is the killer cell of the immune response, the cytotoxic T-cell, eliminating a cell infected with a virus. In this example, as the cell is acting as a breeding ground for the virus it is in the interests of the body to eliminate it. It is also, of course, advantageous for the body not to allow the cell to simply fall apart as this would release the virus to infect other cells. Cytotoxic T-cells, therefore, after recognising the infected cell via a receptor on the surface (the T-cell receptor) that can identify proteins from the virus processed to make them visible to the immune system, gives a signal to the cell to fold in on itself, dying whilst neatly packaging-up the potentially harmful virus. The apoptosed cell remnants are then cleaned up by the scavenger cells of the immune system, such as the macrophages. Apoptosis is also a natural part of human development when tissues remodel themselves. An example is the webbing between our fingers. In utero, developing humans have webbing between their fingers and toes that is a little like a duck's foot. By the time they are born this has disappeared. The cells of the webbing have been programmed to disappear through apoptosis.

Apoptosis of the hepatocytes is the cardinal mechanism for liver cell injury in MASLD. In contrast to the viral example, however, where the signal to the hepatocyte to apoptose is largely delivered directly, in MASLD the signal is likely to be delivered indirectly through chemicals released into the environment near to the hepatocytes by both immune cells and, probably, fat-loaded cells themselves. Called cytokines, these are the communications and action chemicals of the immune response. They include tumour necrosis factor (TNF) which was originally identified, as its name suggests, as a factor, or component, in the blood which could cause tumour cells to undergo apoptosis. We now know that its pro-apoptotic actions are much broader than targeting tumour or cancer cells, and it is a key part of the immune response to infection.

The second, intriguing, potential mechanism for hepatocyte injury in MASLD is senescence. Senescence probably arises as an end-result of a failed attempt by the hepatocytes to cope with injury by apoptosis. When hepatocyte apoptosis occurs, a process of cell proliferation accompanies it where the liver cells divide to increase the numbers of cells and attempt to replace the lost cells. The issue is that almost all cells in the body are limited in terms of the numbers of times that they can divide. This is certainly the case with the hepatocytes and biliary epithelial cells. Exceptions to this rule are the so-called stem cells. The best example of these are bone marrow cells which need to be able to continue to divide to stock the blood with new cells to replace those that are broken down at the end of their life. The liver has its own stem cells which proliferate in the setting of injury and then differentiate (turn into) hepatocytes and biliary epithelial cells. This, together with the response of the remaining undamaged mature hepatocytes and biliary epithelial cells, underpins the regeneration response of the liver to significant injury. In non-stem cells, restriction on the number of divisions a cell can undertake is probably a protective mechanism to prevent unregulated division and, thus, cell immortality, the hallmark, of course, of cancer.

In MASLD, therefore, hepatocyte senescence probably occurs because of a chronic inflammatory response, hepatocyte injury, and the body's response to it. When cells become senescent, they enter a state of limbo where they can neither proliferate any more, nor function properly, yet remain alive. The term "zombie" cells has been used in the popular press, invoking the state of "living death" seen in horror films, and is actually not a bad term. We know that senescence of hepatocytes occurs in MASLD (we can detect it under the microscope). We also know that its development is a bad sign. A possible reason for this is that these cells, in their state of living death, are not benign. They appear to produce lots of cytokines, the precise chemicals that activate the immune system and cause hepatocyte injury in MASLD in the first place. This is probably a natural mechanism to promote the elimination of senescent cells which are no longer useful to the body. The problem is that if you get rid of senescent hepatocytes, and there is no longer any way to replace them, you run out of functioning liver!

**Fibrosis and cirrhosis in MASLD:** This is the aspect of MASLD which is, perhaps, the least specific for this condition as opposed to any other form of liver disease (or at least any other disease type where the primary target for injury is the hepatocytes; conditions in which the bile duct is the main target for injury, such as PBC or PSC, have quite a different disease pathway of fibrosis). As we discussed in **Chapter 1**, fibrosis is a key part of the body's reaction to injury through tissue repair. Fibrotic or scar tissue can develop rapidly following injury, knitting tissues together and sealing off gaps in the cell structure (think of skin healing after a cut or burn). This is important for surviving an injury, but rarely as good as the tissue returning to normal through full healing (going back to the skin, a scar is not as good as skin which has returned to normal). In practice, therefore, fibrosis occurs rapidly in response to injury as "first aid" for the tissue. As the cause of tissue injury disappears (an infection which the body fights off for example), so the fibrotic tissue is replaced by regenerating organ tissue. The fibrous tissue breaks down and disappears. This is the healing cycle. As with the immune response, there are different stages to the process. In response to initial injury, fibrinogen, a protein in the blood which circulates and can be rapidly converted into fibrin, a scar protein, is activated by the signals coming from tissue suggesting that there is injury, and rapidly begins to lay scar down. The second stage of the process in some organs (most classically the liver) is when specialised cells called the stellate cells become activated (again by the signals suggesting local injury). Amongst other things they begin to produce collagen, the long-term scar protein that forms part of the scar tissue in cirrhosis. The activated stellate cells can also play a key role in the breakdown of that scar tissue when the injury process has ended, and it is this balance between scar manufacture and breakdown that is critical to determining whether the outcome is healed tissue or permanent scar. The critical issue is the state of the activation of the stellate cells. If they remain activated, then they will continue to produce and "harden" scar tissue. If the disease process continues to be active in the liver, activated stellate cells will continue to produce scar. This is the beginning of the road to cirrhosis. The answer to preventing fibrosis or scarring in MASLD (and ultimately cirrhosis) is to fully control, and keep under control, the underlying disease processes of fat deposition and inflammation that keep them activated. The problem in MASLD is not the stellate cells but the instructions that they are getting. There is much research interest into developing anti-fibrotic drugs for use in diseases such as MASLD, indeed, as we will discuss in **Chapter 8** regression of fibrosis is a major target of drug therapy in MASLD. Resmetirom appears to have some anti-fibrotic activity but how significant that will turn out to be in practice isn't yet clear.

**Additional disease processes:** There are two additional disease processes that are seen in the liver in MASLD, the significance, and implications for treatment of which remain unclear. These are autoimmunity and bile duct injury.

It is far from uncommon for MASLD patients to have autoantibodies in their blood. Antibodies are one of the body's key tools for fighting infection. They are proteins with very characteristic patterns, and structures, which allow them to recognise and stick to proteins and other molecules from infectious organisms, thereby neutralising them and preventing them from causing harm within the body. Autoantibodies arise when the immune system falsely identifies, for a variety of reasons, the body's own proteins as being foreign and a threat. They are relatively common in the population, suggesting that the immune system is, to an extent, leaky. They certainly do not automatically suggest the presence of autoimmune disease. The most frequently seen autoantibody type in MASLD is **antinuclear antibody (ANA)**, an antibody that is the most frequently seen in another form of chronic liver disease, autoimmune hepatitis (AIH). As the name suggests, the antibodies are directed at the cell nucleus; the structure in the cell that contains the DNA genetic code formed into chromosomes. The target for ANA is thought to be histone proteins - proteins that add the structure to DNA to make chromosomes, although anti-DNA antibodies are also seen (anti-double stranded DNA antibodies (dsDNA)). As with the autoantibodies seen in other diseases ANA are not thought to be, themselves, directly harmful to the liver. Instead, they are a marker of the presence of a disease process.

It isn't entirely clear why MASLD patients develop ANA, given that the disease isn't itself inherently autoimmune in nature (it is a completely different disease process to AIH). The most likely explanation is that the inflammatory environment seen in fat-laden hepatocytes subtly alters the structure of the histones, taking away their invisibility to the immune system and opening them to recognition by the immune system.

What then is their significance in MASLD? There is a significance, but it is not the one that people might imagine! It seems very unlikely that there are actual harmful autoimmune responses present in MASLD patients and, as a result, it is not currently recommended that the presence of ANA should lead to any change in the treatment approach. The significance comes, instead, from the potential for the wrong diagnosis to be made. The presence of ANA and abnormal liver blood tests suggests, to the majority of hepatologists, the presence of AIH. AIH is an important condition and, if left untreated, can rapidly progress to life-threatening liver injury. Timely diagnosis and treatment are therefore essential. Unfortunately, however, first-line treatment for AIH is with steroids, which will dramatically worsen insulin resistance and drive fat deposition in the liver. What this means is that if AIH is incorrectly diagnosed when the actual issue is MASLD, the treatment can significantly worsen the steatosis process. It is essential, therefore, to make the right diagnosis. Ultrasound doesn't help because although the presence of fat in the liver could suggest MASLD it could be that there is pre-existing fat deposition and a new AIH. The ultimate test is liver biopsy, and we would certainly want a biopsy diagnosis before ever treating AIH with steroids. Two blood test features are useful at giving a clue. The first is the level (or titre as it is called technically) of the ANA. High levels of antibody (1 in 320 or 1 in 640) strongly suggest AIH. Lower levels (1 in 20 or 1 in 40) are much more typical of MASLD. The other is the level of IgG (a measure of the total amount of antibody in the blood). This is usually normal in MASLD but typically elevated in AIH. The higher the value the more likely it is that it is AIH. Levels above 30 (the upper limit of normal is 17.5) are almost diagnostic of AIH.

A proportion of MASLD patients (around 10-20%) will also have some evidence of injury to the small bile ducts on liver biopsy (a similar type of picture, albeit at a lower level, to that seen in primary biliary cholangitis (PBC)). The blood tests will reflect this, with an elevation in alkaline phosphatase that is more prominent. As is the case with PBC patients, itch can be an issue. Again, it isn't clear what the significance of this is (other than the itch being a nuisance, although fortunately one that is easy to treat (**Chapter 11**)). It may be that this additional disease process contributes to the speed of disease progression. As we will discuss in **Chapter 11**, the standard treatment used for PBC, a bile acid called ursodeoxycholic acid

(UDCA) has some benefits in MASLD and it may be that this reflects treatment of a bile duct element to the disease.

**Implications for treatment:** Anyone who was watched the film or read any of the many books on the subject will "know" that the problem when the Titanic sank was that it didn't carry enough lifeboats. Whereas it is true that there weren't enough, and people lost their lives as a result, the real problem was hitting an iceberg. If the Titanic hadn't collided with the iceberg in the first place it wouldn't have sunk, and the number of lifeboats would have remained irrelevant.

What is the relevance of this to MASLD? Given the importance of insulin resistance, inflammation, and fibrosis in MASLD there has been a natural and obvious focus on these individual processes when we have looked for treatments. The problem is, as we have discussed in the earlier parts of this chapter, that the inter-relationship between these processes is complicated, probably varies from person to person and is likely to reflect a relatively late stage in the disease process. By the time a person is identified as having clinically important MASLD it is likely that they will already have a complex mix of inter-related inflammation, hepatocyte injury and fibrosis. Altering one aspect of this complex process in isolation may have little or no impact on the overall disease picture. It could be argued that whether to target inflammation or fibrosis in MASLD is a little bit like arguing about whether the Titanic should have had more lifeboats or lifejackets. Relevant, but in danger of missing the point. Not having excess fat in the liver (and elsewhere in the body) would be a little bit like avoiding the iceberg in the first place and make all these processes to a significant degree irrelevant.

The key point, and one that will be the focus of most of the rest of this book, is that it is perfectly possible to remove the fat from your liver and therefore "avoid the iceberg". It isn't easy and it needs hard work, but it is doable and achieving it is entirely in your hands. **Own the problem, own the solution.**

# CHAPTER 4: DIAGNOSING AND MONITORING MASLD

## *The 2-Minute Version*

- Diagnosing MASLD needs clinical suspicion to be followed by the appropriate diagnostic tests. Once the presence of MASLD is confirmed it is essential to determine the severity of the disease (the degree to which fat deposition is accompanied by hepatocyte injury and inflammation) and the stage (how much fibrosis is present and whether this has progressed to cirrhosis).
- MASLD is one of the commonest forms of liver disease and should, therefore, be on the list of possible diagnoses for anyone presenting with liver dysfunction. It is a member of the metabolic syndrome family of linked conditions which includes hypertension, hypercholesterolaemia, ischaemic heart disease and, most of all, type 2 diabetes. Liver function test abnormality in a patient with any of these conditions should make you think automatically of MASLD.
- The presence of elevation of alanine transaminase (ALT) and/or aspartate transaminase (AST) in the context of the presence of fat in the liver on ultrasound is very strongly suggestive of MASLD. The diagnosis can only be confirmed by liver biopsy. Other patterns of liver function test abnormality, including elevation of alkaline phosphatase (ALP) and gamma glutamyl-transferase (GGT) are also seen.
- Liver biopsy is a very important test still in MASLD, both for confirming the diagnosis and for understanding disease severity.
- Degree of fibrosis can be estimated (although not definitively determined) by non-invasive approaches. These include fibroscan (an imaging approach that estimates the liver density), blood-based fibrosis markers and scores (tests that measure the breakdown products of fibrosis) and predictive scores that integrate clinical information that is associated with fibrosis risk. All are useful but not definitive. In all cases the whole clinical picture should be taken into consideration and a single test not treated as definitive.
- Once MASLD has been diagnosed, and treatment approaches instituted, regular follow up should be put in place. This, in essence, repeats the blood and imaging tests used to understand disease

severity and stage. Liver biopsy would not typically be repeated these days.
- In patients where cirrhosis is diagnosed or strongly suspected, screening for cirrhosis complications such as the presence of varices and hepatocellular carcinoma should be put in place.

If you have reached this far in the book then it is likely that you or your loved one will already have been diagnosed with MASLD, or you are concerned about the risk of developing it. This is important as the biggest risk in MASLD, as with many other liver diseases, is faced by people in whom the disease hasn't been diagnosed, and therefore can't be managed. There are more people in the UK with significant liver disease who don't know they have it than do. The presence of liver disease complicates many other, often mundane things (being started on tablets, people having operations, people having car accidents and so on). The additional risk conferred by having liver disease with all these events can be mitigated, reducing the risk. This can only be done, however, if the liver disease is known about.

There are two broad routes to a diagnosis of MASLD being made. These are diagnosis following clinical suspicion of the condition (or investigation of non-specific symptoms) and diagnosis through screening. In the former, the possibility of MASLD, or some other form of liver disease, has been suspected by a clinician based on symptoms, such as fatigue and aches and pains, or the presence of other features of the metabolic syndrome making the diagnosis a possibility. This has led to tests being ordered which have been interpreted as suggesting MASLD. In the latter, tests suggestive of MASLD have arisen in the context of a clinical screening event (such as perhaps hypertension follow up or "well woman" or "well man" screening). The route to diagnosis does not really matter as long as the diagnosis is not missed. Our experience is that diagnosis through screening is sometimes slower than because of clinical suspicion. The moral, perhaps, should be that whenever anyone has screening tests (blood tests, x-rays etc) they should find out the results of all the tests and ask about the significance of any abnormalities.

It is going to become increasingly important that we not only diagnose MASLD but that we diagnosis it as early as possible. Why so? The traditional model in liver disease management has been to manage by risk assessing and risk reduction. In essence, looking for the presence of cirrhosis and its complications and, when present, managing those complications (tablets or endoscopic treatment for varices, lactulose and rifaximin for encephalopathy, transplantation etc). We liken this to keeping a watch for people who have fallen into a river so you can pull them out. It works, but assumes you see everyone and can respond in time. It also feels a little inefficient and reactive. Isn't it better to stop people falling into the river in the first place? This is the direction of travel in liver disease. Effective treatment to prevent the development of fibrosis and cirrhosis in the first place (and thus removing the need to manage complications). We aren't there yet with MASLD; however, we are sure that we will get there. If we are to, however, it is likely that we will need to treat the disease early before the complications develop. If we are going to do this, we need to diagnose it early.

## *SUSPECTING MASLD*

MASLD is a really common problem, and one that is getting commoner in our population for the reasons outlined in the previous chapter. In many western populations it is the commonest of all liver disease. In many low- and middle-income countries rapid development and increase in average incomes is leading to rapid increases in obesity and the features of the metabolic syndrome, including MASLD. It is likely, therefore, that the rapid increases in MASLD seen in Western Europe and the USA will be replicated elsewhere. This is a very real emerging public health problem. Given the rises in both prevalence (the number of people in the population with a condition) and incidence (the number of people developing it for the first time per year) the possibility of MASLD should be thought about in anyone in whom liver disease may be suspected. It is important, however, to suspect rather than assume it is MASLD and make sure that other potential causes for liver disease are looked for and excluded. If we don't, we can miss important chances to treat people. The same trap, of assuming that liver disease always has the most obvious cause, has also applied for many years in relation to alcoholic liver disease.

One important aspect to suspecting MASLD is to not make assumptions as to what a MASLD patient "looks like". Although the archetypal patient will be an overweight man in his 50 to 60s, MASLD can affect anyone in the population. We are, worryingly, seeing increasing numbers of children and young adults with the condition and it can develop at any stage in life. It also affects both men and women. An important trap is also to not assume that someone who is not overweight can't have MASLD. Obesity increases the risk of the condition, but it is fundamentally a condition related to how the metabolism works in the liver and we all have a metabolism!

**In people with suggestive blood tests:** This is probably the commonest route to suspecting MASLD and typically starts with people being found to show elevation of one of the liver enzymes that are released when liver cells are injured. Most often this is an elevation of alanine transaminase (ALT) or aspartate transaminase (AST) (see **Table 1**), although less frequently it can be elevation of alkaline phosphatase (ALP). These are routine blood biochemistry tests which form part of a routine panel of tests ("liver function tests" or "LFTs") done in numerous clinical settings, including, and of huge relevance to MASLD, monitoring people with diabetes, high blood pressure and high cholesterol. They are also measured routinely in the setting of maternity care and in "well woman" or "well man" clinics. When a high ALT or AST is found, it is usually not because the clinician ordering the test suspects that the patient has MASLD (beyond, perhaps, the setting of a diabetes clinic). This, together with the number of different conditions that can result in ALT or AST elevation (they really are very non-specific tests) means that the connection between test elevation and possible MASLD needs to be made after the test abnormality has been found. This is where lack of awareness on the part of many clinicians as to the significance of these test findings can be a real problem. Many patients diagnosed with MASLD have, in retrospect, had abnormalities in their ALT, AST or ALP for years before the diagnosis is made. As we will discuss at length later in this book, it is likely that treatment is most effective, and will be less invasive, when given very early in the disease. Missed diagnosis will, therefore, be missed opportunity to treat.

It is important to remember that elevation of ALT and the other liver enzymes is always non-specific and does not tell you the cause of the liver disease (and thus how you should treat it). Statistically, MASLD is the commonest cause of a raised ALT, but that does not mean that any one individual with a raised ALT has MASLD. Identifying the cause for a raised ALT, and thus making a diagnosing and treating it, needs further information.

**In people with suggestive symptoms:** One of the characteristics of symptoms in liver disease is that, for most of the disease course, they have no characteristic features (odd as it might sound). This is certainly the case for MASLD when it first develops. People tend to think of jaundice and ascites as being the characteristic features of liver disease. Many MASLD patients have symptoms that could lead to a diagnosis being made (and certainly have blood test abnormality) long before they develop jaundice. Ascites should, in an ideal world, never be a reason to diagnose MASLD (and, indeed, should never be seen once the diagnosis has been made) because its presence is a feature of cirrhosis, the prevention of which is the goal of treatment in MASLD. If it is present, it means the condition has been diagnosed late (usually in someone who has not had any prior symptoms at all, meaning that there was no reason to suspect and look for it, although sometimes, unfortunately, the information needed to diagnose is present but is not recognised) or inadequately treated. We will address these issues later in this chapter and in the next chapter.

The initial symptom in MASLD is typically fatigue. In addition to its importance as a symptom raising the possibility of MASLD, fatigue is the commonest symptom in the condition and, across the patient population and throughout the course of the disease, the one with the greatest overall impact on life quality. Experience suggests that it is also the easiest symptom to have its significance missed. The challenge is, of course, the multiple causes of fatigue ranging from physical medical problems (diabetes itself is a common cause of fatigue in the population) to mental health problems (fatigue is a big issue in depression) and life-style issues (working too hard or partying too hard!). There is also the very large group of individuals given the diagnosis of chronic fatigue syndrome (CFS/ME). Given that the diagnosis of CFS/ME is largely a negative one (it is made by excluding other causes for fatigue) it is easy to see how a clinician who doesn't know that liver disease causes fatigue, and therefore doesn't test for it, can end up giving a fatigued MASLD patient the diagnosis of CFS/ME.

If jaundice develops, or darkening of the urine because the jaundice pigment occurs, the possibility of liver disease becomes much clearer and investigation with blood tests is normal. Whether the possibility of MASLD is considered at this stage largely depends on the presence of risk factors for other types of liver disease, and the age and sex of the individual. The other symptom sets that should alert to the possibility of significant MASLD are those of cirrhosis (in addition to jaundice). The clinical features of cirrhosis include ascites, bleeding from varices and hepatic encephalopathy. These are largely unrelated to the cause of the liver disease meaning that, rather as with an elevation in ALT, the pattern of problems doesn't really help us to identify the cause. There can, unfortunately, be an assumption by people, that this pattern of cirrhotic clinical features is suggestive of alcoholic liver disease. It isn't, and that assumption should never be made.

One issue we have come across in clinical practice is a failure to appreciate that cirrhotic liver disease is present when a complication develops, because there isn't a prior diagnosis of cirrhotic liver disease. A circular argument. The key thing is that a number of people have their very first presentation with a complication of cirrhosis. Two patients like this stick in the memory. One presented for the first time with a variceal bleed......whilst flying across the Atlantic. The other was referred by a cardiology colleague who had just seen him with massive ascites which his GP thought was caused by heart failure. Both had cirrhosis and both had never had any medical problems in the past, or symptoms suggestive of liver disease, and, importantly, both did well with management of their complications (making the point that it is never too late to make a difference by diagnosing and managing liver disease).

## *DIAGNOSING MASLD*

There are two distinct challenges in diagnosing MASLD. The first is, as we have previously discussed, suspecting it in the first place. This means thinking about the possibility in "at risk" individuals and appreciating the potential significance of abnormal liver blood tests. The second is identifying the form of the disease, and thus working out the risk it poses.

There are two specific traps that people can fall into in making the diagnosis of MASLD. The first is the tendency to assume that all liver disease is caused by alcohol (a theme we will keep coming back to). This trap is a particularly easy one to fall into with regard to MASLD, because the populations most at risk for MASLD and alcohol-related liver disease are very similar, and a number of the test findings can appear very similar (as we will discuss below). A particular nuance to the issue is that alcohol consumption is obviously common in many parts of our society, meaning that many people with MASLD also drink. This does not mean that alcohol is the direct cause of their liver disease (although as we have discussed in the last chapter, the nutritional load from alcohol can make an important contribution to non-alcoholic MASLD). An easy and obvious way to distinguish the two conditions is the level of alcohol consumption (it is, self-evidently, much higher in patients with alcohol-related liver disease). There is a problem, however, that clinicians almost never believe people when they say how much they drink! One of the things we repeatedly say to doctors in training in relation to liver disease is that repeatedly asking people with liver disease how much they drink when they have told you they don't drink is rarely helpful. They may, of course, be drinkers and not telling you, but badgering them won't, in our experience, get them to change what they say. The more likely possibility is that they in fact don't drink, have liver disease of another cause, and you have just damaged your relationship with them by implying they are lying.......

The second trap people fall into is to think that there is a definitive diagnostic test for MASLD. There in fact isn't any single "smoking gun" type marker comparable to, for example, anti-mitochondrial antibody in primary biliary cholangitis (which is 95% accurate for the diagnosis of the disease). Diagnosis of MASLD is made by a combination of supportive tests (findings which would go along with the diagnosis) and exclusion of other potential causes through a combination of clinical story and tests. MASLD is often, therefore, what is called a diagnosis of exclusion. This always creates a sense of uncertainty (we would love that 95% accurate test) but that shouldn't be allowed to get in the way of diagnosis and treatment (sitting on the fence with diagnosis is, ultimately, almost always counter-productive). It is always worth bearing in mind, however, that little bit of diagnostic doubt that exists with fatty liver and if, down the line, the disease doesn't behave as we would expect, revisiting the diagnosis.

In the clinical investigation for suspected MASLD, it is important to remember that there are tests that help **diagnose** the condition (is it MASLD or something else), tests that help to **stage** the disease (is there fibrosis or cirrhosis or is it early disease) and tests that are used to **monitor** the disease (how is it changing over time, is it getting worse and is there any response to treatment). It is important to understand which test is used for which person, and, in particular, that staging tests aren't seen as tests that confirm the diagnosis. In terms of the diagnosis of MASLD there are three key test types: liver biochemical tests, imaging tests and liver biopsy.

**Liver biochemistry ("liver function tests" or "LFT"):** These are a panel of blood tests that are very commonly done in many clinical settings (hence the discovery of unexpected LFT abnormality as a route to suspicion of MASLD). Within the panel of tests, there are a number that are important for MASLD diagnosis (although none is, as we have outlined earlier, sufficient in isolation). Perhaps the most useful tests are blood levels of two enzymes called *alanine transaminase (ALT)* and *aspartate transaminase (AST)*. These are proteins that are normally present within the hepatocytes, where they play important roles in the function of the liver. In simple terms, when the hepatocytes are injured by a disease process (in MASLD from the dual effects of fat deposition in the cell and inflammation, augmented by the pro-inflammatory actions of fat) ALT and AST are released into the blood. The levels of these proteins can be easily measured. Although it is normal to have measurable levels of these enzymes in the blood (liver cells die and regrow every day of our lives), higher than normal levels suggest extra release, which implies that too many liver cells are dying. Two things are, however, important to make clear at this point. The first is that elevated levels of these enzymes in the blood does not cause any direct harm. They are not in any way toxic, so it doesn't directly matter that the levels are increased. It is the implication that the level elevation holds that is key. The second is that when we talk about too many liver cells dying, this often worries people who, perfectly reasonably, think that this means that they will run out! In fact, it is normal, when liver cells are dying in disease, for the cells that are lost to be replaced by new cells growing. There is thus a balanced loss and regrowth meaning that the total number remains close to normal, and the patient has more than enough functioning liver cells.

There are several cautions in relation to ALT and AST levels and their use in MASLD (and, later in the pathway, disease monitoring). The first is that their release from liver cells is a feature of damage rather than the cause of that damage. Elevation of ALT could therefore be a feature of MASLD, but it could equally also be a feature of other disease processes. The second is that they are not even unique to liver cells. Other tissues such as muscle (both heart and skeletal) and kidney can also release AST in particular, when injured. The final caution relates to levels and their implications for how much liver tissue is being damaged. It is intuitive that the more cells in the liver that are dying the more ALT and AST will be released. In an acute active hepatitis (the generic term for inflammation of the liver) levels of up to 20,000 are not uncommon (the upper limit of normal being 40). These numbers can naturally worry people. A little ALT, however, goes a long way and although the number seems high the actual level of release in relation to the amount remaining in the liver is small. In fact, very high levels of ALT and AST tend to be a feature of very acute liver injury and are rarely seen in the setting of MASLD which is almost always a very indolent condition. In the chronic or long-term disease setting (as is typical in MASLD) the levels are much less elevated. This can sometimes reassure clinicians and patients (lower levels means that the problem isn't that bad). This can lead to false reassurance as in these settings it is the cumulative long-term loss of liver cells that is the issue.

At the risk of causing even more confusion, there is an extra complexity to ALT and AST in the sense that normal doesn't always mean normal. There are two settings in which seemingly normal ALT and AST levels can "hide" significant ongoing liver injury. In very acute liver injury, the presence of normal ALT and AST could indicate that hepatocyte loss has been so extensive that, in essence, the liver is "running out of cells". Therefore, although in most instances the return of an ALT level to normal suggests that liver injury is declining, just occasionally it is going the other way and reaching crisis point. The give-away is that, in this setting, the markers of actual liver function are typically very deranged, something that isn't the case if normal ALT and AST values reflect declining (i.e. improving) liver injury.

The second setting is the emerging evidence to suggest that the values that are routinely used to identify "normal" ALT and AST levels may not be correct and that we have used cut-offs that are too high in the past. This really all relates to how normal ranges for tests are established. It often surprises people that these don't typically come from some deep knowledge about biology. Instead, they come from the test being applied to a very large group of normal individuals and a statistical approach used to define what are outlier values (for the statistically minded it is the mean plus or minus 2 standard deviations). This means that around 2.5% of people will be, by chance, above the upper cut off and 2.5% below the lower cut off, even though they are normal - think about height in the population, there is a huge spread, with the commonest value for men being 5 foot 10 but people being much shorter or much taller than that and being perfectly healthy (they may just come from short families). One of the implications of 5% of healthy people being flagged as "abnormal" for a test (2.5% high and 2.5% low) just by a statistical quirk is that if you do too many random tests you can run into trouble (do 20 tests in someone, each with a 5% chance of being "abnormal" even though you are healthy and then just by chance you will expect one "abnormality"). Do 100 tests (not uncommon these days when we do panels of tests and 5 will be "abnormal" ……all without any actual abnormality). What this means is that we must be very careful in terms of "abnormal tests", especially if they don't fit with the general clinical picture.

With MASLD, this issue of "normal" and "abnormal" becomes even more complicated. When the large group of people had their ALT and AST measured to allow the normal range to be defined, they were "normal" only in terms of their not having any clinical conditions. They weren't excluded because they are overweight, meaning that a good number of them may well have had MASLD but not known about it (all this was done in an era well before it was even recognised as a condition). This means that not all the ALTs measured were truly normal, and we will therefore have to come up with a cut off that reflects "true normal", the level seen if there is genuinely no liver disease. What this means in practice is that we should use a much lower cut off for normal for ALT than the one we are used to (40). The values of 30 for men and 19 for women have been suggested. Using these cut offs, high ALT values are commoner than we ever thought in the population, and most of these are people with MASLD.......

If high ALT and AST are the classical biochemical tests suggesting MASLD, it is important to remember that they are not the only ones that can be elevated. The second type of enzyme released by cells of the liver into the blood, and which can be elevated in AIH, is **alkaline phosphatase (ALP)**. This enzyme is, in contrast to ALT and AST which are released by injured hepatocytes, released by stressed or injured biliary epithelial cells (the cells lining the bile duct). A second enzyme (**gamma-glutamyl transferase (GGT)**) can also be released by injured bile duct cells and is a useful confirmatory test to make sure raised ALP is of liver origin (it can be released by several other cell types in the body, including the bone). In most cases of MASLD the bile ducts are not involved, meaning that bile duct cells are not being injured and ALP is not, therefore, typically raised. In a minority of MASLD patients there is some bile duct involvement (it may be as simple as the swollen, fat-filled cells pressing on the small bile ducts and limiting bile flow). If ALP and GGT are elevated in MASLD, it is usually in addition to ALT/AST, but occasionally they can be elevated in isolation, and this can cause real diagnostic confusion.

Paradoxically, although ALT, AST and ALP are conventionally described as "liver function tests" they do not of course, as we have described them, measure liver function. They measure liver injury. The conventional LFT panel includes two further tests which do measure function of the liver (although both are not pure measures of liver function either and can be abnormal in other clinical situations). These are **bilirubin** and **albumin**. These will be discussed later in this chapter.

**Imaging:** Imaging plays a key role in turning clinical suspicion of fatty liver into diagnosis in most people. The reason for this is that fat deposition in the liver gives very characteristic appearances on all forms of routine scanning. Most commonly the first suggestion is the finding of a "bright liver" on ultrasound. Ultrasound is, as its name suggests, a test where a beam of very high frequency noise (beyond the human hearing range) is released by the probe, and the amount that returns to the probe is measured. Solids reflect the signal better than fluids, which are in turn better than gas. This allows a picture to be built up of the organs underneath the probe. Fat is uniquely effective at reflecting the sound leading to a very high signal indeed. The level of the signal means that there is a very bright appearance coming back from the liver (lots of signal coming back = very bright signal). This means that ultrasound, which is widely available and non-invasive, is very good at alerting to the presence of fat in the liver. There are, however, three caveats to its use in MASLD diagnosis.

The first caveat is that low levels of fat may not be demonstrated using it. A normal ultrasound doesn't, therefore, completely exclude MASLD. The second is that it cannot really distinguish between simple fat and the combination of fat and inflammation which is the key issue (we will discuss this more in a later section). Finally, it doesn't tell you whether that fat is the cause of the liver blood test abnormality that you are investigating. What do we mean? Simply that fat deposition in the liver is common in obesity which is common in the population. Fat deposition can therefore be seen in overweight PBC, PSC, AIH, HCV etc patients as well as MASLD......

Fat deposition in the liver will also be well demonstrated using other investigation methodologies such as CT and MRI, although these tend only to be used a little further down the investigation pathway.

**Liver Biopsy and Histology**: The definitive, and most diagnostic, clinical test is a liver biopsy with direct examination of the liver tissue. In simple terms, the procedure involves using a narrow needle to take a very small sample of the liver. There are three "routes" to get the needle to the liver. The first is directly through the skin on the right-hand side of the upper abdomen (actually going between the ribs because the liver is "tucked up" underneath the diaphragm where it is protected from trauma by the rib cage). The ideal place to take the biopsy is usually identified by ultrasound as part of the procedure, and this imaging-linked approach has important advantages for making the procedure safe. The skin, muscle and the capsule of the liver are frozen using a local anaesthetic and the operator will ask you to breathe in then breathe out all the way and hold your breath (this is to make sure the lung doesn't get in the way). The needle is then quickly inserted, and the sample taken. The procedure usually takes around 10 minutes and has little or no pain associated with it. After the biopsy, people must lie flat for a few hours just to make sure there is no bleeding.

Sometimes it is not possible (or safe) to do a biopsy in this way and in that situation, we use trans-jugular biopsy as an approach. Here a tube is inserted into the jugular vein in the neck and is then navigated through the venous system into the liver (via the hepatic vein). A long flexible needle is then passed down the tube and the biopsy taken through the wall of the vein. The advantage of this approach is that if there is any bleeding after the procedure it is into a vein meaning that blood loss is rare. This means that trans-jugular biopsy as an approach is useful in people whose blood clotting is abnormal (something that can happen as part of the disease process in liver conditions). The disadvantage is that the procedure is more involved and takes longer, and the size of the biopsy is a lot smaller, meaning that it may be less easy to get a definitive answer as to the diagnosis.

The final potential approach to a liver biopsy is the least frequently used in practice. This is via the abdominal cavity in the context of an operation where the abdomen is either opened, or a laparoscope (keyhole surgery camera) is inserted in. This is always a safe approach to doing a biopsy as the operator can see and control any bleeding after the biopsy has been taken. It would be very unusual indeed, however, to do an operation solely in order to do a biopsy.

Once the biopsy has been taken, it is prepared in the laboratory (fixed) and very thin sections are cut, put on a slide and then stained using special dyes for the pathologist to examine down the microscope. There are two information sets that can be gleaned from a liver biopsy. These are features that relate to the diagnosis of MASLD, and then features that stage the disease (as we will discuss later). Determining the presence or absence of MASLD is perhaps the most straightforward aspect. In the fixation process any fat present in the liver cells is dissolved. This leaves behind holes in the tissue section (it looks like Swiss cheese!). The presence of these holes absolutely proves that there was a MASLD process. Occasionally this appearance can occur in people in whom MASLD wasn't suspected at ultrasound (at the end of the day biopsy is a much more sensitive test than ultrasound) but in most people this finding merely confirms what was previously suspected. If this is the case, why do the biopsy? There are two main reasons regarding diagnosis. The first is that it allows us to distinguish between patients who do and don't have inflammation and its resulting injury patterns (MASH as opposed to simple steatosis). This distinction is a really important one and determines almost every aspect of later management. What inflammation means in terms of liver biopsy analysis is the presence of cells of the immune system (lymphocytes, neutrophils etc) both in the portal tract (where they leave the circulation and enter the liver tissue) and infiltrating into the hepatocyte layers. This is accompanied by evidence of hepatocyte injury through apoptosis and senescence, with what are called apoptotic bodies (packaged up cellular debris following the apoptosis process) present amongst the hepatocytes. The nature of the inflammation is actually rather non-specific and doesn't itself direct the diagnosis. It is the combination of this inflammation with fat (or more accurately the holes where the fat used to be) that is key. The traditional visual impression approach (the pathologist observes the biopsy and reaches a conclusion regarding diagnosis) has, in recent year, been complemented by histology scoring systems (such as the HAI or histology activity index). These scores don't really add much in the setting of a one-off biopsy done for diagnosis. They do, however, allow the degree of activity to be quantified. This allows more accurate comparison of biopsies done a length of time apart than does simple description. This is important for looking at change in disease over time and with treatment; something that is essential in trials of new treatments aimed at treating MASLD.

The other value of liver biopsy is, of course, its potential to identify other, perhaps unexpected, forms of chronic liver disease. Remember, fat deposition in the liver is common in the population in general, and that includes in people who have other forms of liver disease.

## ***WHAT ELSE COULD IT BE? THE DIFFERENTIAL DIAGNOSIS***

When doctors are training, they are taught to think of shortlists for potential diagnoses which are then narrowed down to make the actual diagnosis. This is a fail-safe approach because it makes you actively consider, and exclude, the other likely, and frequently important, possible diagnoses. Given the issues with missed and delayed diagnosis in all liver diseases, the concept of differential diagnosis is a key one. The reason why it matters, of course, is that we are increasingly looking to treat liver disease with targeted therapy approaches. Get the diagnosis wrong and at best you miss the opportunity to treat a disease better (give the treatment that is right for another disease, and it probably won't work for MASLD). At worst you can make the condition worse (most obviously giving someone with MASLD steroids which will do nothing to improve the disease but will worsen obesity, type 2 diabetes and thus fat deposition in the liver).

In a way, the increasing importance of differential diagnosis reflects our increasing success in treating liver disease to prevent cirrhosis. In the early days of hepatology, when our only real treatment option was to control the complications of cirrhosis when they arose, it mattered far less to know the cause of the liver disease (as we weren't going to treat it anyway).

We have split this section into two. The first section relates to the "true" differential diagnosis; the other conditions that cause fat deposition with and without inflammation (of which alcohol-related disease is by far and away the most important). The second relates to the other types of liver disease that shouldn't be confused with MASLD, but sometimes are by less experienced clinicians. In practice, the issue is usually the other way around, with other forms of liver disease being assumed to be MASLD just because the patient is overweight and MASLD is common (a modern evolution of assuming that liver abnormality in someone who drinks alcohol must be alcohol-related liver disease).

**Other diseases with fat in the liver:** The name change from NAFLD to MASLD was accompanied by an approach to, for the first time, structuring our understanding of liver diseases characterised by fat deposition. This should help clinicians to think in a structured way about potential diagnoses. In this new approach the categories of liver disease with fat deposition are:

*Metabolic-dysfunction associated steatotic liver disease (MASLD):* The condition previously known as NAFLD (as well as all the alternative terms that came into common usage and which contributed to much of the confusion amongst clinicians and patients). This is the subject of this book!

*Alcohol-associated (alcohol-related) liver disease (ALD):* Fat deposition as part of an alcohol excess syndrome. Other related terms that are used include alcoholic steatohepatitis (ASH). There has been a move away from pejorative terms such as "alcoholic" (which imply addiction which, in reality, often isn't an issue) and towards more neutral terms such as "alcohol-related".

*MASLD and increased alcohol intake (MetALD):* This category codifies a group of people who are increasingly recognised. The concept of MASLD as a "pure" disease state in people who don't consume alcohol ignores the reality that, in western populations at least, the majority of patients with metabolic syndrome, and thus at risk of MASLD, consume alcohol to some degree. Clearly, if both processes are though to be at play, abstinence from alcohol would represent the easiest approach to treatment (in theory at least).

*Specific aetiology SLD:* A group of typically very rare conditions that are characterised by fat deposition in the liver. These include drug-induced changes (for example sodium valproate), a number of rare genetic disorders and fatty liver of pregnancy.

*Cryptogenic SLD:* Fat deposition in the liver without any clear cause. It may well be that many of these patients have atypical forms of MASLD.

By far and away the biggest challenge here is *alcohol-associated liver disease* (a description that includes alcohol-related steatosis and alcoholic steatohepatitis (ASH); exactly the same spectrum of steatotic disease as we see in "classical" MASLD). The reason it is important to distinguish the two is very obvious. If alcohol is driving the problem then there is a very specific and (in theory at least) simple intervention; no alcohol!. There are several complexities and challenges in distinguishing the two disease types.

The first complexity is that in terms of the tests that we do they can look very similar indeed. Imaging reveals fat deposition and the biopsy can show the legacy of fat deposition and a rather non-specific form of inflammation in both. There are some characteristic biopsy changes that are often present in alcoholic steatohepatitis but not in MASH but they are subtle and may be absent in both types of disease. They can also be missed by less experienced pathologists.

A second complexity is the degree of overlap between the lifestyle risk factors. In theory, distinguishing an alcohol-related problem from a non-alcohol-related one is easy. One group drinks and the other doesn't. The problem is that in the real world it is nowhere near as simple as this. Most people with metabolic syndrome-related MASLD (the type this book is focusing on) also drink. In fact, the majority of adults in our society drink alcohol to some degree. You have type 2 diabetes, drink 15 units a week and have MASLD. Is it the diabetes? Is it the alcohol? Is it the fish and chips you eat on the way home from the pub? We have come across a lot of instances where clinicians have really tried to drill down into which aspect or aspects of lifestyle are driving a disease process. In all honesty we suspect that this is probably doomed to fail (at least given the clinical tools we have at our disposal at the moment). It also probably misses the point. All of those aspects are probably contributing and, using our "own the problem/own the solution" model, all could usefully be changed. This is the origin of the concept of *Met-ALD*.

The third complexity is that alcohol-related liver disease itself has multiple different forms. The classical form of alcoholic hepatitis has a significant immune component in which alcohol modifies proteins in the hepatocytes that the immune response then recognises and reacts to. In this sense, the disease almost mirrors autoimmune hepatitis (and is, perhaps unsurprisingly, the form that has been treated with steroids). Interestingly, this is the form of alcohol-related liver disease that has the least steatosis. Alcohol is, however, very energy rich and it can generate a high nutrition load that is absorbed rapidly and goes straight to the liver. It can therefore drive exactly the same process of excess energy fat deposition as glucose or fructose. As we discussed earlier, if you went to the pub and drank 5 pints of a full-sugar soft drink every night you would inevitably get MASLD. It is exactly the same situation with alcohol.

Given all these issues, how do we distinguish a principally alcohol-related from a non-alcohol-related process? There are a few clues. The first is, obviously, the history. Typically, the alcohol history will be more extensive, and prolonged, in people with an alcohol aetiology (although watch the trap about the nutritional load from alcohol). In terms of test results, alcoholic hepatitis typically has lower levels of ALT than MASLD (to the extent that the ALT is often actually normal). The ratio of AST to ALT is another helpful manifestation of the same effect. In most situations that values of AST and ALT are very similar (i.e. the ratio is around 1). If AST is a lot higher than ALT, it can suggest an alcohol aetiology. This occurs because of a direct effect of alcohol on the production of ALT (explaining the strangely low ALT levels). In terms of other blood tests, in our experience, the higher the levels of bilirubin and more prolonged the prothrombin time, the more likely it is that alcohol is the aetiology. Finally, as mentioned above, expert pathologists can distinguish the two.

Another way of looking at it, however, is that if someone is drinking enough alcohol to have abnormal liver blood tests and to make you suspicious that they have alcoholic liver disease, then they are almost certainly drinking too much and, almost regardless of the mechanism by which the alcohol is causing problems, they need to reduce their intake!

The other identified causes of fatty liver, in the *Specific aetiology SLD* category are, in comparison, rare and rarely cause issues in diagnosis. One of the most important in terms of risk (if not frequency) is *acute fatty liver of pregnancy*. This is one of the acute onset liver diseases of pregnancy and is related to stresses in the metabolic interaction of mother and baby. It is said to be commoner with male babies, especially male twins (although this may be more myth than reality). It can be a significant condition requiring consideration of early delivery. It shouldn't cause confusion in terms of diagnosis, in practice, given the pregnancy. However, if liver abnormality occurs late in pregnancy, and fat is seen in the liver on ultrasound, the possibility should always be born in mind that this is another form of acute liver injury in someone with pre-existing and completely unrelated MASLD. The other reasonably frequently seen cause of MASLD is *drug induced liver injury*. The anti-epileptic drugs carbamazepine and sodium valproate can cause steatotic liver disease which is self-limiting if the culprit drug is discontinued. Diagnosis is usually simple (a history of culprit drug exposure) and, as is always the case with suspected drug-induced liver disease, discontinuation of the drug is essential. This can cause issues in terms of epilepsy management and careful thought is needed as to alternative therapies. This lies outside the scope of this book, however.

**Other liver disease not characterised by fat deposition:** The potential for an alternative, or additional, unexpected diagnosis to be revealed on investigation, including at biopsy, is always there. In the case of MASLD, where the evidence for the presence of fat deposition is usually clear cut, the issue is normally one of an unexpected second diagnosis rather than an alternative primary diagnosis.

The commonest "trap" in terms of MASLD (after the issues with alcohol outlined above) is *autoimmune hepatitis*. This is a condition of immune miss-targeting where the immune response causes progressive injury to the liver cells. This arises because of a case of "mistaken identity" as the immune system interprets one of the body's own proteins as being a foreign, harmful protein and tries to get rid of it. It is an important diagnosis because the condition can cause significant liver injury rapidly, leading to liver damage and ultimately liver failure or cirrhosis if it isn't treated. Treatment is highly effective, however, emphasising the importance of accurate diagnosis. It is not associated with fat deposition so, logically, it should not cause problems in terms of confusion with MASLD......but yet it does. The reason is that the characteristic autoantibody seen in autoimmune hepatitis is anti-nuclear antibody; an autoantibody that is also seen in a significant number of MASLD patients. The issue is with mistaking MASLD for autoimmune hepatitis in light of this antibody and then treating for autoimmune hepatitis with the standard therapy of steroids. These, then, make MASLD worse. What is important to realise is that the presence of anti-nuclear antibody in MASLD is for reasons entirely unrelated to autoimmune hepatitis, that there is no element of autoimmune hepatitis in MASLD and that autoimmune hepatitis treatments shouldn't be used in MASLD. It is, of course, possible that the coincidental co-existence of MASLD and autoimmune hepatitis could occur, but it is unlikely.

Another liver disease that should always appear in the differential diagnosis for any liver disease is *drug-induced liver disease (DILI)*. This is in addition to the drug-induced liver changes that cause fat deposition, mentioned on the previous page. The liver, because of its role in modifying and clearing things from the body, is the organ most susceptible to injury by drugs. For most drugs, in the vast majority of people, there is no issue. Problems can, however, arise. Many drugs very occasionally cause issues (but are recorded as causing liver injury in the patient information leaflets, sometimes causing real concern for patients). A much smaller number are the "usual suspects" where the potential for the problem is well recognised. It is worth noting, however, that even for the "usual suspects" most people taking these drugs have no problems at all.

A second important differential diagnosis is with *viral hepatitis*. Included in this category are the "classical" viral hepatitis viruses - hepatitis A, hepatitis B and hepatitis E (hepatitis C is common but rarely presents with an acute hepatitis) and, confusingly, a few other viruses that can infect (or impact on) the liver as well as other target organs. These include EBV (glandular fever), CMV and herpes virus. All these viruses can cause an acute onset hepatitis with lethargy, aches and pains, raised ALT and, eventually, jaundice. All can also cause abdominal pain as well. In practice, viral hepatitis shouldn't cause a problem because all the important viruses can be detected using either specific tests for the virus (looking for and measuring either the virus protein or its DNA or RNA) or the immune features of a recent infection (IgM against the virus). The trap, in our experience, is the assumption that it must be viral hepatitis and a failure to adjust the diagnosis if the specific virus tests turn out to be negative. Of all the viruses it is probably hepatitis E that is the trickiest, and the most likely to catch people out. It is the most recently discovered of the viruses and it is clear that it is commoner than was originally thought to be the case. It is also the cause of virus hepatitis for which the testing is least readily available, and for which the tests often take the longest to come back.

The final important differential diagnosis, *Wilson's disease*, is by some distance the rarest. Wilson's disease is a genetic disorder of copper handling by the body. The body needs very small amounts of copper which is critical for the functioning of some enzymes. Copper can be toxic, however, so the levels are very tightly regulated, with excess copper being transported out into the bile and then out of the body. This acts as a fail-safe if too much is eaten in the diet. In Wilson's, a gene mutation leads to impaired functioning of the transporter and an inexorable, although slow, build-up of copper in the tissues. One of the tissues that is damaged is the liver, with injury ranging from a hepatitis pattern to cirrhosis. Other tissues can also be damaged, including the brain. The deposited copper causes injury to the brain stem (the lower part of the brain essential for basic motor and other functions). There are two reasons why we have included Wilson's disease in our list of differential diagnoses. The first is that it is, by some distance, the condition that can most look like any liver disease. The second is that in its early stages (and that includes the liver disease stages) it is easily and completely treatable. When brain injury occurs, however, it is irreversible, even with treatment, and has devastating impacts. It destroys young people. A challenge with the diagnosis of Wilson's is that it needs specialised tests, and the doctor must have thought of the diagnosis to order them. It is very rare for the tests to be ordered and the significance of the findings not to be recognised. In most instances where Wilson's is missed the tests are simply not ordered because the diagnosis hasn't been considered.

The final condition to mention in this section shouldn't ever cause problems (but does). This is *Budd-Chiari* syndrome. This is one of a family of problems characterised by blood clot formation in the vessels around the liver. In classical Budd-Chiari the clot, and resulting obstruction to blood flow, is in the hepatic veins draining blood out of the liver. The block to drainage can occur rapidly, giving a hepatitis-like picture, or more slowly given rise to chronic injury and even cirrhosis. As with Wilson's, the tests needed to diagnose it are specialised (in this case imaging of the hepatic veins, usually with a contrast CT) and the diagnosis needs to have been thought of before the tests are normally ordered. Treatment is with anticoagulation as soon as the diagnosis is considered. If diagnosed early enough, this can prevent the clot worsening and allow the body the opportunity to break it down naturally. Occasionally, the clot needs to be opened up using radiological approaches. In rare cases liver injury is so severe by the time of diagnosis that the only treatment option is liver transplant. Most people developing Budd-Chiari have some form of underlying clotting tendency, and in most cases, anticoagulation needs to be long term or even life-long. As with Wilson's, unless you think of it you won't diagnose it.

## *STAGING MASLD*

Once a diagnosis of MASLD is made the next step is to stage it (in simple terms to understand "how bad it is"). This matters for the following reasons. MASLD has a very broad spectrum indeed, with disease ranging from simple steatosis (fat deposition in the liver cells but no accompanying inflammation; a relatively benign clinical picture) to more aggressive steatohepatitis, fibrosis then cirrhosis; a high-risk disease state. This notion of severity will dictate what treatment approaches could be tried, what tests will need to be done to monitor the disease and even how frequently you will need to be seen in a clinic and by whom. As the number and types of treatments that are available increase in the future, so the importance of staging will increase. The important thing is that it is the stage that matters much more in practice than just having a MASLD diagnosis written in your medical records. If you know what the current stage and severity of disease is, then you can know if it is improving with treatments (lifestyle, diabetes management and any specific MASLD treatments), or deteriorating.

When considering the stages, they exist in a spectrum, it's not that there is one stage present and not the others. Fibrosis exists at the same time as steatohepatitis, and up to cirrhosis. The stages have been described by a fibrosis stage score, which is useful for drug trials. Simple steatosis and steatohepatitis without fibrosis is fibrosis stage 0. Steatohepatitis with mild, moderate and advanced fibrosis is fibrosis stage 1 to 3 respectively, and cirrhosis is fibrosis stage 4.

What makes staging complicated is that there are several aspects of the disease that need to be considered, and no single test that completely differentiates the stage. Essentially, what you want to know is what has happened to the liver so far (the stage or severity) but also what is currently happening and likely to happen in the future (the activity) to differentiate whether your disease is at low risk of progressing to fibrosis and cirrhosis, or at high risk.

We will describe the different tests available (routine blood tests, specialist fibrosis blood tests, imaging, liver biopsy and predictive scores) in more detail later in this chapter but begin by looking at each stage.

Simple steatosis and steatohepatitis are frequently picked up by an ultrasound scan or other imaging, often being done for another reason. They may also be identified on routine blood tests, with abnormal liver function tests. These tests won't differentiate between steatosis and higher risk steatohepatitis though, although a normal ALT or AST provides a good degree of reassurance, but the only absolute way to differentiate if there is ongoing inflammation is with a liver biopsy. The amount of fat is best measured using Fibroscan with Controlled Attenuation Parameter (CAP) assessment, an increasingly used technique, but not yet readily available. This is likely to become a very powerful tool to help with monitoring the presence of fat, and allowing people to obtain feedback following lifestyle changes. It is very rewarding for people to have a scan that shows that the changes they have made to their lifestyle have effectively treated their disease.

To assess for the more severe stages of fibrosis and cirrhosis, standard blood tests, along with specific blood tests to look for fibrosis, Fibroscan, plus possibly liver biopsy, are used.

One of the challenges of staging and monitoring liver disease is that it is easier to get definite answers for the more severe stages or fibrosis and cirrhosis, but actually what we (doctors and patients) really want to is stop those stages from occurring, by reducing or reversing the steatosis and steatohepatitis stages. The take home message should be, if any fat is present, to try and reverse it and avoid getting to a more definitive, measurable stage.

**Blood Tests:** Blood tests can give limited information in terms of staging MASLD and determining activity. They are, however, readily available. In terms of determining process (distinguishing between simple steatosis and steatohepatitis) LFTs offer little. ALT and AST levels may be higher with the higher risk/higher activity steatohepatitis process, but this is very difficult to determine at the point of diagnosis without a reliable reference point. Bilirubin is elevated, and albumin falls as more significant liver injury develops. Given that progression of liver damage is far more likely with steatohepatitis these changes are a reasonable surrogate for process (as well, obviously, as being a marker for severity).

Bilirubin is a by-product of the breakdown of haemoglobin. Red blood cells have a normal life span of around 150 days. After this, they begin to lose their shape and function and they are replaced by newly maturing red cells produced in the bone marrow. The old red blood cells are broken down in the spleen. At the core of haemoglobin is a chemical group called haem which contains the iron which is necessary for oxygen transfer from the lungs to the tissues (the essential function of red blood cells). When the red blood cell is broken down, the iron is extracted from the haem group and recycled. The rest of the haem group cannot be used and is disposed of. It is converted to bilirubin, which is transported to the liver by albumin molecules, taken up by the liver cells and conjugated ("tagged") for transport out into the bile duct and thence the bowel, allowing disposal from the body. Jaundice, a common feature of liver disease, is a state of elevation of bilirubin. This can occur, in the context of disease of the liver, when the liver is either unable to take up and "tag" the bilirubin molecule because the hepatocytes are injured, when it is unable to transport it out into the bile, or when there is a block to bile flow causing back-pressure of bilirubin into the hepatocyte and back into the blood. In advanced/severe MASLD the loss of hepatocytes and their function means that the whole pathway of bilirubin conjugation and transport can be lost, leading to bilirubin build up in the blood and jaundice. Bilirubin is, therefore, a relatively crude, but easily available marker of disease severity. One point that it is worth noting is that, whereas an elevated bilirubin is suggestive of a certain degree of severity, a normal bilirubin doesn't exclude a high degree of severity as the liver can compensate for injury for a long time. There can, therefore, be a brewing high severity state long before bilirubin is elevated.

There is another potential trap in relation to bilirubin levels and jaundice in any liver disease. This is Gilbert's syndrome, a relatively common genetic abnormality in a gene which encodes one of the enzymes that "tags" (conjugates) bilirubin for transport out into the bile. This abnormality, perhaps even better thought of as a variation in normal, leads to people running a naturally higher bilirubin level than normal individuals. The elevation in bilirubin is with unconjugated ("untagged") bilirubin. The issue with Gilbert's syndrome is not the problems it causes (it probably doesn't cause any, although some people have suggested that it can cause fatigue) but the fact that around 4% of the population have the change. This includes 4% of MASLD patients, as the variant is neither commoner nor rarer in MASLD patients than in the rest of the population. This means that 4% of MASLD patients can have a bilirubin value **which is normal for them** of up to 50µmol/litre compared to the upper limit of normal of 17-20 (the range depends on the laboratory; be really careful with bilirubin values as it is one of the tests where results are expressed differently in different countries (the USA uses a measure of mg/decilitre which has an upper limit of normal of 1.0-1.2)). The difference between 17 and 50 does not sound like a large one but a value of 50 would be enough to worry a MASLD clinician. One of the important messages we give to people training in liver disease management is to look at the patient and all their tests as a whole. If the bilirubin value appears to be too high in the context of the other clinical features and tests, then think about Gilbert's syndrome. Gilbert's syndrome has one additional trick to play on the unwary. The bilirubin elevation is variable and is normally more marked when people are under stress or feeling unwell. It is very common for people with Gilbert's to get a more marked bilirubin elevation (and to become clinically jaundiced) when they have a cold or the flu. The combination of feeling unwell and worsening jaundice can lead to obvious concern that they both result from a worsening of fatty liver disease. This is why it is so important to, if Gilbert's syndrome is present, know about it, record it in the clinical notes and tell the patient so that they can warn future clinicians. This may all feel a little over-emphasised, but we have come across more than one patient referred for liver transplantation on the basis of their bilirubin rise after an operation when it was simply Gilbert's syndrome!

Albumin is, in contrast, a protein which is produced by the hepatocytes and released into the circulation. Hepatocyte dysfunction is, therefore, associated with reduced albumin levels. Although a marker of hepatocyte function, albumin is also dependent on dietary intake of protein and can therefore be low in chronic poor nutrition states or with malabsorption. Provided someone has a normal diet, and no other condition which may lead them to lose albumin, this test is a useful one to provide insight into liver function in MASLD. A normal albumin level is a reassuring sign that the liver is making protein normally and is functioning effectively.

Outside liver function tests, the simple blood test with the greatest value for disease staging is one that often surprises people; the platelet count (a parameter of blood cell numbers). The platelets are very small cells (more accurately cell fragments) that play a key role in clot formation, and thus bleeding prevention. The relevance to MASLD stage is that when cirrhosis develops, and is complicated by portal hypertension (the increase in blood pressure in the portal vein because of interrupted portal vein blood flow through the cirrhotic liver), the increase in pressure causes the spleen to swell. The platelets then tend to pool in the enlarged spleen. This causes the level in the blood to fall. A level below 150 is taken as a very suggestive value. The caveat is that there are a number of other reasons why the platelet count can fall which are unrelated to cirrhosis.

The final easily available blood test that is useful for staging is the prothrombin time (PT). This is a measure of the level of the proteins in the blood that work alongside the platelets to facilitate blood clotting (coagulation). Effective clotting needs platelets that are working, plus clotting factors (the proteins that stabilise the platelet clump that is the origins of the clot) and the natural properties of the blood vessel wall. Clotting factors are largely made by the liver and, rather like albumin, if the liver is not working properly the levels will fall. The levels can be measured as prothrombin time, which therefore makes the test a useful marker of liver function (the normal value can vary slightly from lab to lab, although most have a value of around 12 seconds; the results you get will always have the local normal range to help interpretation). One important point is that the prothrombin time is a measure of time it takes the blood to clot in a lab assay. This means that a higher number means that the blood is taking longer to clot and suggests abnormality. This contrasts with albumin where the actual protein level is being directly measured, meaning that a lower number is worse. PT can also be expressed in a slightly different way which is as an "International Normalised Ratio", usually abbreviated to INR. The INR is, in essence, the ratio of the PT in seconds to the local control value (the normal value the results will give you). If your PT is 12, and that is the local control value, the INR will be one. If the PT is 24 (a value that might suggest liver under-function) the INR will be 2 and so on. Many people will have come across

INR in the setting of monitoring for the use of warfarin, an anticoagulant or blood "thinning" drug used in lots of settings to reduce blood clotting where risk of clot means that an anticoagulant would be helpful (deep vein thrombosis (DVT) for example). Given that it measures PT it is obviously also useful in assessing liver function. The widespread use of INR means that it is sometimes more easily available than PT (odd as it may seem). There are, as always, caveats. There are, again, other reasons for the PT to be high that are unrelated to liver disease (the most obvious one of which is, unsurprisingly, taking warfarin). PT can also be prolonged in people who are deficient in vitamin K. The answer is, yet again, to look at the whole picture before ascribing significance to a single test.

**Liver Biopsy:** As outlined earlier, liver biopsy remains a definitive test for both the diagnosis and staging of MASLD. The direct observation of cirrhotic change clearly makes the diagnosis. Biopsy is also able to demonstrate key changes which predict the risk of progression to cirrhosis. These include degree of inflammation and degree of fibrosis short of cirrhosis. The information from a liver biopsy in this setting is always useful. It has, however, limitations. These are usually manageable in the setting of an initial staging but do come into play in the setting of ongoing monitoring. We will go into this in more detail in the next section.

**Imaging:** This is one of the areas where there has been real progress in the last few years. The imaging approaches really split into two. Standard imaging approaches, where information relevant to staging can be derived, and dedicated staging technologies. Advanced liver disease (especially cirrhosis but, to a degree, progressive disease short of cirrhosis) can have characteristic appearances on standard clinical imaging (ultrasound, CT and MRI). These changes include a nodular, irregular, liver structure, spleen enlargement because of portal hypertension, and the development of varices. All are relatively "soft" changes and experience of the radiologist is critical. In our experience, there can be a tendency to over-report these findings, especially those relating to an irregular liver edge. Unless the centre is very experienced it is better to regard changes on ordinary imaging as suggestive rather than diagnostic of advanced disease.

The area of rapid progress in recent years has been in specialist imaging and quantification approaches. The principle underpinning them is not "imaging" per se (the output is not a picture) but measurement of a value that relates to an aspect of the disease process. The most widely available of these techniques is *Fibroscan* (this is the most widely used proprietary form of a technology called transient elastography or liver stiffness measurement (LSM)). The technique is a variant of ultrasound. The principle is very much like sonar on a submarine. A "ping" is sent out and the machine measures how much is returned. The more of the ping that returns the more solid (i.e., fibrotic (in principle at least)) the liver is. The test can be done in real time as part of a clinic review and is painless, and for this reason it has almost completely replaced biopsy in the staging of MASLD. It, again, has limitations. It cannot, for example, determine the level of inflammatory activity of disease. There are more challenges undertaking fibroscan in MASLD than in any other type of chronic liver disease because of the impact of fat in the liver and under the skin on the signal. This can be compensated for to a degree by increasing the size of the probe (the part of the machine that sends out the "ping" through the skin and measures how much is returned). The technology is also very operator dependent (people doing it need to do a certain number to keep up their skill level). The upfront cost of the machine is also an issue, although once the investment has been made the cost of each individual scan is very low. One important thing to remember is that, although people equate fibroscan values with the degree of fibrosis, in fact what it measures is the density of the liver (the denser it is the more of the "ping" that will be returned). Any other cause of an increased density in the liver will also lead to high values and an over-assessment of the degree of fibrosis.

An emerging "bolt-on" technology to Fibroscan is called Controlled Attenuation Parameter (CAP) assessment. This allows assessment not of likely degree of fibrosis but the degree of steatosis. It is increasing in use, although it is far from universal. Its main value may lie not in the diagnosis of MASLD but in assessment of the degree of steatosis over time. As we will outline in later chapters, an important emerging philosophy in MASLD is the potential value of taking the fat out of the liver (the simple principle being no fat = no MASLD). Fibroscan measures the consequences of fat and inflammation and therefore, it could be argued, tells you that you should have done something in the past whereas CAP tells you how well you are doing now. Given that persistence in lifestyle modification over time is going to be key to taking fat out of the liver, this ongoing progress feedback information is likely to prove valuable to people.

There are a few other emerging technologies that extend the model of change quantification. These include MRI spectroscopy to assess degree of fat and MRI elastography and Acoustic Radiation Force Impulse (ARFI) to assess degree of fibrosis. These are all, however, largely research tools (including in clinical trials) and are not widely used in clinical practice. Time will tell whether they enter ordinary practice. It will be hard to beat the "point of care" utility of fibroscan with CAP assessment, however.

**Fibrosis Blood Tests:** When scarring develops in the liver, the scar tissue isn't fixed and unchanging. Rather, it is constantly "re-modelled" (i.e., existing scar tissue is broken down and replaced by new scar). It is possible to measure the parts of the scar tissue that have been broken down and released into the blood. In simple terms, the higher the levels of these breakdown products, the more scar tissue there is in the body. This measurement can take the form of a single element of the broken-down collagen, such as the terminal peptide of procollagen III (PIIINP), serum levels of which have been shown to discriminate between simple steatosis and MASH, and between early and advanced fibrosis. A slightly more sophisticated (and expensive) approach to this is composite scores such as the *Enhanced Liver Fibrosis (ELF)* and *Fibrotest* assays, which measure multiple collagen breakdown products. They are very useful for risk stratifying patients at disease outset (and are useful for follow up as we will discuss later). One thing to be aware of with all these blood-based fibrosis markers is that it is a marker of degree of fibrosis in the body, and not just the liver (unlike fibroscan where the assessment is directly of the liver). Excessive fibrosis in other parts of the body could therefore conceivably give a high false positive value. As always, they should be looked at in the context of the patient as a whole. These approaches tend to be quite expensive per test and are not widely used in normal clinical practice in the UK, especially in clinics with ready access to fibroscan where the "per assessment" cost is much lower. Blood fibrosis markers are widely used in clinical trials where they add useful additional information.

**Predictive Scores:** Several clinical scores have been developed which take many of the above parameters, especially relating to blood tests, and integrate them into a single scoring system that gives probability of a certain disease state being present. Examples include the **NAFLD fibrosis score** (which hasn't yet changed its name interestingly) which includes age, hyperglycaemia (high glucose), BMI, platelet count, albumin and AST/ALT ratio, **FIB-4** (age, platelet count, ALT and AST) and the **BARD score** (BMI, AST/ALT ratio and presence or absence of diabetes). All were developed in groups of MASLD patients in whom the actual degree of fibrosis was known from biopsy, and then validated in another population (i.e., did the score predict what the biopsy went on to show). The strength of the approach is that it utilizes easily available clinical information (i.e., they are not tests as such, they are ways of making sense of other tests) and it puts the results of multiple tests into a single easily understandable score. The weakness is that, as with all such approaches, they are more accurate at the level of a large population than they are in single individual patients. Because they are so doable, however, they do form a part of the approach used in practice to understand the clinical picture.

## *MONITORING MASLD*

Once MASLD has been diagnosed, and staged, and the treatment options outlined in the next few chapters discussed and instituted, we move to the monitoring phase of the disease. Monitoring goes hand in hand with treatment adjustment (there is no point in monitoring someone if you don't then act on the results of the tests you do). Importantly, when referring to treatment throughout this section we will be meaning both drug treatment (specific MASLD drugs if and when they are licensed, and co-existing diabetes treatment) and lifestyle changes.

Once you have had an episode of MASLD the risk of it returning is always there, meaning that monitoring should be lifelong. When monitoring MASLD there are two very distinct questions that we are asking. The questions are specific, and the answers have their own individual implications. The terminology we use is, deliberately, the same as when thinking about histology findings at liver biopsy as the concepts are similar. Each time we see a patient we ask ourselves both how **active** the disease is and how **severe**.

**MASLD activity:** This is the level of fat deposition and inflammation that is taking place at any one time. We look at the same markers of liver injury (level of ALT and AST), markers of liver function (albumin, bilirubin and prothrombin time (PT)) as we use in the initial staging of the disease. Fibroscan with CAP follow-up may be useful in assessing the degree of steatosis specifically.

**MASLD severity:** This is, remember, the degree of damage the liver has sustained in terms of the amount of fibrosis and the presence of cirrhosis. If cirrhosis is present, then severity monitoring moves towards assessment of the complications of cirrhosis (once cirrhosis is present there is no value monitoring fibrosis level). In practice, we look for fibrosis using liver biopsy and fibroscan, again in the same way as in initial disease staging.

Over the fullness of time, activity and severity will be linked (high activity for a long time will inevitably lead to high severity). At any moment in time, however, they can be independent. Early in the disease, before treatment has been started, activity is typically high, but severity is low. The goal here is to bring down activity to ensure that severity continues to remain low in the future. Later in the disease, after treatment, and especially if the patient presented late in the disease course when cirrhosis was already present, activity can be low but severity high. In this instance severity monitoring moves to assessment of complications whilst activity monitoring and treatment is ongoing to maintain liver function.

**Other monitoring:** The final aspect of long-term disease monitoring and management is to make sure that all other, non-liver aspects of the metabolic syndrome are also being monitored and treated in the best possible way. This includes type 2 diabetes, hypertension, ischaemic heart disease and hypercholesterolemia. MASLD almost never exists in isolation and these additional linked diseases can often be more dangerous to you than MASLD. The hepatologist looking at your liver disease is almost never the right person to look after your heart disease and your type 2 diabetes. Really good management of MASLD requires a team of experts (including you as an expert patient) working together. Many people with MASLD may not actually be under ongoing care from a hepatologist or gastroenterologist and may never have seen one. Unfortunately due to the high number of people being diagnosed with MASLD, and the limitations of service delivery, in the UK at least, they may not be under any specialist teams.

## *WHAT WE WOULD WANT IF IT WAS US*

There has been lots of information in this chapter, and we thought we'd summarise it with this short section of how we would envision the pathway, if one of us was told that we had an ultrasound or blood tests that suggested fatty liver, bearing in mind that this is often identified by non-hepatologists. What we would like, and ask for:

- Referral to a hepatologist or other liver specialist service (in many hospitals it may be a nurse led service following investigation and management protocols, which is a reasonable starting point if the disease is straightforward) to do further tests to confirm that the diagnosis is MASLD, and not another liver disease.
- Staging assessment, using Fibroscan with CAP to assess for the amount of steatosis, and using Fibroscan, but also using fibrosis specific blood tests, to assess for any fibrosis, and rule out cirrhosis.
- HbA1c measurement to look for the presence of type 2 diabetes.
- We would then want to have annual checks, having undertaken lifestyle changes, using repeat Fibroscan with CAP and blood tests, to look for activity and severity. What we would be aiming for would be resolution of steatosis (and no fibrosis) on Fibroscan and normal ALT/AST and alkaline phosphatase in particular on blood tests.
- If steatosis resolves, we will want (lifelong) annual liver function blood tests, which could be checked by the GP or specialist team. If these remained normal, that gives reassurance that steatosis has not recurred.
- If the liver function blood tests become abnormal again, having been normal for a time, we would want reassessment for steatosis and

fibrosis using Fibroscan with CAP, and fibrosis specific blood tests. This will probably require referral back to a hospital specialist team.
- It should be considered that there may be a second disease process that can go along with MASLD, so if liver function tests deteriorate, especially if lifestyle intervention has been previously keeping the disease under control, then it is worth reviewing the diagnosis again.
- If the investigations at any time showed severe fibrosis or cirrhosis, we would want routine hospital follow up six monthly to look for the complications of cirrhosis.

Blood tests used in the diagnosis and assessment of MASLD:

a) LIVER FUNCTION TESTS (LFT)

| | |
|---|---|
| *Alanine Transaminase (ALT) & Aspartate Transaminase (AST)* | Enzymes (forms of protein) that are normally expressed within hepatocytes, and which are released into the blood when these cells are injured. Higher levels broadly suggest higher levels of liver injury. Different laboratories assess either AST or ALT as their "standard" liver injury enzyme. In fact, measuring both is useful in MASLD as they give different information, and values for both are needed for several of the disease severity composite scores. In most liver diseases, elevation in AST and ALT tends to run in parallel (the values are broadly similar). In alcohol-related liver disease AST is disproportionately elevated. This phenomenon can sometimes be useful in distinguishing the two conditions. |
| *Alkaline Phosphatase (ALP)* | Another enzyme that is released by injured cells. Where levels are elevated, it suggests that there is an increased level of cell injury. ALP is particularly produced by the cells lining the bile duct, meaning that elevation is suggestive of cholestatic disease. As such it is the classically elevated liver function test in primary biliary cholangitis (PBC). It is, however, frequently also elevated in MASLD (although it will usually be accompanied by ALT or AST elevation). ALP can also be produced by other organs (especially by growing or diseased bone) so ALP elevation on its own does not automatically mean liver disease is present. Liver disease is suggested if elevated ALP is accompanied by elevation in another liver enzyme (gamma-GT (below)) or if an additional test shows the ALP is of liver origin. |
| *Gamma-Glutamyl Transferase (Gamma-GT, GGT)* | Another enzyme typically released by injured bile duct cells and measurable in a blood test. It can fluctuate more than ALP making it a less reliable test. In a liver clinic it is largely used to |

| | |
|---|---|
| | confirm that elevated ALP is of liver origin. Many doctors believe that GGT elevation suggests high alcohol consumption. It doesn't, and this is one of the sources of the fallacy about alcohol excess in non-alcohol related liver diseases. |
| *Bilirubin* | By-product of the breakdown of the haem group of red blood cells (the molecule that contains the iron essential for haemoglobin function). It is produced in the spleen, carried to the liver by albumin, taken up by the hepatocytes and conjugated (attached to another molecule to allow its ejection out into the bile). Any failure in this pathway (increased breakdown of red cells, disordered transport to the liver, decreased conjugation capacity or blockage to bile flow) can lead to bilirubin elevation in the blood. This can be measured as a blood test and, if high enough, bilirubin is visible as a yellowing of the skin (jaundice). The whites of the eyes (sclerae) are the part of the body where this can be most readily visible. |
| *Albumin* | A serum protein produced at high levels by the liver. It plays a key role as a transporter molecule in the serum and, through the osmotic effect (a natural process whereby more concentrated solutions draw fluid into themselves to dilute their concentration), in controlling tissue fluid flux. It is reduced when hepatocellular function is decreased, as well as in malnutrition states (including those caused by abnormality in absorption of food from the diet). |
| *Prothrombin Time (PT)* | This is one of the measures of the clotting function of the blood. It is very sensitive to reduced liver synthetic function of protein clotting factors, and also levels of the fat-soluble vitamin K which is essential for clotting factor activation. Prolongation (beyond the normal time of 12 seconds), occurs within 30 minutes of the onset of liver failure, making the test a highly useful one in |

| | |
|---|---|
| | monitoring acute liver functional status (once any vitamin K deficiency has been corrected). In the population, the commonest cause of PT prolongation is treatment with warfarin which acts through blockade of vitamin K function! |
| *Immunoglobulin G and M (IgG and IgM)* | Antibodies produced by the immune system in response to an infection or vaccination are immunoglobulins. Total immunoglobulin levels of two types are useful additional tests in liver disease. The IgG fraction is elevated, in the setting of liver disease, in autoimmune hepatitis (AIH). IgG levels are typically elevated at presentation and reduce rapidly with treatment, mirroring the change in ALT. The target is normalisation of the IgG. Along with ALT, IgG is a key part of ongoing disease activity monitoring. The M fraction (IgM) is almost always elevated in PBC (although the level of elevation is not associated with disease severity). Occasionally, although it is not one of the classic diagnostic tests in PBC, high IgM can help in making a diagnosis when other tests are inconclusive as there are few other causes of IgM elevation. IgG and IgM levels are both typically normal in MASLD and these normal levels are a useful piece of information to help distinguish MASLD from AIH and PBC. |
| *Autoantibodies* | Autoantibodies (antibodies produced by the immune system that react with the body's own structures) are frequent in MASLD, although typically only seen at low levels. The most frequently seen autoantibody type is anti-nuclear antibodies (ANA) which have a diffuse nuclear staining pattern. The same autoantibodies can also be seen in lupus and, of most relevance in liver disease, AIH. Anti-smooth muscle antibody can accompany ANA. IgG is normally elevated in AIH but is typically normal in MASLD, making it a useful test to help determine whether ALT elevation with an ANA is AIH or MASLD. |

# CHAPTER 5: **TREATING MASLD 1: *INTRODUCTION***

The next five chapters in this book will cover the treatment of MASLD. In the previous books in the series this has been covered, each time, in two chapters. This difference is very telling indeed. Treatment in MASLD is a very complex, and rapidly changing, area. There is complexity in terms of individual specific therapies. Over and above this, however, there is complexity in terms of different approaches to drug treatment and when, and in which patients, they should be used. There is also the critical issue of ensuring that the other conditions of the metabolic syndrome are also effectively treated, in ways that are cognisant of, and sympathetic towards, liver disease. MASLD is most definitely not a disease where "one size fits all" in terms of treatment. This chapter will try to explain the thinking behind different treatment approaches (thinking that can sometimes be muddled in clinical practice) and put the chapters detailing specific treatments into context.

### *THE GOALS OF TREATMENT IN MASLD*

This may seem like a strange, and somewhat unnecessary, thing to discuss. Isn't it obvious why we treat a disease? Right at the outset it is worth, however, taking a step back and asking ourselves what we are trying to achieve. What is the problem that we are trying to solve? The first and easiest thing to say is that curing the disease (most peoples' answer to the question "why we treat a disease") is the thing that is least likely to be achievable. Because MASLD represents the culmination of a complex series of physiological and pathological changes, complete reversal is, for most people, going to be unattainable. It may be possible, through extensive lifestyle modification (the diet and exercise changes that each have their own chapter) to reverse the disease changes. The tendency towards MASLD will, however, always remain (rather as diet control of type 2 diabetes controls diabetes but doesn't make it go away; loss of diet control will be accompanied by rapid return of the disease).

Given that cure is almost impossible, what are we trying to achieve through treatment? As is the case with every disease, we are trying to do two things. The first is to reduce the risk that that disease will shorten a patient's life, whilst the second is to make sure that the quality of that patient's life is as close to normal as is possible by controlling symptoms (think of someone having a heart attack; we use clot busting drugs and stents to open up the coronary arteries to ensure that the patient doesn't die, but at the same time give pain killing drugs for the severe pain). For any patient, with any disease, the balance of priority between length of life protection and quality of life improvement will be personal. Doctors, as a rule, tend to focus more on length of life and under-appreciate the importance to patients of quality of life (sometimes even making quality of life worse through the side-effects of the drugs that they use).

In the case of MASLD, risk to life comes in two broad categories (over and above the risks to life that patients also experience for reasons unrelated to their fatty liver). The first, and obvious, one is the risk of progression of the liver disease to cirrhosis and the development of the complications of cirrhosis that can shorten life (variceal bleed, hepatocellular carcinoma, etc). This is the traditional view of liver disease; try and stop cirrhosis if you can, but if you can't, look for the complications and manage them as best you can. The second risk to life, and a key one in MASLD, is the risk that comes from the other components of the metabolic syndrome that are almost always present in MASLD patients. The key ones are ischaemic heart disease, type 2 diabetes, and their complications (including ischaemic heart disease as a further diabetes complication, and chronic kidney disease). Patients with MASLD are actually statistically more likely to die of the complications of these conditions then their liver disease. To focus on MASLD to the exclusion of these linked conditions and, even worse, to use therapies to reduce MASLD risk that worsen these other, even more risky, conditions is clearly a false economy. Treating MASLD is therefore a real balancing act. One of the challenges we face in clinical practice is the tendency towards siloed working (hepatologists look after the liver, diabetologists look after the diabetes and cardiologists the heart etc). One of the areas we discuss later about the future is thinking about ways to integrate, or at least harmonise, clinical care.

Symptoms can be a major issue in patients with MASLD and are an issue that tends to be under-appreciated by clinicians. For some patients they can be the major issue. They come in three forms. The first and most obvious one is the symptoms associated with cirrhosis and its complications. People with cirrhosis often feel rotten. Fatigue can be a problem, as well as specific issues related to encephalopathy (confusion) and ascites (abdominal distension, pain, and difficulty in breathing). In addition, cirrhosis is associated with muscle loss, meaning that people can become weaker and less mobile. This can contribute both to a spiral of physical decline and increased risk as people become less able to cope physically with a complication of cirrhosis. Clearly, if we could prevent people from ever getting cirrhosis it would reduce the burden of these symptoms as well as reducing risk to life (even more reason to focus on cirrhosis avoidance).

The second is, again, the symptoms related to the other features of the metabolic syndrome (chest pain from ischaemic heart disease, fatigue from diabetes and kidney impairment etc). This further emphasises the importance of managing all aspects of the metabolic syndrome, and not just MASLD.

The final symptom type is the most enigmatic. These are the symptoms that MASLD patients can develop even though they don't have cirrhosis. The most prominent of these is fatigue, a problem that is very poorly understood in MASLD. An area of particular uncertainty is around the inter-relationship between the fatigue seen in type 2 diabetes (also poorly understood) and that in MASLD. Are they in fact the same process being given different labels? We will explore symptoms in MASLD in another chapter. Our feeling is, however, that if we can control the underlying metabolic abnormalities in MASLD (especially through diet and exercise) it will go a very long way to controlling symptoms.

## *TREATMENTS TO IMPROVE PROGNOSIS*

This is the essence of the treatment challenge in MASLD, partly because it is the major challenge experienced by patients and partly because, as mentioned in the previous section, if we crack this challenge, it will probably go a long way to cracking the symptoms as well.

The key thing to think about in approaching prognostic treatments in MASLD is, as is the case with the whole treatment approach, to think through what we are trying to achieve in any particular patient. What would the perfect treatment look like and how close to achieving it are we? There are three broad treatment approaches for prognosis in MASLD: management of existing advanced liver disease, reversal of steatohepatitis and fibrosis in high-risk patients and reversal of steatosis.

**Management of cirrhosis:** One of the ways of thinking, that we teach medical students and doctors in training, is to understand why people with any disease die, and then find ways of stopping that from happening. People dying of MASLD (and, again, it is important to remember that they are more likely to die of other aspects of the metabolic syndrome than their MASLD) do so usually because of decompensation of cirrhosis (variceal bleed, liver failure etc) or the development of hepatocellular carcinoma, itself a complication of cirrhosis. The traditional model of hepatology is, therefore, to screen people with cirrhosis for these complications and then intervene to reduce the complication risk. There is also the option of transplantation for when the risk becomes excessively difficult to control. Where someone has developed cirrhosis, these approaches are incredibly important and can support people for a long time. This model is, however, far from perfect. First, it assumes that we know who has cirrhosis. A number of people actually have their cirrhosis diagnosed when they develop their first complication (for example a variceal bleed) ….something that can really limit our capacity to manage that complication. Second, the person might have a complication managed, but they still have cirrhosis, meaning that the intervention does not reduce the risk of future complications (the classic example is hepatocellular carcinoma, the risk for which goes up progressively with the duration of cirrhosis). Finally, and crucially for us, as we have discussed earlier, cirrhosis per se is associated with significant impairment of life quality. Supporting people long term with cirrhosis therefore means leaving them with long-term life quality reduction. Then there is transplantation. We will dedicate a whole chapter to transplantation later in the book but suffice to say at this stage the benefits of transplantation aren't quite as clear cut as people sometimes think they are. We have managed many people up to and after liver transplantation and are yet to meet anyone who wouldn't have much rather avoided the need for it in the first place if that had been possible.

**Reversal of steatohepatitis and fibrosis in high-risk patients:** We don't think that anyone would disagree with the idea that it would be good to be able to stop people developing cirrhosis if possible, and thereby avoid the risk of its complications, symptom burden and potential need for transplantation. It would also save the NHS and other health care systems a lot of money! An attractive model for treatment would, therefore, be to identify people who are at high risk of developing cirrhosis in the future and treat them to stop or even reverse the damaging disease process, preventing progression to cirrhosis. This approach is the one that most drug treatments under evaluation in MASLD are taking (again, we will cover this in detail in a full chapter). We are at an exciting point in the story of MASLD with the approval for use of the first drug to reduce risk of disease progression of MASLD to cirrhosis. Although this approach to therapy appears highly intuitive (we only treat people who are at risk and therefore "need" treatment and avoid over-treating low risk patients with simple steatosis) it has three important limitations.

The first practical limitation is that it assumes that we can, and in practice are able to, identify those patients who are at risk. There are several clinical tools available, as discussed previously, that can help with this, but they are only really accurate at a population level. They become less accurate when you start looking at single patients (our earlier "how representative is one person in a football crowd of the whole crowd" question). Biopsy is, of course, valuable but it is resource heavy, unpopular with patients and has its risks. The second, linked, limitation is that an active decision step such as secondary identification of high-risk patients is exactly the type of approach that can "fall through the cracks" in pressurised health care systems. We only have to look at the impact on structured long term condition care in COVID to see how easy the "wheels can come off". Sensitivity of an approach (targeting the therapy to only the people who need it) and complexity (the steps that need to be taken to achieve this) tend to go hand in hand. There is a further important dimension to this which is health inequality (the concept that everyone in a population has the right to the same degree of health and health care), the founding concept of the NHS in the UK. The quality of health care varies far more than it should between different locations, as does the confidence and awareness that people have to navigate the system. Disadvantage tends to co-map, meaning that areas with the greatest social disadvantage often have the greatest amount of chronic disease, and the most limited health care provision. A sophisticated decision-making step is most likely to fail in practice in just those disadvantaged areas, yet the populations in those areas will include the people at greatest risk of MASLD. The final limitation is that we don't really understand the dynamics of MASLD and the points in the disease process where therapy will be most effective. It may be (and experience with other liver disease suggests this may well be the case for MASLD as well) that waiting for the development of the higher risk forms of the disease misses the opportunity for therapy to be most effective.

**Reversal of steatosis:** Given that the presence of fat deposition in the liver is the *sine qua non* of MASLD, its prevention or, if present already, reversal would seem to be the perfect approach to treatment ("no fat = no MASLD"). This concept underpins lifestyle intervention as a treatment approach in MASLD; approaches that look to "re-balance" the pathway of nutrition handling in the liver through dietary change, exercise, or a combination of the two. It also underpins the concept of bariatric surgery which is, in essence (although in practice it is a little more complex than this), a surgical approach to limiting nutrition intake. There is little doubt from research and real-life experience that the approach can work in practice and we have experience of many people who have managed to completely reverse MASLD, especially in its milder forms, using these approaches. The problem is the effectiveness of these approaches in the real world. People are human and usually struggle to put into practice, and then sustain, significant changes to their diet and exercise patterns (the whole business model for gyms assumes that a percentage of people will stop coming after they have paid for a year's subscription at New Year and think of how many weight loss books there are on the market……). One of the authors of this book has struggled with his weight all his life and has very much "been there, done that and bought the T-shirt" in this area. One of the things that we will go into in detail in the chapters on diet and exercise in the book is practical hints and suggestions as to how to do it. One of the things that people can find dispiriting is being told what to do by super-thin and super-sporty people who don't really have any insights into how difficult all this is for some people. One of the questions that has fascinated us for years is why motivation can be such a problem when it comes to lifestyle modification. One interesting idea that we will explore is that this is a manifestation of the disease (one of its symptoms if you like). People struggle to get going with diet and exercise because the disease makes them struggle. It therefore isn't their "fault". This is a really interesting concept, and we will go into it in more detail. Perhaps one of the areas where drugs might be useful in the future is short-term courses to help people "get going".

## *MANAGEMENT OF LINKED CONDITIONS*

MASLD almost never exists, as we have discussed, in isolation. Patients will almost always also experience one or more of the other features of the metabolic syndrome. Patients frequently have other conditions, and treatments for those conditions, which need to be managed in the context of liver disease. What this means is that MASLD cannot, and must not, be managed in isolation. The whole picture needs to be born in mind, not just one part of it. The detail of current thinking on the management of conditions such as type 2 diabetes and hypercholesterolaemia is beyond the scope of this book and, to be honest, beyond our areas of expertise. What we will do in this section is introduce some of the key concepts.

## *CONCLUSION*

Perhaps the take home message from this chapter is that we may have been guilty as a scientific community of rushing in with approaches to treatment without really thinking through the strategy. Focusing on the answer without being clear in our minds as to the question. We believe that greater clarity of thinking will really help make the next period of treatment development in MASLD more successful than the last.

## CHAPTER 6: **TREATING MASLD 2:** *DIET*

### *The 2-Minute Version*

- Dietary advice for MASLD has evolved over the last few decades and is very likely to continue to evolve. This is an area where experts can have strongly held, and often contradictory, views. In truth no one knows the definitive answer. Always remember this! There is no right and wrong. Find out what works for you.
- There has been recognition that not all fat is bad, some fats are healthy and beneficial. Trans-fats and added fructose are particularly high risk for causing MASLD. Processed foods are more likely to lead to MASLD development than unprocessed foods.
- Snacking and breakfast are not essential to keep the blood sugar up. There has been increasing use of intermittent fasting to improve MASLD and blood glucose control.
- Vegetables should make up the majority of carbohydrate intake, rather than refined starches or sugars.
- There are advantages and disadvantages of many "diets". The best ones for avoiding or reducing MASLD are the Mediterranean diet, with avoidance of too much starch, or a low carbohydrate diet, ensuring plenty of vegetables are eaten.
- Joining a programme or following a website guide can be helpful to motivate you to make, and maintain, change in your dietary lifestyle. Embrace technology – there are website resources, apps and monitors that can help you.
- You do not have to be overweight to have MASLD, and you can get metabolic benefits from lifestyle changes using diet and exercise, even if you don't lose weight. What is more important than actual weight is what is going on metabolically inside the cells.
- Bariatric surgery (operations such as gastric banding which reduce the volume of food you can eat thus reducing the appetite) may have short-term benefit for MASLD, but with a risk of further deterioration later. Orlistat, a weight loss drug, has no benefit for MASLD.
- Medicines for diabetes will need reviewing before making significant changes to reduce carbohydrate intake. Blood pressure medication may also need reducing.

This chapter will start by talking about diet, and "diets". The second half of the chapter has a slightly different theme, but is very relevant to diet, and so is included here. This section is about obesity, bariatric surgery and altering medication with dietary change.

It's useful to start this chapter by looking at what is meant by the word "diet". There are two definitions describing what a diet is in the dictionary. Firstly, it can mean the kinds of food that a person, or community, habitually eat. Secondly, it can mean a special course of food to which a person restricts themselves, often to lose weight or for health or medical reasons. There is no "diet" for MASLD, as such, with the second meaning of the word above. It's important, however, to understand the types of food that can cause liver disease, what can be helpful and what the national guidelines suggest, so that you put it into the context of your own life. What we are aiming to do with this chapter is to give you the knowledge to have a healthy diet in the first meaning of the word, something that you habitually eat, that will ensure long-term good health.

It is, however, useful to look at some types of diet ($2^{nd}$ meaning) as many of these have elements that contribute to good health, and in particular, good liver health. They have also been widely publicised, and you may well have heard of some or all of them. If you are trying to change your diet to improve your liver's health, which given that you are reading this book is a significant possibility, it's useful to understand these diets, as many websites or recipe books use these dietary labels, so you can pick and choose what fits with your needs and your likes.

There is an irony in medicine that, as doctors, we are able to prescribe and administer macronutrients and micronutrients intravenously but have minimal training on what makes up a healthy diet, and would therefore provide these nutrients by the oral route – i.e., what we should eat! Other than telling people to eat less, as a profession doctors are not very skilled in giving dietary advice. This situation has been made worse by the many changes in dietary advice over the last few decades, which has confused doctors as well as patients. There is still much debate about the advantages and disadvantages of various foods and diets, but here are a few where the consensus has been recognised to have changed.

## *CHANGING PERSPECTIVES*

One area where dietary advice can be confusing is where guidance, expressed with a high degree of certainly at the time, is subsequently changed. The revised guidance is then expressed with a seemingly identical level of certainty. Confusion all round!

**From bad to good:** Some foods which were previously demonised are now thought of as either being not be as bad as previously thought, or actually as being good for us. These include –

*Eggs:* previously blamed for causing high cholesterol, something that is now recognised not to be correct. They can be a good source of protein, as well as a useful ingredient in cooking.

*Fats:* previously considered to be the cause of many problems, especially heart disease. It is now recognised there is a much more nuanced risk to benefit profile. Animal, fish, and plant fats that are not highly refined, such as the fat on meat, olive, coconut and avocado oil, and minimally refined dairy products have some health benefits. Fat is high in calories though, so it's best to have it in moderation if you are overweight or have MASLD. It is only the trans-fats that directly lead to MASLD.

**From good to bad:** By the same token, some foods and concepts around nutrition have gone from being perceived as helpful to unhelpful.

*Refined carbohydrates:* Having previously been told that "pasta makes you faster", some now argue instead that "pasta makes you fatter". Calorie dense carbohydrates, such as foods made from processed (white) flour or white rice are more likely to lead to accumulation of fat in the liver and type 2 diabetes mellitus.

*Fruit:* A bit of fruit is beneficial, but high fruit consumption, particularly in the form of processed smoothies, contributes to MASLD.

*Fats:* Highly processed fats such as some seed oils and margarine, and especially trans-fats, are harmful for cardiovascular and liver health. Margarine was previously marketed as being good for the heart, but the processed fats in it cancel out the other benefits.

*FODMAP Fibres:* Fibre is beneficial for gut microbiome health. However, as with everything in nutrition, it's more complex than previously thought. Many people with irritable bowel syndrome (IBS) in the past were told to eat more fibre, only to find that their symptoms got worse. It's now recognised that some fibres (FODMAPs) may cause or worsen IBS symptoms.

*Frequent snacking:* Rather than staving off low blood sugar, regular snacking means it is not possible to use the fat that is stored in the liver.

*"Breakfast is the most important meal of the day:"* Many experts advocate fasting, or delaying the first meal of the day, to help reverse the process of storage and encourage release of energy from fat and glycogen.

**Different countries, different guidelines:** A further source of confusion is the fact that there is a significant degree of variation between the guidance from different countries, and the sense that they can't all be right. What all national guidelines agree on is that too much sugar and processed food in the diet is harmful, and that eating a variety of, and plenty of, vegetables is good.

The "UK Eatwell Guide", a government guidance document, still recommends that a third of the diet is made up of starchy carbohydrates. It is, however, increasingly being recognized that these contribute to type 2 diabetes mellitus and MASLD.

In **Chapter 3** we explored the food types that contribute to the development of MASLD, and those that are probably beneficial. As we said at the start of this chapter, there is no specific "diet" per se for the prevention and treatment of MASLD, and it is notoriously difficult to get evidence in terms of clinical trials for the benefits of different diets for different diseases (it is inherently difficult to have effective control arms in a trial in an area where belief sets play an important role, and blinding (the technique of making what people are doing or taking in a study unknown to them) is impossible). That said, avoiding those foods that are more likely to cause MASLD, and eating more of those that provide health benefits, are likely to reap rewards in terms of improving liver, and overall, health. It's just we may never be able to "prove" the benefit.

To recap from **Chapter 3**, foods that are recognised to contribute to the development of MASLD include:

- Highly processed foods, which are often high in trans-fats and sugar.
- High amounts of processed fats containing omega-6 fatty acids, such as from seed oils, margarine.
- Foods with added fructose, and high amounts of fruit intake.
- High intake of starchy carbohydrates.
- High intake of sugar

Foods we need to ensure adequate amounts of intake are:

- Protein – plant, fish, or animal
- Omega-3 fatty acid rich foods such as oily fish, nuts and seeds
- Fibre – from plant sources
- Micronutrients – from a mixture of plant and animal sources

## *"DIETS"*

This section will describe commonly used diets, in the 2$^{nd}$ meaning of the word as outlined above. We would emphasise here that we are clinicians giving our views on the different diet types rather than dieticians. These are our opinions and should be taken as such rather than fact.

**The Mediterranean Diet:** There is no strict definition of what the Mediterranean diet consists of. It is based, not surprisingly, on the types of food eaten in European countries bordering the Mediterranean, as it was identified that people in those areas had a low risk of many chronic health conditions. Studies have associated the Mediterranean diet with health benefits for cardiovascular disease, type 2 diabetes and MASLD.

The general principles is a high intake of vegetables, fruits, whole grains, legumes, nuts, seeds and healthy fats, especially olive oil, fish and poultry. There is the greatest consensus worldwide for the health benefits of a Mediterranean diet.

*Advantages:* Good evidence, plenty of information and recipes available, provides a wide range of valuable nutrients, tea, coffee, and a glass of red wine a day are allowed, easy to follow for omnivores, vegetarians and vegans, you don't get weird looks for saying you are following it.

*Disadvantages:* Some recipes can include significant starchy carbohydrates, e.g., pasta, which if you have MASLD or type 2 diabetes it is best to restrict. It's also important to ensure you are getting enough protein.

**The Nordic Diet:** This is the Scandinavian cousin of the more well-known Mediterranean diet and is designed to reflect foods that are locally available in Scandinavia. It emphasises eating berry fruits, vegetables, legumes, whole grains, nuts, seeds, rye breads, fish, seafood, and high-quality meat (food from seas, lakes and the wild). It uses rapeseed (canola) oil instead of olive oil, which is not naturally available in the Nordic countries.

*Advantages:* Has been shown to contribute to a reduction in obesity, advantages are likely to be similar to the Mediterranean diet.

*Disadvantages:* High quality organic or wild food is not cheaply and easily available in the UK. Unlike in Scandinavia there's not very much reindeer roadkill in the UK, and although there is plenty of badger roadkill here (at least near where we live), badger doesn't taste good.

**Low Carbohydrate Diet ("Low Carb"):** As with the Mediterranean diet, there is no definition for what constitutes a low carbohydrate diet. It tends to be lower in carbohydrates by avoiding starches (grains including rice and flour products), high glycaemic load vegetables (this is predominantly the root vegetables like potatoes), sugars and high glycaemic load fruit (such as bananas). There may be higher protein and fat intake, although most people following the diet will use minimally processed fats such as butter, olive oil, coconut oil.

*Advantages:* Many people find this effective for weight loss, there is plenty of information and recipes available, there is considerable overlap with the Mediterranean Diet. It is possible to adapt conventional meals and eat out without too much difficulty.

*Disadvantages:* If you follow this you need to ensure a good amount and variety of vegetables to provide micronutrients and fibre. May have a higher intake of processed meat than is generally recommended.

**Ketogenic Diet ("Keto"):** This is the more extreme end of the low carbohydrate diet spectrum, where intake of carbohydrates, including from plants, is severely restricted. This results in energy being provided from release of fatty acids from fat cells which are turned into ketones. These can be used by many cells in the body instead of glucose, which can be helpful in certain circumstances, including drug resistant epilepsy in children, and for long distance runners.

*Advantages:* Very effective for weight loss.

*Disadvantages:* This diet can be lacking in the micronutrients and fibre that are gained from vegetables and may result in an increased intake of processed food. It usually involves intake which is high in protein, which is more difficult with vegetarian or vegan diets. It can be difficult to maintain over long periods of time as it requires planning and preparation.

**"Atkins Diet":** This is a form of low carbohydrate diet, initially starting with very low carbohydrate intake for 2 weeks, then increasing intake to include low carbohydrate vegetables, nuts, and fruits, then gradually increasing carbohydrate intake until desired steady state weight is achieved. Protein and fat are unlimited.

*Advantages:* A popular and effective diet to achieve weight loss.

*Disadvantages:* It may be lacking in the micronutrients and fibre that are gained from vegetables and may result in an increased intake of processed food. It usually involves intake which is high in protein, making it more difficult with vegetarian or vegan diets, and can be difficult to maintain as it requires planning and preparation.

**Palaeolithic Diet ("Paleo"):** This diet is based on eating only foods that were available before the agricultural and industrial revolutions, based on the principle that that is what our bodies evolved to use. It includes meats, fish, seafood, eggs, vegetables, fruits, nuts and seeds. It excludes grains, legumes, and some dairy products.

*Advantages:* Ticks the box for avoiding highly processed food! Little evidence so far of health benefits, given the difficulties of doing trials on dietary practice, but provides a good mix of nutrient-dense food.

*Disadvantages:* Requires planning and organisation, particularly for vegetarians and vegans. Large chunks of the modern diet are excluded e.g., legumes, which includes beans, peas, lentils, soy products and peanuts, and cheeses.

**Low Glycaemic Index Diet ("Low GI"):** The glycaemic index is an indicator of how quickly foods increase the blood glucose level. A low GI diet avoids foods that rapidly increase blood glucose level, such as sugary drinks and processed starchy foods. However, the glycaemic index is not a very good indicator of the actual total amount of carbohydrate in a meal, which is better represented by the glycaemic load (GL). A particular problem

with the low GI diet and MASLD is that fructose has a low glycaemic index, but this is at the expense of causing accumulation of fat in the liver. The low GI diet only applies to carbohydrates. While there is some logic to following a low glycaemic load diet, the differentiation between low GI and low GL diets is vague.
*Advantages:* Inherently avoids some of the worst causes of blood glucose rises.
*Disadvantages:* Could actually worsen MASLD by encouraging fructose intake and doesn't give useful guidance on other nutritional constituents.

**Low Fat Diet:** Low fat diets have been advocated since the 1970s by the healthcare profession. Despite, or maybe even because of this, obesity related problems have increased. Although some trials show evidence that low fat diets can be effective for weight loss, they are not as effective in the real world. They may lead to an increase in intake of processed food and refined carbohydrates.
*Advantages:* Some evidence of effectiveness in weight loss, although that may not transfer well to the real world.
*Disadvantages:* Increased intake of other unhealthy nutrients, and lack of intake of healthy fats.

**5:2 Diet ("The Fast Diet") and Intermittent Fasting:** This is less about what you eat, but more about having prolonged periods of not eating (fasting) or restricting calorie intake on certain days, such as 2 days a week in the 5:2 diet. It's important to also eat healthily on the remaining days. It is an eating pattern that can be combined with any other diet that you are following and is often also used by people who are following a low carbohydrate or ketogenic diet. In a medical context, fasting is defined as a voluntary abstinence from food. Intermittent fasting is between 12 and 48 hours without food, while long term fasting is for longer than 2 days. It's important to maintain fluid intake and electrolytes, some people take supplements or use bone broths for this. If you are planning to fast for longer than 24 hours, we would recommend reading up about it first so that you understand completely what it entails.
*Advantages:* It can help with weight loss, and improves insulin sensitivity, which is a key underlying abnormality in type 2 diabetes. There is a lot of interest in other health benefits, with small scale studies suggesting that fasting may help with heart disease, prevention of cancer and regulation of inflammation. Once you get over the initial hurdle of thinking it's not possible to survive without breakfast (and lunch) many people find it easier to resist that biscuit in the cupboard when they are fasting, compared with when they've just eaten. It's become popular because many people find it effective, and it fits in easily with their lifestyles.
*Disadvantages:* Diabetes medication may need to be tailored, and anyone on

treatment for diabetes should monitor their blood glucose closely, with a plan to reduce medication if needed. This doesn't mean they shouldn't do it, on the contrary, this should be seen as a positive thing if less medication is needed. Similarly, it can reduce blood pressure so home blood pressure monitoring may be helpful to ensure there isn't a drop to levels which are too low. It isn't healthy to black out because of really low blood pressure when crossing the road in front of a bus, no matter what other health benefits the diet may bring.

**NHS Soup and Shake Diet:** This diet approach has had a lot of publicity, and a high level of uptake for the treatment of early type 2 diabetes in the UK. It is, in essence, a supported ultra-low-calorie diet. It can result in significant weight loss. It has not, as far as we are aware, been specifically applied in MASLD, although liver function test improvements have been reported in type 2 diabetes patients following the diet. It probably has its impact through nutritional restriction rather than any specific mechanism.

**'Diets' – Conclusion:** As we said at the outset, this area is complicated and one lacking in robust evidence on which to make recommendations. While there is no trial that can prove it, it seems like the Mediterranean diet is the best eating pattern for the prevention of MASLD. However, for those who already have MASLD, it may be that somewhere between a Mediterranean diet with less starchy carbohydrates, and a low carbohydrate diet with plenty of vegetables and other plant foods is the best regime. It's important to avoid highly processed food, whatever you choose to do. A good diet for MASLD prevention and treatment does not have to be expensive. On the contrary, by eating a lot of unprocessed food it can be very economical. It can also be very tasty and satisfying, with a variety of natural food sources, including a moderate amount of health fats, which enhances the flavour of food, and it doesn't require any calorie counting. It does require a bit of thought, planning and cooking, so that you don't succumb to buying whatever food is available in the shop at lunch time.

It can be easier to make small changes at a time, we get used to our regular recipes, so one trick is to substitute the higher carbohydrate foods for lower carbohydrate vegetables of a similar texture or appearance, e.g., vegetable rice or spaghetti, or an alternative vegetable mash, instead of rice, pasta or potato mash.

## *GETTING STARTED*

One of the dangers of the whole area of diet modification for MASLD is that it, very rapidly, becomes very complicated indeed with lots of often contradictory views that are frequently strongly held (and equally strongly expressed) by "experts" who may, coincidentally, have products to sell (which we don't). This can make it very difficult indeed for people to even begin to know where to start. For this reason, we have decided to go back to the very beginning and keep it really simple.

At the end of the day, MASLD is a disease of too much fat being deposited in the wrong places and having unhelpful effects. It's as simple as that. We can talk about different genes that regulate metabolism and the degree of inflammation and environmental co-factors such as the gut microbiome but at the end of the day it boils down to too much nutrition of the wrong type for the way that your body works (and there is no point comparing your situation to other people who seemingly can eat what you eat and get no problem; everyone's metabolism is different) and/or too little consumption of that nutrition by exercise. Once we think about it this way, diets become easy. Eat less overall and avoid those food types that will make MASLD worse (the "bad guys" such as fructose and the trans-fats). Drugs will undoubtedly have a role to play. However, they can't make excess harmful food intake "go away". They are therefore best thought of as an adjunct to diet modification.

Once you have decided on the diet approach you are going to take (and there is no "magic bullet" right answer (other than eating less and eating better of course)) then it is worth thinking about the three key steps. These are getting started in the first place, keeping going until you are in a steady state (a couple of weeks) and sustaining it long-term. As we will talk about in later chapters, keeping it going longer term will be helped significantly by your being able to see and feel the improvements yourself. This is called "secondary gain" and is the key point at which you believe that making the change is helpful, because you can feel the impact or see it with your own eyes, rather than just believing it because a clinician has told you. The fundamental challenge is getting to that point.

**Top Ten Tips for Getting Started and Keeping Going:** In this section we will outline our "top tips" for getting started with a diet in MASLD, and keeping going.

*1) Small changes may be better than big changes.* The important thing is to make changes to your diet that are going to be achievable and long-lasting. This doesn't happen overnight. It may seem overwhelming to give up all carbohydrates and go keto, but perfectly manageable to swap a lunchtime sandwich for a salad with (unsweetened) dressing, four days a week.

Give your body, and tastebuds, time to adapt before trying to change too much. You may find that changes in your diet, and your body's metabolic response, can continue to improve over several years. The picture below gives a rough idea of the priorities, which may help you decide what area of your diet you want to change as a first step, aiming to gradually more from left to right.

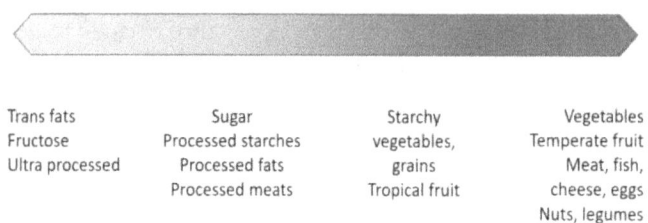

| Trans fats | Sugar | Starchy | Vegetables |
| Fructose | Processed starches | vegetables, | Temperate fruit |
| Ultra processed | Processed fats | grains | Meat, fish, |
|  | Processed meats | Tropical fruit | cheese, eggs |
|  |  |  | Nuts, legumes |

***2) Keep it simple (at least at first):*** Find some simple exchanges that fit into your normal recipes or meals. Here are some examples:
- Use chopped vegetables instead of rice or pasta, or use a spiralizer to make vegetable spaghetti, boiled or fried in butter or olive oil. Supermarkets often sell frozen cauliflower or broccoli rice ready to microwave, or you can chop it yourself using a food blender.
- Many vegetables can be used to make a lower carbohydrate mash as a replacement for potato mash.
- Make pizza bases from vegetables (there are many recipes with a variety of vegetables, usually with egg and mozzarella).
- Use lettuce leaves as wraps around favourite sandwich fillings, which gives all the flavour without the starchy carbohydrates.
- Vegetables can be used in smoothies, along with fruit.
- Swap higher carbohydrate fruit (frequently tropical fruit) for lower carbohydrate ones, especially berries.
- Eat fresh fruit with plain (preferably live) yoghurt, rather than processed fruit yoghurts.

***3) Snack healthily:*** Have a supply of healthy snacks for when you have the munchies. Nuts and seeds, cheese, vegetables, unsweetened vegetable dips like hummus or guacamole, dark chocolate or hard-boiled eggs can be helpful to stave off hunger without affecting glucose or insulin levels much. Take lunch in with you to work. Apart from salads, it's virtually impossible to find appropriate food in shops, cafes and most definitely, in the hospital canteen!

***4) Realise there is no right and wrong:*** Find out what works for you, and your family, rather than slavishly following expert advice. Remember this may well change from day to day, or year to year. Every day is a new day, every meal is a new meal. Every calorie you eat is not accumulative, that's not the way the body works. The body is hugely adaptable, think of the example of the pre-operative two-week liver-reducing diet in the earlier chapter. What this means is that, if you feel your diet has gone haywire, don't worry, don't give up, just think again about what small changes you can start with that will have the most impact, and how you can avoid the pitfalls.

This is dietary change for life, but it doesn't have to dictate your life.

You can still go out and enjoy a meal, or a celebration. If you're going out for a meal, you can choose to avoid some of the more problematic dishes, or just enjoy it, and know that one meal doesn't ruin a lifestyle. It's much more important to cut out the daily biscuits, cakes, crisps, and smoothies, than to cut out a restaurant meal with family or friends once a month.

**5) *Alcohol in moderation:*** You can enjoy red wine in moderation (this is not an instruction, just a suggestion!), but overall, you should aim to reduce alcohol, for both its calorific value, and direct effect on the liver. The more severe your liver disease, the more strongly we would recommend that you avoid alcohol completely, however.

**6) *Use the internet (wisely):*** Use the internet but be aware of its pitfalls (there is no regulator to ensure that the information on it is correct and safe in the way that medicines are regulated). There are many individuals as well as organisations with great ideas on how to adapt your diet to reduce the risk of MASLD. There are many Mediterranean recipes and diet websites, along with low carb websites, with great ideas for how reducing processed and high carbohydrate food can become part of your life for the entire family. Many of the organisation websites focus on type 2 diabetes, but are equally relevant for those people with, or at risk of, MASLD. We will include a description of some individual websites in the next section. This is not an exhaustive list but are some websites that may be useful. There is a focus on low carbohydrate diets, as there are already plenty of books and websites with information on the Mediterranean diet. Some of them have subscriptions for meal plans, but there is still useful information to be gained without a subscription.

**7) *Consider signing up to a diet programme:*** There are many websites, including some of those listed below, that can help keep you motivated, in addition to giving helpful guidance and resources, including meal planning and menus.

**8) *Don't be a slave to calorie counts:*** It is not necessary to count calories, or even to worry about the nutritional content of food. However, some people may find it helpful and motivating to do so. There are apps that can be used to record a food diary and provide a breakdown of the nutritional content. Look for ones that provide a breakdown of macronutrients, as a minimum, rather than focusing on calories, which is not helpful. One example is Carb Manager. Despite its name, it can be used to target a variety of dietary plans.

**9) *Don't set yourself up to fail.*** Aim for pragmatism, not perfection or purism. It would be great if we could all cook from scratch organically grown, ethically sourced food. For most people, that is not going to be possible all the time, or possibly ever. Don't let "the perfect be the enemy of the good". Frozen, dried, or tinned food is fine if that's what's going to be sustainable for your lifestyle. Work to improve your diet, not to make it perfect. Also, read the section below about functional foods. Sometimes we don't have time to cook, and having an appropriate snack or meal replacement may help keep us away from the biscuit tin.

Perhaps the most important advice in this section is to realise that tomorrow is a whole new day. Anyone who says that they stick to the perfect diet day in day out without fail is probably a liar (or more perfect than anyone we have ever met). You will have bad days, stressful days when you eat the wrong thing. The key thing is to get back onto the plan the following day. One day of bad eating isn't a problem. It happens. It is if this sets you off eating badly every day afterwards that is the problem.

**10) *Embrace technology:*** Knowledge is power. One of the most useful developments of the last few years has been in glucose monitoring devices. In the past, it was only possible to know your blood glucose level by stabbing your finger, not something that anyone enjoyed. Now there are sensors that leave a tiny piece of tubing under the skin for two weeks, which measure the glucose in the tissues below the skin (interstitial glucose) and is attached to a plaster on the skin. You can use a phone app to read the glucose level at any time, and the newer generation of devices give constant information to your phone, allowing alarms to be set. There is a slight delay in change of the interstitial glucose from the blood glucose, which means that Type 1 diabetics and type 2 diabetics using insulin may still need to do finger prick tests at times. However, it has revolutionised our understanding of how our bodies react to what we eat, which is something that varies from person to person, and by time of day, and with what food combinations we eat. Both authors have used the Freestyle Libre device, which is available on Amazon amongst other places, and learnt far more from using it than they did in medical school, or post-graduate exams. The monitors are not cheap, at just over £50 for a fortnight at current prices, but a short period of using them can be invaluable in providing feedback. In our opinion, everyone diagnosed with type 2 diabetes should be given a monitor for a couple of months on first diagnosis; it could be a very cost-effective way to remission. One caveat to be conscious of is that the blood glucose may not rise with high intake of some sugary foods, particularly fructose, but this is not reassuring, as the fructose is not getting beyond the liver into the blood. As of Autumn 2022, the NHS has agreed to provide Type 1 diabetics with a continuous glucose monitoring device. There may be a small number of patients with type 2 diabetes who are also provided with a continuous glucose monitor by the NHS, but this is not widespread, despite those making up a much larger proportion of the population with morbidity from diabetes and contributing to the huge costs to the NHS due to the complications it causes, as well as the medications which are prescribed. As type 2 diabetes is effectively a surrogate marker of the metabolic syndrome and associated with MASLD, this is relevant for many readers of this book, and worth the investment.

**Websites, books, and other resources:** As we explained above, there are lots of websites and resources that can really help. The ones listed below are just some websites and resources which we think may help to give ideas and motivation to get started. There is a strong emphasis on diabetes, as there are still not many websites or books dedicated to MASLD (which is, of course, why we're writing this book!). The resources listed below share an international theme of moving towards lower carbohydrate diets to improve health. There is also a recurring theme in the narrative by many of the healthcare professionals involved, which is something we as clinicians also share, of having seen many patients over several decades who are "doing the right thing", following the national dietary guidance, and yet having worsening obesity, raised insulin and glucose. This leads to a dawning recognition, a revelation even, that the status quo of dietary guidance may be part of the problem, not the solution.

*Low Carb Program* (lowcarbprogram.com)
This is a UK-based low carbohydrate diet program, which has been shown to help people lose weight and improve diabetes management. It is a subscription service, but it is possible for patients to be referred on the NHS, if their GP or local Integrated Care System has commissioned the program.

*Public Health Collaboration* (phcuk.org)
A UK charity, formed from a collaboration of healthcare professionals amongst others, aimed at providing information on healthy diets, based on the concept of 'Real Food', which is a term it uses to describe foods that are naturally nutrient dense and minimally altered from their natural state. There are some useful visual graphics within the free resources.

*Real Meal Revolution* (realmealrevolution.com)
Led by Tim Noakes, a South African sports scientist, it also uses the term 'Real Food' as above. There is a website with subscription options, but he has also published several books which cover useful background science about low carbohydrate diets, along with recipes. These books include 'The Real Meal Revolution' and 'Super Food for Superchildren', which concentrates on child friendly food for different ages, and are easily available online. They also use the term "Banting" to describe keto diets, which is explained in the history section of The Real Meal Revolution book.

*Diet Doctor* (dietdoctor.com)
Dr Andreas Eenfeldt is a Swedish family doctor. His website also provides useful free resources, as well as membership options.

*Diabetes.co.uk* (diabetes.co.uk (not to be confused with diabetes.org.uk))
This website is aimed at people with a diagnosis of diabetes, both type 1 and type 2 diabetes. There are plenty of useful resources, particularly regarding management of diabetes alongside reduced carbohydrate diets.

*Dr Michael Mosley and The Fast 800*
Dr Mosley was a British journalist and doctor who died unexpectedly in 2024. He wrote many books, including, of relevance to MASLD, 'The 8-Week Blood Sugar Diet', 'The Fast Diet', 'The Clever Guts Diet' and 'Fast Exercise.' The Fast 800 online programme provides nutritional, exercise and lifestyle advice. It also sells meal replacement shakes (see functional foods section below) which are described as being based on the Mediterranean diet.

*Dr Jason Fung*
Dr Fung is a Canadian nephrologist, who developed an interest in nutrition after looking after many diabetic patients with end stage kidney failure. Books include 'The Obesity Code: Unlocking the Secrets to Weight Loss', and 'The Complete Guide to Fasting. Heal your body through Intermittent, Alternate-Day and Extended Fasting.'

**Supplements, superfoods and functional foods – helpful, or money down the drain?** To start with, we will consider what is meant by a food, dietary or nutritional **supplement.** It is a product taken in addition to the diet, usually by mouth, and which typically contains one or more dietary ingredient, such as a mineral, vitamin, herb, amino acid, or enzyme. These may come from natural or synthetic sources. They are not regulated in the way that drugs are, with a licensing process requiring evidence of safety and effectiveness. As they are not licenced drugs, they can be bought freely by consumers. There is, therefore, little point in manufacturers trying to spend money doing research to prove their effectiveness. Even if there were trials to look at effectiveness of supplements, as with food trials, it is virtually impossible to be able to demonstrate effectiveness.

This does not mean they are not effective. Some may actually contain powerful chemicals. It's a very grey line differentiating what is a supplement and what is a drug. To give two readily available examples, iron and vitamin D are frequently prescribed by doctors to their patients when they have a deficiency. However, it is perfectly easy to buy iron supplements and vitamin D supplements online, in the pharmacy and even the supermarket. These, therefore, are both drugs, licenced and regulated, and food supplements. The difference is that the food supplements are not regulated in terms of quality control.

It is often said that, if you eat a healthy varied diet, there is no need to take supplements. However, many people do not manage to eat a healthy varied diet for a whole host of reasons. It's also impossible to get adequate vitamin D for people living in the UK during the winter months. The NHS advice currently is that women planning a pregnancy should take folic acid, everyone should take a vitamin D supplement from autumn until spring, and all year round for those at risk (people not getting adequate sun exposure), and that all children between 6 months and 5 years should take a daily supplement of vitamin A, C and D. There is also some suggestion that Vitamin C and E may be helpful in MASLD. It's probably sensible to take a multivitamin supplement that contains vitamins C, D and E.

As we're said, it's virtually impossible to collect evidence in a trial of effectiveness of supplements. However, many people take them, and anecdotally claim to feel some benefit. One of the author's grandmothers died contentedly at the age of 105, having run out of things to do with her life. She swore by the benefits of cod liver oil (which contains omega-3 fatty acids, vitamins A and D) and apple cider vinegar (which decreases blood glucose level and increases insulin sensitivity) which she had taken for all of her life, although if you asked her what they did, she wouldn't have been able to explain, just that she felt they worked!

The question then moves to, if effectiveness can't be proved, is there any harm to taking supplements, other than to the wallet? There needs to be an element of caution in taking supplements, particularly the lesser-known brands, as it is not always clear what chemicals are in the supplement, or at what doses. It's also probably best to avoid taking multiple supplements that contain the same or a similar substance, to avoid excess intake.

One important thing to be aware of is the difference between food supplements and Chinese herbal or traditional medicine. Some Chinese herbal medicines have been found to contain drugs, toxins, and contaminants, and have caused liver failure in people with previously healthy livers. We would not recommend any use of Chinese herbal or traditional medicine for this reason.

In conclusion, supplements may be beneficial, (indeed vitamin D is recommended), but be cautious in avoiding taking multiple different sources at once and look for sources that appear to be reliable and consistent.

The next thing to look at is **superfoods**. Unlike supplements, these are actual foods that have been arbitrarily identified as having valuable nutritional benefits. However, there is no actual definition of what constitutes a superfood, nor a list of what foods count as superfoods. There is very much an element of journalistic and marketing hype, with trends as to what counts as a superfood. The nutritional values that are felt to be important are very subjective. Many of the foods that are described as superfoods have that label because they are relatively high in vitamins, minerals, antioxidants, protein or fibre. A healthy diet includes multiple and varied food sources, especially amongst the plant family, where different types and colours of plants provide a variety of beneficial substances. It is no bad thing to include some of these foods in your diet, but not worth spending a lot of money on, or restricting your intake of other similarly healthy foods, to try and get your intake of 'superfood'.

A third category of foods to consider are '**functional foods**', which overlap with another category of foods known as 'nutraceuticals'. Functional foods are foods that naturally contain bioactive components which can provide health benefits beyond the traditional nutritional value of the food. Nutraceuticals involve the bioactive compound being used for fortification or supplementation, rather than in the direct food form. We will just talk about functional foods here, to cover both groups. Functional foods can be categorised into conventional and modified foods. The conventional foods are those foods that we know to be beneficial, including those "superfoods" mentioned above, and should be making up an important element of your diet anyway, if you are following a varied diet based on the Mediterranean diet or something similar. There are multiple definitions of functional foods, and descriptions of categories. These include foods that have added fibre, known as prebiotics, as they provide food for the gut microbiome, and probiotics, which are foods or supplements that contain live microorganisms to improve the "good" bacteria in the gut.

Fermented foods are foods that naturally contain live bacteria, or probiotics. It's noteworthy that cultures around the world developed their own naturally fermented foods, which have been used for hundreds, or maybe thousands, of years. These include live yoghurt, kefir, kombucha, sauerkraut, miso, tempeh, kimchi, sourdough bread, some cheese and some alcoholic drinks. These have become very popular, and may help the gut health, including with some evidence for a benefit in MASLD. These can be bought, although it's remarkably easy to make some of them yourself at home for very little cost and with little or no equipment. It's possible to make continuous kefir or yoghurt, starting with just one batch, for example a supermarket purchase of natural live yoghurt, which then can be used in the next generation and so on.

It's also possible to take probiotic supplements as tablets or drinks, which provide live bacteria to the stomach. How many of these bacteria can live beyond the stomach, which is naturally very acidic, is not clear. There is a suggestion that probiotics taken in the form of fermented foods are more resistant and likely to survive the acidic environment of the stomach that those from supplements.

Other modified functional foods include some of those foods specifically designed and marketed to aid and enhance health, or, frequently, for weight control. One example of this is the many drinks, meal replacements or shakes that are available. Whilst in an ideal world we would be able to prepare all the healthy food we need at all times; the reality is often very different. Using such products may be a pragmatic, helpful way to keep up the healthy lifestyle. What's important is to check out what the foods or drinks include very carefully, and to try and use food replacements that are similar to the diets we have recommended above, i.e., based on the Mediterranean or low carbohydrate diet. As a rough guide, and this is very much based on our opinion rather than any guidelines, we would suggest you look for meal substitutes that, when made up, contain less than 10g carbohydrate per serving, at least 10g protein per serving, and some fat and fibre to aid fullness and satiation, as well as providing the many benefits of fat and fibre. If you can't find a list of ingredients and nutritional information on a product, don't buy it. Be conscious that foods that are advertised as high protein may also be high carbohydrate in content and should therefore be avoided.

Continuing with the functional foods theme, there are some products that have been designed to have reduced carbohydrate, alongside increased protein, and fibre, either as readymade foods, or as ingredients. Many people use flour alternatives in baking which are naturally lower in carbohydrate, such as almond or coconut flour, or make their own seed flour by grinding up seeds in a blender. However, there are also manufactured alternatives. One example is FiberFlour (longjevity-foods.com), which was developed by a retired cardiac anaesthetist, with the intention of reducing starches and sugar and replacing them with fibre and other nutrients, to improve metabolic health and insulin resistance. Another brand providing products that are lower carbohydrate and higher in protein and fibre is Carbzone. There are many others, and we are not endorsing these products in particular. They are just some that we have tried and found to match our recommendations for people with MASLD.

To conclude and answer the question at the start of this section, are superfoods, supplements and functional foods helpful, the answer is, probably, but it all depends on your individual circumstances. And cooking skills.

## *OBESITY AND BMI*

Obesity is a very emotive subject. Nobody wants to be described as obese, as it is seen as some kind of judgement on people. There is good evidence that obese people experience discrimination and disadvantages due to their weight, which can have a negative impact on their opportunities throughout life. Due to the increased awareness of this in recent years, there has been a move towards being more sensitive in healthcare, to avoid any discrimination. This is very much to be welcomed.

However, obesity still has huge health implications. If we don't feel comfortable talking about the consequences of obesity, it becomes the elephant in the room. Just because we don't talk about it doesn't mean it isn't there and isn't important. There is a danger that, if healthcare professionals act as if it doesn't exist or doesn't matter, we are doing our patients a disservice, and denying them the chance to make changes that would improve their health. We have flipped 180 degrees, patients are now being discriminated against because they are obese and because doctors are terrified of the consequences of telling them this, so they do not get appropriate care.

We need to eliminate this emotional overlay and put it into an objective medical term.

What is meant by obesity? Overweight and obesity are defined as the abnormal or excessive fat accumulation that presents a risk to health. It is most commonly categorised by the body mass index or BMI. This is a calculation of your weight in kg divided by your height in metres, squared.

i.e. $BMI = \dfrac{\text{weight (kg)}}{\text{height (m)}^2}$

There are plenty of websites, including the NHS, that work it out for you. When BMI is used to define obesity, the categories, based on the NHS website, are:

| BMI | Category |
| --- | --- |
| <18.5 | underweight |
| 18.5 – 24.9 | healthy |
| 25 – 29.9 | overweight |
| 30 – 39.9 | obese |
| >40 | severely obese |

The BMI has some limitations as an indicator of obesity, which is supposed to be describing excess fat. People with a lot of muscle will also have a high BMI, but without the same obesity related health risks. A 2009 report on the All-Blacks New Zealand rugby players described how all of them were overweight with many of them counting as obese on the BMI scale, but clearly without carrying any surplus fat. The article also illustrates another problem with the BMI scale, which is that the categories also vary by race, so in the example of the New Zealand rugby players, the overweight category was 25 - 30 for those of European descent, but for the Māori and Pacific Islanders it was 26 – 32.

Although the NHS website only gives the categories in the table above, there is a recognition that other populations and races have health risks with different ranges, and whereas the range for the Māori and Pacific Islanders was higher, for Asians it is lower. For Asians, therefore, the BMI ranges are 18.5 – 22.9 healthy, 23 – 27.5 is overweight, and greater than 27.5 is obese.

The healthy BMI range for children also varies with age, so BMI for children (boys and girls) charts should be used, rather than adult ranges. The BMI is a useful screening tool, but not infallible. Alternative ways to measure for excess fat i.e., obesity, is using waist circumference, as a screening for risk. A waist circumference that is more than half a person's height has been found to be a useful indicator of increased health risks from obesity. This leads on to the importance of fat distribution, whether it is central or peripheral. People have often categorised themselves as being apples or pears, based on whether they tend to carry fat around their abdomen, or around their hips and thighs. Those people who are pear shaped have more subcutaneous fat. Whilst there are still some health risks associated with this kind of obesity, subcutaneous fat provides a safer storage site than visceral fat, the fat that is stored in and around the abdominal organs, which is a feature of the apple shape.

Whether people are more likely to store fat in subcutaneous or visceral sites is determined by a combination of factors, including genetics, diet (both calories and content) and activity levels. It is visceral fat that is most strongly associated with MASLD. It is also not necessary for people to be overweight to have MASLD as there are some people who are within the normal weight range who have the condition. For these people, reducing carbohydrate intake rather than calories, and increasing exercise, may be even more important.

Using weight and BMI does have some value. However, as clinicians, we find that there is an even more useful indicator of people's health and nutritional status, and that is simply by looking at them. Many people we see have, what can be termed, obesity malnutrition. Many doctors are surprised when we point out that an overweight person has malnutrition, but malnutrition simply means "bad" nutrition, that is, not having the good nutrients that their body needs. Whilst it's not possible to look at someone and know if they are deficient in the micronutrients mentioned in the earlier chapter, it is possible to look at them and get an idea as to whether they have a relative deficiency in protein. We are always much more concerned about people who are overweight, but with little muscle mass to see. This is usually due to a combination of lack of protein intake and lack of exercise (especially resistance exercise). As is discussed in the following chapter, muscle is important for healthy glucose and insulin control, and lack of muscle therefore is associated with increased risk of type 2 diabetes and MASLD.

One marker of muscle mass, which is not usually thought of as such, is creatinine. This is one of the two main tests of kidney function, and is a compound continuously produced by muscle as part of its maintenance process, which is then removed by the kidneys. Doctors and nurses worry about high creatinine levels, as this is usually an indicator of a degree of kidney failure, as the kidneys are not removing the creatinine from the blood into the urine. However, a low creatinine should not be considered as reassuring, it is a sign of lack of muscle mass, and sometimes of lack of protein intake. Seeing a patient who is obese, but with a low creatinine, suggests someone with a high caloric intake but low protein intake and reduced muscle mass, and highly likely to have some elements of the metabolic syndrome.

It's important to remember that all we have discussed in this chapter (and in the book) is aimed at improving the metabolic health of the body, and in particular the liver cells. Losing weight in order to achieve a healthy weight may occur as a result of these changes, but weight loss (or more accurately weight optimisation) should be seen as a secondary gain, rather than the primary objective. Weight optimisation can be unpredictable, and healthy weight optimisation does not occur quickly, but can continue over several years of healthy lifestyle changes.

## ***BARIATRIC SURGERY***

Although this chapter is about diet, we have also included bariatric surgery, as this causes a profound reduction and alteration in dietary intake. Bariatric surgery is surgery that reduces the volume of the stomach, with the intention of causing weight loss in obese people. Two of the most common operations are a gastric bypass, where the top of the stomach is connected directly to the small bowel, bypassing the rest of the stomach, and a sleeve gastrectomy, where part of the stomach is removed. Bariatric surgery is effective in causing weight loss and improving obesity related diseases such as type 2 diabetes and heart problems. However, it is major surgery, with some significant risks, and with long-term consequences. These include vitamin and mineral malnutrition, and dumping syndrome, where food is deposited rapidly in the small bowel, having not had time to start digestion in the stomach, which can make people feel very unwell, and can be disabling. People need to change what and how they eat. The question, therefore, is whether it works "enough" for MASLD to justify the downsides and risks. There is evidence that both gastric bypass and sleeve gastrectomy result in an improvement of MASLD at 12 months. However, and concerningly, around one in five people develop worsening liver fibrosis following bariatric surgery at later follow up.

A less invasive bariatric surgery is gastric banding. This is a band that is put around the upper stomach, narrowing the stomach down to a much smaller 'upper stomach', which slowly drains into the rest of the stomach. It is done using keyhole surgery, and the band is removable, meaning that this can be reversed. It also has complications, and requires a change of eating behaviour. It is less effective for weight loss than the more invasive gastric bypass or gastrectomy, and is less likely to have any effect on MASLD.

Newer techniques are being developed rapidly, and these include gastric balloon insertion and endoscopic sleeve gastroplasty. These are both techniques which are done using an endoscope down the oesophagus, so don't involve any cutting open of the abdominal wall. The gastric balloon works by occupying space in the stomach, therefore reducing the remaining space available for food. The endoscopic sleeve gastroplasty involves a section of the stomach wall being stapled off or closed by stitching, therefore reducing the stomach cavity size. These are recent developments, so the evidence of benefit in MASLD hasn't has time to be fully developed, but there is a suggestion that both techniques reduce fat in the liver, with possible benefits on fibrosis with the gastroplasty technique. As with the other techniques, they require lifelong changes in eating patterns.

In conclusion, bariatric surgical techniques and procedures may improve MASLD, but all have complications, and all require lifelong changes in eating pattern. It's therefore better, if possible, to change eating patterns to those that benefit the liver and metabolic health, without going through the complications of bariatric surgery.

## *ORLISTAT*

Orlistat is a drug that stops the digestion and absorption of dietary fat, therefore resulting in fat being retained in the bowel content and lost in the stool. It can help with weight loss. Side-effects include abdominal pain, diarrhoea and malabsorption of fat-soluble vitamins, especially vitamin D. It has been reported to rarely cause severe liver failure. Although effective for weight loss, there have not been any trials to demonstrate effectiveness in MASLD, and it is not therefore recommended for this purpose.

This lack of effectiveness is not that surprising, given that the fat in the liver is not significantly derived from the fat that is ingested as food, but from the liver processing of the carbohydrate that it receives from the bowel. As carbohydrate absorption is not affected by orlistat, excess carbohydrate will continue to be stored as liver fat, regardless of whether any fat is absorbed from the bowel.

## *GLP-1 AGONISTS*

In the UK there are now several GLP-1 agonists licensed for weight loss. These include semaglutide (Wegovy), liraglutide (Saxenda) and tirzepatide (Mountjaro). These were initially used as medication for type 2 diabetes, but have also been found to aid weight loss, and are now additionally licensed for management of obesity. They are discussed further in Chapter 9. Please note that, at the time of writing, Ozempic, which is another brand of semaglutide, is licensed for type 2 diabetes but is not licensed for weight loss.

## *ADJUSTING MEDICATION WITH CHANGING DIET*

Modifying your diet is an essential part of improving MASLD. However, for two groups of medication in particular, which people with MASLD are commonly taking, it is important to be aware that dietary changes may influence your medication requirements. In simple terms, the improvements that result from reduced dietary intake mean that you may need less treatment. A good thing, but one you need to be mindful of in the short term (adjusting doses down to take account of reduced dose requirement) and in the medium term (putting doses back up if weight regain occurs). These two groups of drugs are diabetes medicines and blood pressure medicines (anti-hypertensives). In each case you may need extra monitoring when changing your diet to ensure that you are on the correct dose and should discuss this with a relevant doctor or nurse. It is important, however, that you aren't put off trying to improve your diet because it's considered "unsafe" or "too complicated" to do so. That would be completely the wrong message to take away.

Sadly, however, this response is all too common. We have come across diabetes nurses telling obese patients with type 2 diabetes, i.e., too much glucose and too much insulin, that they must make sure they eat an extra slice of bread with their meal, or have some apple crumble, because they've just had their insulin, and it could be unsafe if their blood glucose drops. Pointing out that they could eat less carbohydrate, and possibly not need the insulin, has led to a response that that's not the steady and safe option. Given that we, as hospital consultants, struggle to get this dogma changed, we fully recognise that it may not be easy for patients to get the response and support they want, need, and deserve. This is one of those occasions where you must remember the mantra of this book – own the problem, own the solution. It's your body, your health, and your future, and you have the right to persist until you get the support you need to monitor and reduce your medication safely.

It may be that the doctor or nurse you discuss this with may not feel confident to advise you on how to adapt medication when reducing carbohydrates. There is a useful article in the British Journal of General Practice which gives guidance on this. It is freely available. The title and link is below:

Adapting diabetes medication for low carbohydrate management of type 2 diabetes: a practical guide
Murdoch C, Unwin D, Cavan D, Cucuzzella M and Patel M
https://bjgp.org/content/69/684/360

If you are reducing medication, it's important to monitor your glucose, particularly if you are using medication like insulin. This could either be with a continuous glucose monitoring or intermittent blood glucose monitoring. The other group of medicines where you may need to reduce your requirement is blood pressure treatment, anti-hypertensives. This is usually a slower change than that which happens with glucose. Again, this should be discussed with your doctor. Which medicines can be reduced, and in which order, will depend on your individual risk factors, combination of medicines, and other co-existing conditions. What you need to look out for, though, are the signs that your blood pressure may be over-treated and seek a review. The most noticeable sign you may get if your blood pressure is falling includes dizziness on standing up. You can also check your blood pressure at home with an automatic blood pressure machine, which can give you a trend over time.

# CHAPTER 7: **TREATING MASLD 3:** *EXERCISE*

## *The 2-Minute Version*

- Exercise is an important aspect of self-management of MASLD. It is something that can have a really meaningful impact on the disease, and it is in your hands as a patient. It is a key part of "owning the problem and owning the solution".
- Although muscle will "burn" fuel (glucose and fat), the benefits in terms of MASLD go far beyond this simple impact on the metabolic "balance sheet". Exercise will alter metabolism, increasing energy consumption, and shifting the pathways that are used, beyond the specific period of exercise.
- That you actually do exercise is more important than doing the perfect exercise programme. It is helpful to find ways to include exercise in everyday life (walking to work, walking the dog, climbing the stairs rather than taking the lift etc).
- If you want to develop your programme, look to do exercise three times a week for at least half an hour. Look for an intensity of exercise that leaves you a little bit short of breath. As you do more and more exercise so you will get fitter and need to step up the exercise levels. If you really want to go for an optimum programme combine cardiovascular (bike, treadmill, fast walking etc) with resistance (weights) elements.
- Think of using technology to support your exercise. Technologies such as heart rate monitors and activity monitors can really help you keep a check of how much you are doing.
- Be ready to cope with the downs as well as the ups. A nice walk in the country in summer is easy, jogging on dark streets in the middle of winter is less easy. Think through how you are going to keep it going.
- Exercise in MASLD will really improve fatigue as well as the disease. It will get easier to keep going when you directly feel the benefit.

Exercise therapy is perhaps the great paradox in the treatment of fatty liver disease. It is a treatment that both clearly works and clearly doesn't work. How so? As we will discuss, there is very clear evidence that a structured and sustained programme of exercise is highly effective at reversing hepatic steatosis (i.e. it works). In practice, however, people struggle to start exercising and then struggle even more to sustain it (i.e., all too often it doesn't work in practice).

In drug trials we use the concept of "intention to treat analysis". If we are comparing a drug with a placebo or dummy tablet, and the participant decides to stop taking the treatment (usually because of side effects) we don't then leave that person out of the comparison as if they didn't exist. We continue to include them in the drug-treated group as we "intended to treat them". What this means is that the failure to take the treatment is treated in the same way as if the participant took it and it didn't work. This is, of course, entirely logical as a treatment that people decide not to take is clearly not a very effective one. Oddly, in clinical practice we tend to think in a different way, only "seeing" the effects of treatments that people take, and disregarding people who don't take them from our thinking (this is called "per protocol analysis" technically) as we only include in that analysis those people who followed the protocol in full. A good example is liver transplantation. The "success" of liver transplantation is always quoted in terms of the outcomes of people having the operation but tends to exclude the often large number of people who are never referred for consideration of transplantation, are referred but turned down because they aren't suitable, or who die on the list, waiting for an organ. For these people, transplant has "failed" as a treatment just as much as if they had had the operation and died of a complication. Exercise therapy is another perfect example of this paradoxical thinking. In people who start and complete exercise programmes, exercise is highly effective. Most people advised to start an exercise programme, however, will not start it let alone sustain it and therefore don't derive benefit. Exercise in MASLD is highly effective on a per protocol basis but much less so on an intention to treat basis.

In this chapter we will explore the biology of exercise therapy, explore the types of exercise you should be considering and then make some suggestions on the tricky topic of how to get started and how to continue.

## *THE CONCEPT OF EXERCISE THERAPY*
Fundamentally, the metabolic syndrome is an imbalance between the amount of energy people take in (food) and the amount of energy they use (exercise). The balance is modified to a degree by the genetics of energy use and the nature of dietary intake, as well as baseline activity levels, but the basic concept is key. This simple balance gives rise to the aspect of exercise that is, perhaps, least important in reality; the calories you burn during the exercise

period (who amongst us hasn't looked at the "calories used" readout on the bike at the gym and thought "only 100 more and I can have a Mars Bar!"). Although clearly exercise does "burn calories" it has a much more profound impact that really adds to its importance.

**Resetting metabolism:** Exercising on a regular basis leads to an improvement in capacity to undertake exercise. This has been known about for thousands of years and underpins all the concepts around "training" to improve sporting performance. What exercise does in the setting of training is, essentially, twofold.

The first aspect of the response to exercise, i.e., the repetitive contraction of the muscles, is that it triggers their growth. This is in part a repair phenomenon (repeat contractions cause low level damage to the muscles which needs to be repaired; think of "stiff" muscles after a brisk walk). There is also an overshoot aspect with this, with the muscles growing back slightly larger than before as a protective response (stronger muscles will be less vulnerable to damage). As we will discuss in the next section, this underpins the whole concept of weight training in the world of body building.

The second aspect is an alteration in the metabolism of muscle (i.e., the process by which the muscles generate and use energy). Again, the world of sport tells us that repeat exercise increases the capacity to do exercise. Many of us will have experience of building-up over time to the point when we can do a half marathon for charity; something that is unthinkable at the beginning of training. There are now excellent and structured programmes to help with this such as the BBC "Couch to 5k" app. As we have discussed, part of the benefit of training is muscle strengthening. There is, however, another aspect that anyone who has been through the process will be familiar with, energy levels.

For muscle to function, its cells need to have energy. This comes from the processing of food molecules (in all their different forms). There are, in essence, two types of energy generation, anaerobic and aerobic. Anaerobic metabolism is very inefficient but will generate large amounts of energy very rapidly. Its inefficiency means, however, that it can't be sustained for any length of time. The essence of anaerobic metabolism is that it does not rely on a balanced process in which oxygen is used at the same rate as energy generation. It builds up an oxygen "debt" that needs to be paid back after the exercise episode has ended. Think of a sprinter running the 100 metres. Their muscles generate a vast amount of energy very quickly. This is all done anaerobically and there is, in fact, no attempt by their bodies to balance nutrition and oxygen consumption. Anaerobic metabolism generates large amounts of lactic acid in the muscle. This acid load means, of course, that they can't carry on exercising at the same level. In fact they normally collapse onto the track breathing hard. This over-breathing is to allow a high oxygen delivery to help metabolise the lactic acid (and pay back the oxygen "debt").

Aerobic metabolism is completely different. This is metabolism that is in balance, with food consumption being fully in step with oxygen delivery. This form of metabolism generates lower levels of energy but does so in a sustainable way. Think not of a sprinter but a marathon runner. They are not as fast as a sprinter, but they can keep going for hours at the same pace! At the heart of aerobic metabolism is the function of the mitochondria; structures within all cells that contain linked enzymes that process nutrition molecules and oxygen to generate energy in a sustained fashion.

What is the link to MASLD and exercise therapy? Exercise training can build up the capacity to utilise each of these types of metabolism. Anaerobic metabolism is essentially all about converting glucose into lactic acid (and back again). In contrast, aerobic metabolism can utilise a number of different energy sources, most relevantly free fatty acids (part of the fat that is deposited in the cells of the liver in MASLD). Aerobic training (increasing the amount of exercise that you can do without crossing into anaerobic metabolism) both "consumes" fat and switches the preferred fuel type in the body towards fat. A double win that directly reverses fat deposition.

Does this mean that only aerobic training (e.g., cardio exercise such as an exercise bike, jogging or swimming) is useful in MASLD? The answer is no, as it is, perhaps inevitably, not as a simple as that. Anaerobic exercise training also has real benefits. As well as increasing the capacity to undertake anaerobic exercise (in essence you train to sprint faster by sprinting) by increasing muscle blood flow and developing better mechanisms to transport lactic acid out of the muscle cells, anaerobic exercise restores insulin sensitivity. As we discussed in **Chapter 3**, the metabolic abnormality that lies at the heart of MASLD is insulin resistance. The cells of the liver don't "hear" the signal given by insulin in response to eating a meal. This means that, rather than converting glucose into glycogen (the physiological storage form that is easily accessed between meals), it is converted into fat. The other tissue that normally expresses insulin receptors at high level is muscle (and muscle cells can also convert glucose into glycogen as an energy store). The principle physiological role of insulin signalling in the liver is, however, to allow uptake of amino acids and their conversion into muscle protein. Insulin signalling is, therefore, integral to the repair of muscles after exercise and the growth of muscles after training. Insulin resistance, however, doesn't impact muscle cells in the same way as it affects the liver, with the net result that muscle can continue to function in an insulin sensitive fashion even when liver insulin resistance is occurring. In a simplistic sense, muscle can take over some of the normal metabolic burden in MASLD, provided it is stimulated to do so. This is why exercise matters so much in MASLD.

**"Owning the solution":** Throughout this book we will keep returning to the mantra of "own the problem: own the solution". Ultimately, MASLD is a health challenge where there are solutions that lie in your hands. This sadly isn't the case in many other disease types such as cancer. You therefore owe it to yourself to be given the opportunity to help yourself. Although we now have the first drug licensed for use in MASLD its effects are not comprehensive. This makes it doubly important that you undertake the steps which are proven to benefit. Exercise and dietary intervention. "Owning the solution" is also something which is incredibly beneficial at a psychological level; empowerment comes from achieving something which isn't easy but is very worthwhile.

**Improving wellbeing:** Owning the solution clearly is, as we have outlined, something that can give a sense of wellbeing in MASLD through a perception of self-empowerment. There is, of course, the broader physiological benefit that comes with regular exercise. People who exercise regularly have a greater perception of wellness than people who don't exercise, irrespective of whether they have underlying health conditions. It is often ascribed to endorphins (the body's own natural opiate painkilling molecules). Whether this is true or not the effect is clearly there. Exercise makes you feel better. It is as simple as that.

**Reducing cardiac risk and improving diabetes:** Another issue we will keep coming back to in this book is that in MASLD the risk to health does not just come from the complications of liver disease. MASLD is strongly associated with type 2 diabetes and cardiac disease. Exercise intervention also benefits both conditions. There is unequivocal evidence that exercise benefits type 2 diabetes control through restoration of insulin sensitivity. There are likely to be multiple contributing processes. Weight loss, and in particular loss of fat tissue, inherently improves insulin sensitivity as adipose or fatty tissue drives the whole process of insulin resistance. An effective exercise programme over a period of time will almost without fail be associated with weight optimisation. There is then the more specific effect of muscle insulin responsivity outlined earlier in the chapter.

Perhaps the most striking impacts of exercise in diabetes come in very early disease where effective exercise can reverse the whole process, rendering people non-diabetic again. A colleague of ours did a study around the Great North Run (a large half-marathon which takes place annually in the north of England). He recruited a group of people with early type 2 diabetes, who didn't usually exercise, several months before the race. Half got general health advice and half got a structured exercise programme with lots of support to help them train. Of the general health advice group, none got to finish the race (or even, in fact, start it) and all remained diabetic. Of the structured exercise programme group all started the race, most finished it, and most were non-diabetic by the time of the race. This gives pretty clear cut evidence of the benefits of exercise, but also of the challenges of starting and maintaining exercise without support.

The other health improvement area relevant to MASLD is heart disease, and specifically ischaemic heart disease (angina and heart attack risk). Here, again, exercise is known to be very effective at both reducing risk of developing heart disease and improving outcomes after a heart event. Again, there are likely to be a number of contributing processes including reduction in diabetes impact (diabetes directly contributes to atherosclerosis, the key disease process in heart disease) and reduction on blood pressure elevation (again a common association with MASLD and a major contributor to heart attack risk). It may well also be the case that, rather as exercise improves the metabolic "health" of skeletal muscle it also directly helps improves the function of cardiac muscle.

The key thing is that exercise in MASLD is a win, win, win situation. Improvement in MASLD itself, improved sense of well-being and reduced impact from other important linked diseases. What is not to love!?

## *EXERCISE THERAPY IN PRACTICE*

The problem with exercise therapy, however, is not the concept but the practice. We suspect that most people with MASLD are quite accepting of the idea that exercise is going to be good for them. It makes complete sense given everything we know about exercise and fitness. The issue is converting that acceptance of benefit into what is often a significant lifestyle change. We are all familiar with New Year's resolutions…... Each year we commit to making changes in our lives that we know full well will be good for us, yet each year willpower fails…….

In this section of the book, we will talk really practically about what you can do, and how you can get going and keep going. We will talk about the different types of exercise, building on some of our earlier discussion about how exercise improves insulin resistance, but only in quite general terms. In our experience, exercise as a therapy is vastly more likely to fail because people don't start (or if they do start, they don't sustain it), than because they do the "wrong sort of exercise". If fine tuning of your exercise programme is needed to get the most benefit from it, then congratulations are in order. You are 90% there!

**What exercise to do:** Having said we won't dwell on the potential types of exercise it is important to start by thinking about the options. This is because worry about what to do is, in our experience, one of the real barriers. In simple terms the answer to the question "what is the right sort of exercise" is simple. It is the type that you start and then carry on doing..........

As we will discuss in the next section, it is worth thinking right at the outset about the reasons why people who have started an exercise programme then stop. In our experience there are three reasons. These are injuries to muscles and joints, a sense that it isn't working and, perhaps most importantly, time. The last aspect is important if we are thinking about what exercise to do. There is no point in devising the best exercise programme in the world if you are simply not able to do it because of time constraints. If we had a pound (or dollar!) for every time someone had said they would love to exercise but they are working full-time, as well as looking after children and/or elderly relatives we would be very rich indeed. One of the traps that doctors and other clinicians can easily fall into is to expect that people take on simply undeliverable lifestyle changes, and then blame them if patients aren't able to do it. The authors of this book are, in contrast, most definitely "inhabitants of the real world".

If exercise is to be effective (and it needs to "challenge" muscle if it is to be effective) then you need to do enough of it, frequently enough, to change the biology of muscle. In simplistic terms, people with MASLD are "energy hoarders" rather than "energy users". They are efficient at eking out the energy they take in through the diet and storing up for the future as much of it as they possibly can. Exercise prevents that from happening because the need to repair and strengthen muscle trumps the need to energy hoard. Remember, insulin drives amino acid uptake into muscle to repair it and so the body can't "afford" to have insulin resistant muscle. Exercise once a week and this allows the body to slip back into the hoarding pattern. Exercise every day and it can't (but, then again, you can't fit that into everyday life). The sweet spot is exercising three times a week, ideally spaced out on roughly alternate days. More frequently is great if you can do it, less frequently runs the risk that the effect is lost. Three times a week is therefore the benchmark.

How much and for how long are the next questions. In terms of duration, we conventionally think of 30 minutes as being ample to effect metabolic change (provided, of course, it is regular; remember the three times a week!). This isn't a hard and fast rule and, without question, 20 minutes three times a week is vastly better for you than not exercising at all. The question of what exercise is enough is both difficult and easy to answer at the same time. Let us explain. It is difficult in the sense that we can't "see inside" muscle to understand its metabolism. It is easy in the sense that we don't need to because your body can do it for us by the way it responds to exercise. Our heart rate is a really good way of monitoring how your body is responding to exercise. If exercise is placing a burden on the body, then your heart rate will go up (through the effect of adrenaline which pushes the rate up to improve the blood flow delivering nutrition and oxygen). Conversely, if exercise doesn't put your heart rate up at all then it is probably at a level where the body isn't "feeling it". What this means is that your heart rate is a natural "monitor" for the amount of exercise you are doing. This makes it important in planning and monitoring your exercise programme.

There are two important questions about heart-rate controlled exercise. The first is how do I know what my heart rate is in the first place? The second is what rate should I aim for? Both are easy to answer. You can, of course, take your pulse rate by feeling for the artery at your wrist (just up the arm from the base of the thumb). This is, however, not terribly convenient to do when doing your exercise. Technology has, however, come to our aid because there are simple and easy to use heart rate monitors that can be bought online and from sports shops. These are really accurate to use and have transformed exercise therapy in practice. The simplest form is just a heart rate monitor (i.e., it tells you your heart rate at any time and, usually, includes an average heart rate and a stopwatch to help you time your exercise). A step up from this is the exercise monitor itself ("Fitbit" is both the term people tend to use and one of the first companies in the field). Such monitors both record heart rate and count the number of steps that you take. As we will discuss later, this is a useful additional bit of information. The important point is that for a few tens of pounds (or dollars) you can use heart rate monitoring to determine if you are exercising enough.

What about the second question in relation to heart rate. What heart rate levels constitutes "enough" exercise. This is where the concept of maximum heart rate comes in. Our hearts all have a rate which is the very maximum level they can go at. This declines with age as older hearts beat less frequently. You can estimate your maximum heart rate (MHR) from the formula **220 beats per minutes (bpm) minus your age in years**. A 20-year-old has a maximum heart rate of 200 bpm whilst in a 60-year-old it is 160 bpm. The target heart rate with exercise is a percentage of your personal maximum heart rate. Above 90% of MHR (180 bpm for a 20-year-old, 144 bpm for a 60-year-old) is performance training and is a level that you really shouldn't be exercising at. Conversely, a level of below 50% of MHR (100 bpm for a 20-year-old, 80 bpm for a 60-year-old) is likely to have no health benefit at all as it is too low for the body to notice. Between 50 and 90% are four exercise bands that you will gradually begin to explore.

**50-60%** (80-96 bpm for a 60-year-old):   Very light exercise, good for warming up and cooling down. A good level to start at if you haven't exercised for a long time.

**60-70%** (96-112 bpm for a 60-year-old): Light exercise. Good for fat burning and switching on the metabolism. This is the level you should aim for after a couple of weeks at the lower level. This will really build your endurance.

**70-80%** (112-128 bpm for a 60-year-old): Moderate exercise. At this level you are really boosting your aerobic capacity (mitochondrial energy generation). This type of exercise promotes use of stored fat as an energy source and is the absolute bedrock of exercise therapy in MASLD.

**80-90%** (128-144 bpm for a 60-year-old). Anaerobic (sprint-like) training. Short bursts of this are potentially useful once you are very comfortable with your training, especially if you are including some resistance training ("doing weights") to boost insulin sensitivity in the muscles.

With this information you can begin to see a programme emerging. Start at 50-60% of MHR for 30 minutes three times a week and take it from there, gradually stepping up the heart rate as you get fitter. Three 30-minute sessions a week at 70-80% of MHR will make a major difference to your MASLD. Own the problem and own the solution.

The other advantage of heart rate monitoring is that it provides reassurance about safety. People are always concerned about the risk of starting exercise, especially if they haven't done it for a long time (you should **check with your own doctor that there isn't any reason for you not to do it** (especially around heart problems which can be linked with MASLD)). Monitoring your heart rate and ensuring that it stays comfortably within the low risk zone below your MHR should provide you with reassurance that you are benefitting yourself rather than putting yourself at risk.

**Getting started:** You will by now be aware that we haven't actually talked about the type of exercise you should take yet. This may seem odd but there is a purpose behind it. By far and away the best exercise type is....... the one that you can actually do. There are two "danger periods" for an exercise therapy programme failing. The first is the difficulty in ever getting started. The second is the challenge of sustaining it in practice. We will give some practical thoughts on these in turn.

In terms of getting started with exercise, there are two things that can get in the way. The first is inertia (literally and metaphorically) and the other is a genuine concern about being able to exercise. In a sense inertia is easy to deal with. It is about deciding, at a particular time on a particular day, to start. There are two sayings that we use in the clinic which are potentially helpful. The first is "even a journey of a thousand miles begins with a single step" and the second is "tomorrow is the first day of the rest of your life". The meaning behind each of them is that it is that first step, and deciding to take it, that is critical for the future. Once you have taken it you have crossed the line into someone who is taking an exercise therapy programme. "One small step for man etc". As to when to take the step, that is up to you. New

Year resolution time can be useful (but don't feel guilty about "another failed year" if you fail the first time around). Any day is as good as the next for this, however. An important personal or family milestone may also help with starting with the right mindset (a birthday for example). Partners and family members are likely to be worried about you having liver disease so perhaps starting exercise would be a great Christmas or birthday present for them. In our experience it is helpful to kick this off at a time which gives you the best chance of keeping it going. The beginning of a week off work in the summer when you can do a little exercise every day is a really good time. In the middle of winter when you don't know when you will have time to do another session over the next couple of weeks is less likely to be successful.

In terms of being able to do it, we know from research that people can really lack the confidence to embark on an exercise programme with concerns about the safety of it, about whether they will be able to do it and about looking silly all being common. Let's take them in reverse order. We are in a world where many people have taken up exercise for their health. All ages, sexes, levels of fitness. Who cares what other people think! Think of all the people doing their local half-marathon dressed as a rhinoceros! There is also a misconception that gyms (if that is where you would like to exercise) are full of incredibly fit people with honed bodies. In fact, they are full of people just like you. You may well have heard of "Parkrun", one of the most inspiring examples of community-led exercise programmes. We have been the unfit people who are running at the back. The thing is everyone cheers you on and encourages you. They have been there themselves and remember it. There is also a "tail runner" from the organising team who runs at the back.... guaranteeing you aren't last and left behind.

In terms of confidence to exercise, this is an important aspect. This is where heart rate monitoring, and using the rate to understand your exercise level so that you can build it up, is so very useful. If you heart rate monitor, you can absolutely start exercising at a level that will put no pressure at all on your body. See how it feels and then gradually build up. If you don't have a heart rate monitor, you can start by exercising up to the point when you become out of breath. There are useful tips for exercising with heart disease on the British Heart Foundation information and support website page.

Another area where people are concerned is about their joints and muscles. They are worried that they will cause joint damage. It would be wrong of us to say this doesn't ever happen. It does, and the risk of it is an ever-present issue for exercise programmes. The art is to minimise the risk. There are three aspects to think about.

The first is the type of exercise you choose to do. The highest impact on your hips and knees comes from running (which we don't advise you to start with). The lowest comes from swimming. If you do have knee troubles, get going with a type of exercise that is gentle on your joints. Remember, your heart rate allows you to integrate different types of exercise whilst making sure you exercise to a high enough level. A pulse rate of 120 is a pulse rate of 120, no matter what type of exercise you did to get to 120! It is good practice to ring the changes with your exercise type to avoid chronic injury.

The second is to warm up properly. It is key to gently stretch the muscles before you exercise. This helps you avoid muscle tears. A torn muscle won't cause you long-term harm, but it will stop you exercising. This can be a negative when it comes to the real challenge with exercise, that of keeping it going once you have started. The third aspect is footwear. An important thing to minimise musculoskeletal injury is to get the best possible footwear you can if you are aiming to walk, jog or run (less of an issue for swimming!!). The biomechanics of your feet is a whole science in its own right. Properly fitted shoes (replaced before they wear out) is a key thing is you are going to start and then maintain an exercise programme.

The third barrier to starting exercise is concern about safety. This is, of course, a really important issue but one that is surmountable. It is advisable to discuss the safety of an exercise therapy programme with your doctor or nurse before you start to ensure there are no reasons why this isn't appropriate. The main issue is usually around cardiac disease, although given that exercise is part of the rehabilitation and risk reduction approach in patients with ischemic heart disease this is unlikely to be problematic. The key issue is, of course, that you will be starting gently and, ideally, monitoring your heart rate so that you gradually increase the work that your heart needs to do. Another safety aspect is in relation to diabetes, especially if you are using insulin to control it. Although exercise will ultimately be hugely beneficial in terms of diabetes control (it is a therapy for type 2 diabetes after all), it can complicate things a little whilst your programme becomes established. If you have a fixed dietary intake, and don't alter your insulin doses, then significant new exercise will tend to cause your sugars to fall, even resulting in hypos (the exercise "burns" glucose). The key thing ideally is to monitor your glucose level around exercise, adjusting insulin doses as needed. Fit the diabetes management around your exercise rather than fitting the exercise around your diabetes management (with the obvious risk that you don't exercise). The new generation of continuous glucose monitors (such as "Freestyle Libre") make this vastly easier than it used to be in the days of finger prick blood testing. This is another example, like heart rate monitors and step counters, of technology making it much easier than it used to be to manage your own disease. The final area of risk is around musculoskeletal injury. The key here is to always "warm up" before exercise and to listen to your body. If you are getting joint pains then just ease back a little on the exercise, let the pain settle and then build back up again.

**Keeping going:** Of all the areas we are discussing in relation to exercise in MASLD this is probably the most important. Failing to keep up a pattern of exercise that you have successfully started is the biggest single reason why exercise therapy in MASH doesn't work in practice. What we want to do here is to talk through the reasons why this happens and to come up with common sense ways to avoid this happening. There is very little science here, just a lot of common sense and understanding human nature. It is easy to list reasons why people fail to "keep it going", indeed some or all of these apply to the authors of this book just as much as anyone reading it.

1) **Work:** Exercise takes time and people are busy dealing with all the pressures of day-to-day life.
2) **Travel:** You get out of the habit when you go on holiday or travel for work and never get back into the habit.
3) **Illness or Injury:** You are doing fine but get a knee injury or a bad cold. You get out of the habit of exercise and never get back into it.
4) **Weather:** You start an outdoor exercise programme in the summer and really enjoy being outdoors during nice summer evenings. This is all less attractive on icy winter evenings.
5) **Daylight:** Outdoor exercise makes you feel a little vulnerable on dark winter evenings.
6) **Cost:** If you go down the gym line the costs can be significant.
7) **Boredom:** Exercise has just become a bit repetitive and boring.
8) **It isn't working:** It feels like hard work and yet you don't seem to be getting any real benefit.
9) **Injuries:** That joint or muscle injury that never seems to settle down and gets worse again every time you exercise.

These potential issues are all, to a degree, predictable and avoidable. The following is our practical advice.

***Develop a range of exercise approaches that give you resilience:*** This is probably the single most important piece of advice. A single approach to exercise (jogging round your local park) puts you at real risk of a number of these issues arising. The park isn't there when you go on holiday, it is cold, icy, and lonely in the winter and it gets, to be honest, a little boring. Take different routes, mix it up with swimming or cycling or, of course, join a gym where there are lots of options for indoor exercise. Over all the years we have been advising people about exercise, cold weather and ice in the setting of an outdoor exercise programme is the single commonest reason for people giving up. Having an outdoor walking or jogging aspect element is, however, useful because you can take your shoes and kit and go out when you are travelling. It is only then that you notice all the other people doing the same thing. Hotel swimming pools are also useful!

***Build exercise into daily life:*** Another important trick is to not assume that exercise has to be a discrete event, distinct from day-to-day life. A colleague of ours uses the term "movement as medicine" to encapsulate the concept of daily life activity being your health-promoting exercise. Meetings with him consist of walking across a park to a coffee stand (fast) and then walking back sipping on the coffee. Same meeting length but with 30 minutes of exercise built in! Walk to work if you can. If you can't, park further away and walk the last bit. If you get the bus, get off a couple of stops further away and walk the rest of the distance. You will find that it adds remarkably little time! This is, of course, where step counters come in. If you know that your standard 30-minute fast walk (the one that gets your heart rate up to the right level) means you take a certain number of steps in that half hour, then as long as you add that number of steps through the day via additional activity the impact on your body will be just the same.

***Use feedback to keep you going:*** In medicine we use the term "secondary gain". It is an important concept in those settings where people need to change behaviour. Take stopping smoking as an example. Most people who smoke want to give up, but they know that they will feel immediately worse when they do give up. We can persuade them of the benefits (indeed they can persuade themselves) but willpower and determination come up against short term cravings etc. Importantly, before too long they will feel better from not smoking (able to breathe better and feel better). At this point they don't need to be convinced that it is a good thing to do, they will know it is, because they have directly benefitted. This is secondary gain. The key thing is that you don't have to be convinced it's a good thing to do for ever, just long enough to reach the point where you get the physical benefit. A much easier task. The same principle applies to exercise in MASLD. It will be hard to start if you haven't exercised for a long time (although the approach to starting gently that we have outlined will undoubtedly help). After a couple of weeks, however, it will really start to help you feel less fatigued and better about life. Grit your teeth for those 4 weeks and reap the reward.

One way to get you to the point where you get secondary gain is to use other forms of positive feedback to prove to yourself that you are getting better. This is where step counters and heart rate monitoring are, again, useful. You can prove to yourself that you are doing more steps in your half hour, or your heart rate isn't going up as much for the same exercise programme; all signs that exercise is working. Being able to feel that it is working will really help you keep going.

***Avoid boredom:*** There is no avoiding the fact that the same exercise three times a week can get boring. Some people like the quiet time to reflect on the world and think about things but for others this is a negative. The answer is music or some other form of audio entertainment. Try some running playlists on Spotify to help keep up the momentum. Do watch out for the traffic if you have earphones in and never cycle using them! All the pro-health good work is rather undone if a bus hits you!

***Teamwork:*** The final tip is to try and not do this alone. Exercising with someone else can be helpful. This is one of the ways that Parkrun is so helpful. There is a ready-made group of people with whom you can join up and who are just like you. Parkrun also operates, literally, around the world so it is a great way of exercising if you are travelling. If you are exercising alone then something like the BBC "couch to 5k" app can be useful.

## *TAKING IT TO THE NEXT LEVEL*
You are doing well. You got started and then navigated the danger times as the nights got longer and the roads less enticing. You then reached the point where it wasn't just the doctors telling you this is really good; you are feeling it yourself (secondary gain); buzzing with energy. You have also been to the clinic and they have told you that your liver function tests are improving…….You have therefore reached the point where exercise isn't just something you manage to fit into day to day life, it is becoming a key part of your future life. As such you want to "take it to the next level". What, therefore, should you do? There are four aspects to look at, duration, frequency, intensity, and nature.

**Duration:** In many ways this is the aspect that people find most difficult to step up because of the everyday time pressures of work and family. Trying to increase sessions to 45 minutes is quite time effective (a greater period of "peak" exercise between the warm-up and cool down elements). To aim for much more is to set yourself up to fail. The key thing is to make these periods as energetically "good value for money" as you can.

**Frequency:** Again, this can be a challenge for many people given time constraints but stepping up to 4 sessions a week is good if you can manage it. Much more frequently than this and you don't allow the muscles to recover and grow (remember the integral part played by insulin in driving muscle growth) in between bouts of exercise. It also increases the risk of developing the low-grade joint and muscle injuries that can be the bane of exercise therapy programmes and which are the other reason why people end up stopping exercise, and running the risk of having to go back to square 1.

**Intensity:** This is where the real gains are to be made. As you exercise more, so you become fitter, and your heart rate will rise less for the same amount of exercise. As we have discussed, however, we are using heart rate as an exercise intensity monitor. You therefore need to step up the exercise level to reach the same heart rate. This is, of course, a virtuous circle. As you do more, and get more confident, you are likely to also want to go for a higher target heart rate. As we discussed earlier in this chapter you will have started with a target of 50-60% of your maximum heart rate (220 bpm - your age in years). This is a safe level and allows you to get going without causing problems. You will then have moved to 60-70% of MHR. Now is probably the time to go to 70-80% of MHR, if you feel ready.

**Nature:** This is the point where what you do starts to become important. Up to this point it was more a case of doing anything than being prescriptive about exercise type ("don't let the perfect be the enemy of the good"). Once you are up and going it is helpful to think about exercise type. In essence, you want to have a balance of cardiovascular training (heart rate targeted, sustained exercise such as running, jogging, or swimming) that drives aerobic metabolism, and resistance training (using weights that drive insulin responsivity in the muscles). How you mix these up slightly depends on the facilities that are available to you. By this point you may well have thought about joining a gym. If so, this makes life easy as they will have cardio machines (treadmills, exercise bikes and cross-trainers) and weights, either "free weights" (dumbbells in essence) or weight machines; better to go for the latter until you are a real exercise expert. The cardio aspect is fine outside the gym setting (running, cycling, and swimming as you have been doing all along) but the weights are more complex. Home weights are available, as are things like pull-up bars that you put on the door frame that have the same effect. A boxing bag also works well. If you are going to combine cardio and weights, then the optimal arrangement is to mix the two together in a single 45-minute session 4 times a week. If you do decide to join a gym, then they all have fitness instructors who will design your programme for you.

## *DECONDITIONING AND REHABILITATION*

These are two related areas that are worth mentioning as they can have a profound effect on people's health outcomes, and of which many people are not aware. Firstly, what is deconditioning? In health terms, this is a complex process of physiological changes, including loss of muscle, lung, and heart function, which occurs after a period of inactivity, bedrest, or sedentary lifestyle. It can result in reduced physical function, poor mobility, and impacts on mental health. We saw it happen to a whole nation following the government restrictions put in place in response to Covid19, with a generally reduced level of physical activity for many people. It can also happen when people have had to reduce their activity due to injury or other chronic health condition, such as arthritis. This is the opposite of getting fit, and can result in permanent loss of function, and reduced lifespan. It is important to recognise when this has occurred, because it can be minimised and reversed....but only if this is thought about. There are now campaigns to reduce the deconditioning that occurs to patients during hospital admissions in some hospitals. On an individual basis, readers of this book may recognise how they have reduced fitness and function due to some change in life. Again, covid restrictions were a major cause of deconditioning for many of us, and the authors also have personal experience of how arthritis can cause gradual deconditioning over time. We adjust our lifestyles to what we feel we can do, essentially moving the goalposts. The importance of this is to recognise this is happening, and try and maintain as much fitness as possible, for example by participating in other physical activities that may not use affected joints. It also leads onto the related topic of rehabilitation.

Rehabilitation is a process to restore abilities that have been lost due to an illness, injury, or disease, in order to regain function to normal, or as close to normal as possible. This is an active process, usually involving some kinds of physical exercise, including targeted physiotherapy, to regain function beyond that which is part of the natural healing process.

Let's take the example of arthritis of the knee, and subsequent knee replacement surgery to illustrate the effects of deconditioning and rehabilitation. Arthritis usually develops gradually over many years. During this time the person may have increasing pain and instability, resulting in a reduction of physical activity. This leads to reduced cardio-respiratory fitness, alongside a reduction at the level of cellular metabolic function that happens with fitness training. It also leads to loss of muscle and weakness, not just around the affected knee joint, but elsewhere throughout the body due to overall reduced muscle use. This situation may progress over several years, especially in a system such as the UK where there are prolonged waits for elective surgery, often for many months. By the time people get their surgery, they may be very deconditioned, which puts them at increased risk of complications from surgery, and poorer outcome. Following surgery or illness, many people are given advice on rehabilitation from physiotherapists, but the amount of hands-on input may be limited. Engaging fully with physiotherapy and rehabilitation advice can make a huge difference in outcome.

In summary, the importance of this section is to be aware of and spot if you have become deconditioned, and think how you can reduce the consequences of it. All the principles for physical activity that have already been covered in this chapter are relevant, but the mantra "own the problem, own the solution" is so important here. Exercise, increased physical activity, and rehabilitation with physiotherapy after injury, can reverse these effects, but you are the most important person to recognise the need, and take charge of reversing these changes. With positive action and realistic expectations, these changes can be reversed.

# CHAPTER 8: **TREATING MASLD 4: *DRUGS***

### *The 2-Minute Version*

- We are at a landmark point in the history of MASLD treatment with the approval, (in the USA) in 2024, of the first drug therapy for the disease (resmetirom (trade name Rezdiffra)).
- Resmetirom, a completely new agent, appears to offer promise, improving both fibrosis and steatosis/inflammation. It works by activating a thyroid hormone receptor that is only expressed in the liver. This switches up metabolism, increasing the burn rate for glucose and fat.
- Given the scale of the problem with MASLD, and the relatively limited response seen to resmetirom (some improvement in some patients), there is still significant unmet clinical need and a huge amount of research looking at new drugs.
- Most current trials use liver biopsy change as their key endpoint (the "test" that is used to assess whether the drug has worked). Two histology endpoints are used. These are: improvement in fibrosis by at least one stage with no worsening of steatosis (MASH), and MASH resolution with no worsening of fibrosis. Liver blood test improvement is useful for early assessment of drugs but is not likely to be sufficient for proving an effect. In due course, definitive outcome data will be needed (the ability of a drug to reduce risk of death or need for transplant). Given the slowly progressive nature of MASLD these trials will be challenging to do within a reasonable time frame.
- Semaglutide acts as a GLP-1 agonist, stimulating the release of insulin. It both reduces steatosis and inflammation, and cause significant weight loss. At least part of this effect is caused by actions on the brain to reduce appetite. It is, however, an injected medicine which can limit its attractiveness to patients. It also has significant side effects including nausea, vomiting and muscle loss. It is currently licensed for type 2 diabetes and obesity, but not for MASLD.
- A number of other drugs developed for the treatment of type 2 diabetes also seem to reduce MASLD severity. None of these effects are significant enough to warrant the use of them in patients who

don't have diabetes. Where patients also need treatment for type 2 diabetes it makes sense to choose anti-diabetic therapies that also improve MASLD.
- The challenges in conducting clinical trials in MASLD has meant that there has been a high failure rate for new therapies for the condition.

This chapter is, at the same time, both the easiest to write in the whole book and the most difficult. The explanation for this apparent contradiction is simple. It is easy because, at the time of writing, there is a single drug treatment licensed for the management of MASLD which is likely to be recommended in clinical guidelines. This drug is called resmetirom. It is difficult because the journey to reaching even this single approved drug has been long and very painful, with a significant number of drug and company casualties along the way. A number of these drugs have shown real evidence of benefit, but have failed to reach the standard of evidence needed for them to be approved for licensing. We suspect that this evidence challenge reflects both the limitations of the drugs trialled to date and, dare we say, flaws in the regulatory pathway.

In this chapter we will try and make sense of the very complicated picture regarding drug development and evaluation, and give some pointers as to where we think drug treatment may be going. It is quite detailed and a complex subject, so many readers may find that the 2-minute version has all the information they need, or may just wish to read the sections about any drugs that they may be taking.

**_DRUG LICENSING: TRIALS, LICENSES & LABELS:_** One thing that is important to understand, if we are going to explain the drug therapy landscape in MASLD, is the process by which drugs come to be deemed useable in clinical practice. It is important to note that all the hurdles that have to be crossed in this process **do not apply to operations, diets or exercise regimes**. Perhaps counter-intuitively these can all be used in practice without any evaluation, proof that they work or oversight by regulators. This is something that you should keep in mind when you read about fantastic new treatments in these categories on the internet.

In order to be prescribed to patients, a drug must be licensed by the relevant authorities for the country that you live in (there are different rules for over-the-counter medications available in pharmacies, and for "off the shelf" medicines available in supermarkets). Over time, treatments often move across the categories. An example is the proton-pump inhibitors which are the most effective drugs for suppressing acid production in the stomach. Once only available on prescription, now they are available over the counter, and even off the supermarket shelf.

The licensing process ensures that new treatments are both safe for use in people and are likely to be effective. Different parts of the world have different licensing bodies. In the USA it is the Food and Drug Administration (FDA), in Europe the European Medicines Agency (EMA), and in the UK the Medicines and Healthcare products Regulatory Agency (MHRA). All such bodies use the data from clinical trials to decide whether drugs should be licensed. In many ways, safety is the primary concern as the licensing process in its current form arose in response to drug injury scandals, such as that linked to thalidomide, where unsafe drugs were made available to vulnerable patients. Effectiveness is clearly important as well, as a safe but ineffective drug would indirectly harm you by not treating the disease. Drug licensing implies that a high bar has been cleared for both safety and effectiveness; something which should give patients confidence. A licence per se does not mean that a drug will be available to all patients, however. Depending on the health care system there will typically be a second stage of assessment of a drug by the body that will pay for it, if the patient isn't paying directly (the NHS through NICE in the UK and the insurance companies in the USA). In this second stage, the licensed drug will be assessed as to whether it is effective enough to justify the cost.

For a drug to be licenced it will need to have been shown to be effective and safe in clinical trials. The process of evaluating drug effectiveness and safety in clinical trials involves several stages or phases. In **Phase 1** trials the drug is given to healthy volunteers to assess blood levels for given doses (starting with very low doses), and to ensure that there is no toxicity (in cancer, Phase 1 trials are sometimes done in patients). **Phase 2** trials are where the drug moves to patients. These are small trials with a short duration, principally to show that the drug is safe in patients who might be very different in their age and physical status to healthy volunteers. We are also looking, in Phase 2, for evidence that the drug is effective for the disease, typically through improvement of an aspect of the condition, which is meaningful and measurable, and might reasonably be expected to change in the often-short time frame of Phase 2 trials. In MASLD the phase 2 endpoint is usually liver blood tests. If a drug is safe, and there is evidence to suggest that it is effective, then it moves to **Phase 3**. These are the larger and longer clinical trials with an endpoint, or trial question, that is highly relevant to patients (ideally survival or avoidance of a major and meaningful endpoint such as, in the case of liver disease, liver transplantation; this is, as we will discuss below, the challenging area in MASLD drug trials). A typical phase 3 trial might still only involve the patients getting the drug for a couple of years, so it is common to have what is called a long-term safety extension where the drug is, if participants in the trial want it, available for, typically, another 5 years, during which the longer-term effects are monitored.

In all good quality trials, the effect of the new drug needs to be compared directly with either a dummy or placebo (if there is no currently available treatment in the space) or with the current most effective treatment ("standard of care") if such a treatment is available. Trials include a high level of monitoring of participants. This is partly to ensure safety but also to ensure that all the possible evidence to support the drug being licensed is collected (it would be a disaster if a drug clearly works but the tests collected don't manage to show it because they are the wrong ones; it happens!). To license a drug, the FDA, MHRA or EMA will typically want to see that the drug is safe and that it is effective in a minimum of 2 Phase 3 trials.

Once a drug is licensed it will be provided with a "label". This is a description of the situations in which it is approved for use (the disease area, the types of that disease and, importantly, the situations when it shouldn't be used). This is all important in practice in MASLD where some of the drugs being evaluated are brand new (i.e. they are not licensed for use yet and thus don't have a label), whilst other drugs (in fact the majority in MASLD) are already licensed for a disease other than MASLD (in this setting the drug is licensed, but not labelled for use in MASLD).

If a drug is licensed and labelled for use in a disease, and the patient meets all the conditions for use (typically around kidney function being normal/acceptable, pregnancy, breast feeding etc) then a doctor can prescribe it with full legal protection (the issue of whether the health authorities or insurance companies in their country will pay for it and thus "allow" it to be prescribed is a slightly different question). At the other end of the spectrum, an unlicensed drug can only ever be used as part of a clinical trial that has gone through all the approvals to check for safety and which is being monitored closely (the route to the drug becoming licensed).

The grey area is where a drug is licensed for use in another disease area but not MASLD. Although the fact it has been licensed in patients gives a basic level of information about safety, the situation in a MASLD patient may be very different. What do we mean by this? A hypothetical example might be that a drug that has been licensed and labelled for use in a condition that only affects young, otherwise fit adults may have very different properties in elderly patients with diabetes and kidney disease. An extreme example might be the oral contraceptive pill which is licensed and labelled for use as a contraceptive in women. Technically we could, as doctors, prescribe it in men because all licensed drugs are prescribable. It wouldn't be a great idea though……. The concept of using drugs licensed for one disease in another is called "repurposing". It can be very powerful indeed (think about aspirin which started out as a pain killer but now saves literally millions of lives repurposed as a clot reducing drug in heart disease) but it shouldn't be done without the same level of clinical evaluation with regards to safety and effectiveness as a brand new drug.

## ***WHY ARE THERE SO FEW LICENSED DRUGS IN MASLD?***

We will, in the next few sections, outline the status of the drugs that have been evaluated, or proposed for use, in MASLD. As we explained at the beginning of the chapter, however, only one has, as yet, reached approval. Why so few? In simple terms there are three potential explanations. The first potential explanation is, obviously, that the other failed drugs don't work for the condition. The second is that they do work, but not to a sufficient degree to allow them to be used in MASLD. The third is that they do work but have too many in the way of side-effects to allow their use. Although there are examples of all three of these situations in MASLD, overwhelmingly it is the second situation that is at play. There are lots of drugs that are typically safe, and which improve some aspect of MASLD, but which fail to "get over the bar" that is set by the licensing authorities. Ultimately this all comes down to trial endpoints: the aspects of disease that we actually measure in the clinical trial.

All trial endpoints represent a trade-off between certainty and missed opportunity. Let's take an easy example. Death. If a trial shows that a drug reduces the chances of someone dying, then that is as strong a form of evidence as you will get and absolutely supports licensing (provided the drug is safe of course). Should we therefore only license drugs with this level of certainty? Absolutely not is the answer. This is because of the limitation of trial designs. Most chronic diseases, such as MASLD, cause harm over a long period of time. Furthermore, and this is really the case for MASLD, the time when you are most likely to be able to intervene is early in the disease, before the damage is done. In practice this means before significant fibrosis has developed, and certainly before progression to cirrhosis. If you had a treatment that really reduced the chances of dying several years in the future, to show benefit you would either need to do the trial over many years to ensure enough events happened (in the field of trials we use the concept of event rate: the number of the "events" (in this case death) that you would expect to happen per year if you did nothing) or, if the trial cannot be done over many years, do a trial with a very large number of people in it. Fundamentally, this is about another important concept which is "person years", the number of people in a study multiplied by the number of years they have been followed up. To get a reasonable event rate you need a lot of patient years, which means either lots of people or lots of years (or both). Very large trials massively increase the complexity and cost (and can act to prevent other treatments "getting a look in" even if they might be even better), so we would probably be looking at long trials. The problem with this is a question that you can ask yourself. How many years would you be prepared to be in a trial and getting the placebo or "dummy drug" when there are other treatments potentially out there.......

So, we need to get the event rate up using a different approach. How could we do that? One way is to broaden out the definition of a significant event. A first and obvious one is liver transplantation given that, as we will discuss in **Chapter 10**, to an approximation people only have a transplant in MASLD because otherwise they would have died. The problem with this is that factors over and above "need" for transplant come into play. Say you have the active drug in a trial, progress to the point where you "need" a transplant but have bad heart disease that stops you having that transplant.

In a short trial, where someone has not had a transplant because they are too high risk but haven't yet died of the disease (sorry to be morbid) has the drug "worked" or not? They are alive and not transplanted (i.e., it would count as the drug working), but they needed a transplant and only didn't get it because of issues unrelated to the action of the drug (it didn't work). What about people who are listed for transplant but haven't yet had it because they have an odd blood group (again nothing to do with the drug). Has it worked or not?

We could also include what are called "clinically meaningful endpoints"; things that really matter to patients. Immediately in liver disease everyone thinks of variceal bleeding, resistant ascites, and chronic encephalopathy. A treatment that meaningfully reduced the risk of these would undoubtedly be useful. However, what about varices that haven't bled, small varices (that may not even be varices because the endoscopist is inexperienced). What about ascites that is only resistant because people don't take their water tablets. We are not trying to bamboozle people here. We are making a really important point that even what feel like obvious endpoints in trials can be complex. We see trial protocols all the time that talk about these endpoints without ever seemingly appreciating the complexity. This may be why trials have been negative in many cases.......

Most trials in most disease areas, and basically all of those in MASLD, use a different approach which is that of utilising "surrogate markers". These are things that can be measured which do not themselves present a risk to people, but which predict the presence of risk now or in the future. Think about a raised temperature in someone with an infection. It is clearly linked to having an infection, and if the temperature is returned to normal with antibiotics it suggests that the infection could be being controlled (a good thing). The temperature is not, however, itself harmful and therefore control of the temperature is not inherently advantageous. The temperature is a surrogate marker for infection. The temperature analogy can be taken a step further, however, to explain the potential risks of using surrogate markers. What if you have an infection but took paracetamol (acetaminophen). That would reduce the temperature (it is why you took it) but would not have any impact on the infection and its risks to your health. The connection between temperature as a marker and infection as the key part of the disease process has been lost.

All this really matters in liver disease because almost all trials are done using surrogate markers (although we don't tend to think of them as being surrogates). The most obvious are liver function tests. Tests such as ALT, bilirubin and albumin are clearly associated with liver disease activity/severity. The higher the ALT and bilirubin and the lower the albumin, the more active or severe the disease. We can therefore use these blood values as markers in trials, with improvement suggesting a response to treatment, can't we? Well, yes and no. If you put someone with jaundice caused by raised bilirubin on dialysis the bilirubin would fall (it is pulled out of the circulation with dialysis) but this wouldn't improve the liver disease. Likewise, we frequently give liver disease patients drips containing albumin (often when draining ascites). This will result in the albumin value going up but, again, has no implications for outcome. These traps are, of course, obvious. The potential, however, for more subtle issues with marker improvement that is unrelated to actual liver disease severity change is always there.

So why, at the end of the day, are there so few licensed drug therapies for MASLD? In essence it is because although many drugs improve liver function tests (as we will discuss below) there is no evidence that they improve survival and little evidence that they reduce complications. There is some evidence of impact on liver biopsy changes, as we will discuss, however there is much debate about the extent, relevance, and significance of those changes. On this basis they haven't "got over the bar" to be licensed (yet).

When we discuss all this with patients, people often make the very reasonable point that, if the alternative is taking no treatment, why can't I at least take a treatment that makes my blood tests better. There are several important reasons why not. The first is that all drugs have side-effects to some degree. You would, therefore, be being exposed to the risk without clear evidence of benefit. Given that all drug approval and use has to be on the basis of an acceptable trade-off between risk and benefit this skews the balance. The second reason is opportunity cost. If a drug with weak evidence of benefit is approved and widely used it will disincentivise the development of newer and better drugs that might, in the future, have a substantial beneficial effect on MASLD. The history of medicine is full of examples where the first drug developed for a disease was rapidly and completely replaced by better drugs. The third and final reason is actual cost (and its close relative, cost-effectiveness). The step beyond licensing of a drug is approval for use in the health care system. In essence, this is the decision by whoever pays for your drugs (the NHS in the UK and insurance companies elsewhere in the world) as to whether they will pay for the drug. In making these decisions the benefits of the drug in terms of improved survival and quality of life are weighed against its cost. A critical part of the benefit calculation is the reduced health care costs that might result from effective treatment (in simple terms a drug costs £x, but we will save £y in reduced health care costs as people won't go on to develop the costly complications of cirrhosis or need the even more costly procedure of liver transplantation). If we end up using a drug and incurring the costs of it, but don't go on to save anything though reduced complication rates, this equation goes out of the window.

There are then two final issues to factor in. The first is the scale of the problem with MASLD. If the condition affected a few hundred or thousand people, then the risk of allowing the use of a drug that ultimately had limited benefit in terms of incurred cost would be relatively acceptable. If we were to use a drug, potentially at high cost, in millions of people who still went on to develop complications, it could bankrupt health care systems. The final issue is perhaps the most controversial. Many politicians (and healthcare provision is, at the end of the day, a political issue) see MASLD, rightly or wrongly, as a lifestyle disease; a condition that arises because of peoples' actions and one which, crucially in their minds, can be controlled through a change in actions (diet and exercise). Is it appropriate (the politicians ask) to give people "permission" to continue their unhealthy lives by giving them a tablet that compensates for damage? There is a story (possibly true, possibly apocryphal) that one of the drug companies developed a drug that could reverse the effects of alcohol so that you could go out and drink heavily and then instantly "sober" up by taking a tablet. Its development as a useable treatment was deemed politically unacceptable and it never made it to market.

What this all means for drug treatment in MASLD is that we need better drugs, assessed in better ways and which are used more creatively. We will discuss this in more detail **Chapter 14** where we look into the future of MASLD care.

### *DRUGS USED IN MASLD (Licensed, unlicensed and experimental)*

The majority of drugs evaluated to date in MASLD, and showing some evidence of effect, fall into two loose categories, metabolic/diabetic drugs, and antioxidants. There has, as yet, been little work on combining the two drug types, although there might be real logic in doing so. The sole licensed drug, resmetirom, falls into the metabolic category.

**Metabolic/diabetic drugs:** Given the almost complete overlap between type 2 diabetes, the metabolic syndrome and MASLD it is perhaps not surprising that drugs that are effective in managing metabolic change have been developed and explored in MASLD, and show some evidence of benefit. One question, however, is the degree to which there is a true benefit on MASLD per se and not just an effect on liver involvement in diabetes (an important, if subtle, distinction). There are also drugs under evaluation that, although not anti-diabetic per-se, also probably exert their effects through modulation of metabolism. Paradoxically, given the investment in anti-diabetic drugs as an approach to MASLD, it is one of the metabolism modifying but non-anti-diabetic drugs that is the first to be licensed.

*Resmetirom* works in a way that is completely different to the other drugs that have been evaluated in MASLD to date, and this may explain why it has been successful (it doesn't run into the same traps that the other drug types do). It works by activating a receptor for thyroid hormone that is specifically expressed in hepatocytes. Activation of this receptor mimics the signal that thyroid hormone normally gives to cells to increase their metabolic activity and "burn more fuel". People with overactive thyroid glands because of disease increase their metabolic rate and actively burn fat. The increased thyroid hormone level, however, has lots of other effects on the body, giving rise to lots of clinical problems. Because resmetirom only works on the receptor in the liver, people taking it get the increased "fat burn" in the liver but none of the other effects elsewhere in the body (in theory at least). The key phase 3 trial of resmetirom showed 26% of patients had a reduction in fibrosis by 1 grade and 26% had MASH resolution. Both differences were statistically significant, although this shows that it only gives improvement in around a quarter of patients, and around ten percent of the patients in the placebo group also showed improvement. It cannot, therefore, be considered as the 'cure' for MASLD as yet. There are, so far, no data relating to survival. The evidence of improvement of liver biopsy features, in the context of a very good safety profile, led to it being approved by the FDA in early 2024. At the time of writing (late 2024) it is not yet licensed in Europe or the UK, although some people may be receiving it as participants in a trial. It is also not a cheap drug, and it may be that there will be limitations on prescribing approval if it is licensed in the UK.

In the first edition of this book we identified two drugs as being the front-runners for licensing in MASLD. One of these was resmetirom which has, as we have outlined, "made it" to licensing (in the USA so far). The second was **obeticholic acid**. In contrast to resmetirom, obeticholic acid failed to be licensed and is now no longer being developed as a therapy in MASLD. This black and white outcome highlights absolutely the challenge of drug development in this condition. Apparent complete success versus apparent complete failure. When you look closer, however, this contrasting black and white just morphs into slight variations in grey. The differences in effect between these drugs are relatively small, but if they fall on different sides of an outcome line this makes an absolute difference to regulators. A 10% difference in effectiveness in a trial can lead to a 100% difference in licensing. People like to think in terms of drugs "working" and "not working". In reality, almost all the drugs explored in MASLD, including obeticholic acid and resmetirom, "work". The question is do they work "enough" to gain approval to outweigh any side effects.

The story of the lost front-runner obeticholic acid is informative. It was evaluated, as was resmetirom, in trials using an approach that is emerging as the consensus approach (albeit one that is not without its issues). This approach involves enrolling patients with active MASH (i.e. MASLD with the features and sequelae of inflammation) and fibrosis in the moderate to advanced range (F2/F3 to use the technical terminology). The trials used the same dual primary endpoint of MASH resolution (complete reversal of MASLD or resolution of inflammation returning MASH to simple steatosis) and/or improvement of fibrosis by 1 stage (i.e. F3 to F2 or F2 to F1) with no worsening of MASH. In terms of our understanding of the disease process, these dual endpoints reflect the potential value of either an improvement in fat deposition and inflammation (remember they are linked) or a reduction in fibrosis (or, of course and in an ideal world, both).

Obeticholic acid (trade name Ocaliva and frequently referred to by the abbreviation OCA) was one of the most intensively studied therapies in MASLD. It has a number of potentially key actions relevant to MASLD. These include reducing both inflammation and fibrosis and several metabolic actions. It also significantly reduces cholestasis by suppressing bile acid production and, on that basis, has been licensed for use as a second line therapy in primary biliary cholangitis (PBC). This has given us a great deal of experience of its use in practice and it is clear from this setting that it is a very safe drug. In MASLD it has a clear effect on improving liver function tests and there was some evidence from earlier trials to suggest it improved liver fibrosis. On this basis it went forward into larger scale trial evaluation. The key phase 3 trial suggested that it did indeed reduce fibrosis by at least one stage (without worsening MASH) in a proportion of patients (22.4%). However, there was a much lower level of MASH resolution (6.5%). It is also important to note that some improvement was seen in the placebo group as well. The improvement in fibrosis was significant, but not the rate of MASH resolution, and it wasn't felt to be effective enough to be licensed.

It is difficult to directly compare trials because of differences in the approach, trial design and the location where they were carried out (people differ!). With this caveat, comparing the outcome data for resmetirom and OCA is interesting. In both trials, improvement was seen in people not actually taking the active drug (the placebo groups). This may represent subtle lifestyle changes that people made because they were taking part in a trial, or a sampling issue (you inevitably don't sample the same part of the liver in the two samples taken before and after a treatment and there may be subtle differences in the disease process in the two sites sampled). In neither trial is there any data on actual survival or complication development (i.e., the outcomes that really matter to patients). Whereas both drugs showed benefit in terms of fibrosis over and above that seen in placebo, only resmetirom showed improvement in MASH. This difference, perhaps logically, follows the difference in metabolic activity of the two drugs with resmetirom having the more overt anti-metabolic action.

What about other candidate drugs? The other drug class which has a relatively strong evidence base is the GLP-1 agonist group of diabetes medicines. The best known is *semaglutide*, which is given as a weekly injection. These drugs, which have entered the popular zeitgeist since the first edition of this book was published as weight loss drugs (Wegovy, Ozempic) mimic the action of a natural peptide called glucagon-like peptide (GLP-1) which appears to have two important actions that are relevant to MASLD. The first is that it stimulates the islet cells of the pancreas to produce increased levels of insulin. The second is that it seems to act on the brain to give a sense of "satiation" (i.e., people feel full and therefore don't feel like eating). Experience of the drugs in the clinic is that they both reduce insulin resistance and help with weight loss through reduced dietary intake. Both are very attractive effects in MASLD management. In terms of specific clinical trial outcomes in MASLD, in the trials to date they significantly improved liver function tests and promoted resolution of MASH on liver biopsy. Preliminary data from ongoing trials suggests there may also be a benefit to fibrosis. There are words of caution, however. These drugs can cause injection site discomfort, and nausea is a common issue because of delayed gastric emptying. More significantly they can, rarely, be associated with serious complications including pancreatitis. Finally, there is some evidence that although they can give rise to significant weight loss (at face value a good thing), this is more marked for muscle than it is for fat tissue. Given our desire to build muscle for metabolic reasons in MASLD and, as we have previously discussed, increase exercise capacity, this may be somewhat counter-productive.

Another category of drug that may have value in MASLD is the ***sodium-glucose co-transporter inhibitors (SGLT2i)***. These are a relatively new class of anti-diabetic treatments which reduce blood sugar by increasing sugar loss into the urine. Given their mode of action, any benefit in MASLD would be expected to be indirect, through reduction of blood glucose driven steatosis development. Clinical observation in MASLD would fit with this, with some impact on liver steatosis and inflammation but, to date at least, no evidence of reduction in fibrosis.

Before the emergence of the drugs described in the previous paragraphs, the focus in MASLD was on the potential benefits of more conventional type 2 diabetes drugs. These include the ***glitazones*** and ***metformin***. The glitazones (for example rosiglitazone and pioglitazone) are members of the PPAR agonist family of drugs and are thought to reverse insulin resistance in fatty tissue. Given the importance of insulin resistance in the biology of MASLD this gives an obvious potentially valuable mode of action. As with many of the other drugs explored in MASLD, they improve liver function tests. They also improve liver biopsy features of hepatic steatosis and inflammation (although not fibrosis). As with all other drugs trialled to date there is no evidence in relation to directly relevant clinical endpoints such as death or transplant. There have also been concerns about their safety in MASLD. There are concerns regarding worsening of pre-existing heart failure, and possibly weight gain. They are not licensed for MASLD. Other PPAR agonists have been explored in MASLD with very limited evidence of efficacy. The exception (possibly) is *lanifibranor*, a trial drug (i.e. not yet licensed for any other treatment) which has MASH resolving activity. It is currently (in 2024) undergoing further evaluation. One aspect that does appear to be favourable is improvement in overall cardiac health in MASH patients receiving it. Given the importance of cardiac risk in MASLD patients, this is potentially important.

Metformin is a drug that is widely used in the treatment of type 2 diabetes. It has several actions around appetite reduction but appears to mainly function through restoration (to a degree) of insulin sensitivity. Unlike other oral anti-diabetic therapies, it does not cause weight gain (indeed it can result in weight loss). Given its mode of action there has been a great deal of interest in it as a potential therapy in MASLD. The data from the numerous, frequently small, clinical trials suggest that, although liver function test improvement is seen (especially alanine transaminase and aspartate transaminase), and weight loss is consistently seen, there is no apparent improvement in liver biopsy changes. Metformin can also have significant, albeit rare, side-effects such as lactic acidosis. It is not licensed for use in MASLD and therefore shouldn't be used purely for this indication.

One further experimental drug with proposed metabolic effects, this time on fatty acid synthesis, is *icomidocholic acid* (Aramchol), a bile acid (cholic acid) based agent. It is a partial inhibitor of an enzyme called stearoyl-CoA desaturase, an important enzyme in the pathway of synthesis of unsaturated fatty acids. Its application in MASLD is therefore intuitive. In its phase 2 trial it showed significant reduction in liver fat levels when assessed using Magnetic Resonance Imaging. In terms of the conventional MASH trial endpoints it showed significantly greater MASH resolution without fibrosis worsening and fibrosis improvement without MASH worsening, as well as significant improvement in LFTs.

**Anti-inflammatory drugs:** For a condition in which inflammation is a key feature, treatments that reduce inflammation, and the damage caused by inflammation, would seem to be logical options. In this setting two different drugs with antioxidant properties have been evaluated. These are *vitamin E* and *ursodeoxycholic acid (UDCA)*. Vitamin E is, as its name suggests, a vitamin. It has been formally evaluated in MASLD, in one of the earliest of the key trials, and shown to have benefit in terms of MASH severity as well as improving liver blood biochemistry. More extensive study has suggested significant side-effects when it is used at high dose. These include cardiac problems, bleeding, and an increased risk of prostate cancer. On this basis it is not currently recommended for routine use in MASLD.

UDCA is widely used in cholestatic liver disease and improves liver biochemistry and (probably) survival in PBC. Its use is less intuitive in MASLD given that it is not overtly cholestatic (involving the flow of bile out of the liver) in most patients. It does, however, improve liver biochemistry in MASLD and is very safe. There is no evidence, however, to suggest that it improves liver histology or survival.

**Anti-fibrotic drugs:** As outlined in the previous sections, assessment of anti-fibrotic activity has been included in the evaluation of all drugs in MASLD as part of their complex actions. There is a single agent (to date) that has been explored as a specifically anti-fibrotic drug, independent of any actions on steatohepatitis. This is ***Belapectin***. Belapectin inhibits galectin 3, which plays a key role in driving fibrosis. Animal studies suggested a significant anti-fibrotic effect in MASH models, with human trials ongoing, and no license as yet for treatment of any condition.

## *SHOULD I TAKE RESMETIROM?*
At the end of this long discussion of potential drug therapies we return to the single licensed agent, resmetirom. At the time of writing, this is still only licensed in the USA, but hopefully will become available elsewhere in the world soon. The obvious question to a MASLD patient (assuming they are able to access the drug) is, should I take it? As with any drug there are pros and cons. It certainly appears to "work", at least in terms of the biopsy and blood changes that we know are important predictors of poor outcome in MASLD; it will be a long time before we find out whether it lengthens life or reduces the likelihood of needing a liver transplant. It also certainly seems to be safe (with the caveat that it has only been used for a relatively small period in relation to what is a life-long disease). However, it is important to be realistic that this isn't a miracle drug or any form of cure. It improves important features of MASLD to a significant degree in about 1 in 4 patients. It is also expensive (around $50,000 dollars a year in the USA; something that will impact on how widely available it is in practice) and is only licensed for a relatively narrow sub-group of MASLD patients. It therefore is best thought of as a good start rather than the whole answer. The search for other approaches to treatment needs to go on.

## *CONCLUSIONS*
Where does all this leave us, if anywhere, in terms of MASLD treatment. We think it is possible to draw the following conclusions.

1) There are a number of drugs which have a beneficial effect in MASLD, with one drug (resmetirom) showing enough benefit to warrant its being licensed for use in MASLD. None, however, are absolute "game-changers"

in the sense of having a significant effect on meaningful endpoints in most patients. There is, accordingly, real unmet need in the condition and we need to explore future options.

2) There are a relatively large number of drugs that improve liver blood tests, a smaller number that improve liver biopsy features of steatosis and inflammation (MASH), an even smaller number that reverse fibrosis, and none that have been shown to improve survival or reduce the need for transplant. Given the options, we must target MASH and fibrosis (typically separately) and we therefore need to clarify our thinking as to which drugs we look at using in which patients at which stage of the disease. Intuitively we should be targeting MASH early in the disease and fibrosis later.

3) Given the different modes of action of drugs it is likely that combination of different agents will be an interesting option to explore in the future. Again, we need to think this through rather than expecting all drugs to work in all situations.

4) It is important to distinguish between the options in MASLD patients with and without type 2 diabetes mellitus. Clearly, patients without type 2 diabetes can't get the benefit of a drug-driven improvement in their diabetes. Any drug used in patients without type 2 diabetes therefore needs to justify its use in terms of benefit balanced against risk purely for MASLD. On this basis no drugs currently get over the line. In patients with type 2 diabetes, where type 2 diabetes drug treatment is required, it clearly makes sense to choose the drug in the context of potential additional MASLD benefits. Try and "kill two birds with one stone".

# CHAPTER 9: **TREATING MASLD 5:** *CIRRHOSIS MANAGEMENT*

### *The 2-Minute Version*

- Cirrhosis is the end-stage of all forms of chronic liver disease and avoidance of progression of disease to the cirrhotic stage is at the heart of all approaches to management in MASLD as in diseases of other aetiology.
- Limitations in our currently available therapies for MASLD, and late presentation and diagnosis limiting the time window to use therapy, mean that cirrhosis remains an important practical problem in MASLD management.
- The focus in cirrhosis management is to mitigate the risks posed by the complications that arise and which can be life threatening. The most important of these are portal hypertension with its risk of variceal bleeding, hepatic encephalopathy, ascites and hepatocellular carcinoma.
- Additional risk comes from progressive failure of liver function as cirrhosis damages the liver and impairs its ability to perform the essential functions needed for life.
- Even if the disease has progressed to cirrhosis, it remains important to make every effort to reduce further damage to the remaining liver cells. Cirrhosis is very unlikely indeed to reverse, but people can live for many years without any problems provided the remaining liver cells are healthy.
- Cirrhosis development can be associated with a significant additional reduction in quality of life. This is partly through the symptom burden of the specific complications, and partly because of the degree of liver cell dysfunction. This is another important reason to try and avoid cirrhosis from developing, for effectively treating complications, and for trying to maintain remaining hepatocyte function if progress to cirrhosis has occurred.
- Liver transplantation is an effective treatment for cirrhotic MASLD, as it is for many forms of end-stage liver disease. The need for it is normally in patients with the MASH form of the disease where risk of progression to cirrhosis is the greatest.

- Progression to cirrhosis without any complications is not, in and of itself, an indication for liver transplantation. There must be a specific reason (a problem that will be solved by the transplant) to ensure that the risk/benefit ratio is favourable. Examples of a reason to consider transplant include intractable ascites, chronic encephalopathy, and the development of hepatocellular carcinoma.

The principal goal of therapy in MASLD is prevention of the type and scale of chronic injury that gives rise to the development of cirrhosis. In practice, cirrhosis is the end-stage of a pathway of progressive injury with increasing levels of fibrosis or scar formation within the liver. If fibrosis or cirrhosis develop this does not mean that any less attention should be paid to control of the disease process. The reasons for this are two-fold. Firstly, maintaining the health, and thus function, of the remaining hepatocytes is critically important in the damaged liver. Secondly, there is emerging evidence to suggest that, in some instances of chronic liver injury, fibrosis, and even early cirrhosis, can reverse over time. The possibility of this (and it is just a possibility) is critically dependent on complete control of underlying disease activity, as progression rather than reversal of fibrosis will occur if the disease is not controlled. This is likely to remain a real challenge in MASLD for the foreseeable future because of the limitations of the available therapies. If we are honest, we are a little sceptical as to the extent to which this fibrosis regression really happens in practice (especially, in MASLD) but it does further emphasise the potential benefits of striving for complete disease control.

Many patients with cirrhosis have no problems at all and often don't even know they have it. It is always said that there are more people in the UK with cirrhosis who don't know they have it than do know. Of course, just because a person has cirrhosis without any current problems doesn't mean that problems won't arise in the future……. Where problems do arise in cirrhosis they fall into three groups - cirrhotic complications, hepatocellular failure, and symptoms impacting on quality of life. We will discuss these in turn.

## ***CIRRHOTIC COMPLICATIONS***

It is not cirrhosis, per se, that puts any chronic liver disease patient at risk, but the consequences of cirrhosis in all their forms. If the consequences and complications of cirrhosis are avoided or managed, and the level of ongoing liver injury controlled to the greatest extent possible, then people can live an entirely normal life. The message with cirrhosis is, therefore, **don't panic**, but work as hard as you can on getting as good control of your disease as you can (through diet, exercise and any medication options) and work with your clinical team to minimise risks. Patients with definite or likely cirrhosis (and the approach to determining this is outlined in **Chapter 4**) should be screened for the following complications on a regular basis. If it is not possible to be certain as to whether someone has cirrhosis (and the clinical and test findings can be more subtle than people sometimes imagine) then it is correct to err on the side of caution and screen for and manage complications.

**Porto-systemic varices:** Rather as cirrhosis, in general, is feared by patients, this is the complication that worries patients the most. This is because of the risk of bleeding. The reality is that significant variceal bleeding in patients with managed MASLD is a relatively rare occurrence these days. Why the low impact of variceal bleeding? The answer is the same one that will be repeated throughout this chapter, a combination of improving management of the underlying disease and good management of the complication risk is effective in practice.

There are two aspects to varices management; bleeding prevention and managing a bleed if it happens. Prevention is, unsurprisingly, preferable to managing an actual bleed. Screening for varices is done through endoscopy (fibreoptic camera tube down the oesophagus) which is a quick and well-tolerated procedure to visualise the common sites for varices. This should be done in all patients with proven or suspected cirrhosis on an annual basis. If significant varices are found, then the standard approach is to start treatment with a beta blocker (especially propranolol or carvedilol), tablet medicines normally used to manage conventional hypertension, but which also reduce portal venous pressure in portal hypertension. Very rarely, if the varices are big, thought to be at high risk of bleeding, or if the patient can't tolerate beta-blocker, we may use some of the invasive management approaches, such as banding, which are normally reserved for managing a bleed, in a preventative way.

A patient with proven or possible cirrhotic MASLD who vomits blood or passes black tar-like stools containing blood which has been digested as it passes down through the bowel (melaena) should be treated as if they have had a variceal bleed until proven otherwise (the precautionary principle). A variceal bleed is a medical emergency. In a newly presenting patient with liver disease, in whom assessment for the presence of cirrhosis hasn't taken place yet, bleeding should, again, be assumed to be variceal until proved otherwise. If there is a possibility of variceal bleeding, then it is essential to get urgent medical attention. This is one of the times when it is correct to call for an emergency ambulance. Variceal bleeding can sometimes occur without any overt signs of blood loss (vomiting blood or passing blood in the stools). In these situations, the bleeding is typically in the upper bowel and the blood is in the process of passing down the bowel but hasn't yet emerged in the stool. In a bleed of this type, the signs of bleeding can be more subtle and include light-headedness from a falling blood pressure, palpitations, or a fast heart rate.

When a variceal bleed is suspected, the critical first step to treatment is, irrespective of the type of bleeding seen, to put a cannula into a vein to allow the patient to be given fluid to replace the blood loss. This needs to happen quickly and can only be done in the hospital setting or by a paramedic. If bleeding continues it can become more difficult to insert a cannula because the veins collapse. Early attention is therefore key. Initially, the fluid will be clear fluid (saline or an equivalent). In hospital, once blood has been cross-matched, it may be blood and plasma. Once fluid is being given it is usual to give an intravenous drug called terlipressin. This causes the bleeding vessels to clamp down on themselves, applying pressure to stop the bleeding. This allows the situation to stabilise.

The mainstay of initial treatment is through an endoscopy, this time done to treat rather than look for varices. The current state of the art is to apply small rubber bands onto the bleeding vessel, which pinch it off (an approach called "banding"). This is highly effective. Once varices have been banded the bleeding should stop and things can be allowed to settle down. It is then normal to repeat the endoscopy and banding every couple of weeks until the varices have been completely obliterated.

Rarely, banding and terlipressin don't control the bleeding. In this case, most liver units would use a procedure called TIPSS (trans-jugular intra-hepatic porto-systemic shunting). In this procedure a cannula is put into the jugular vein in the neck and navigated down into the liver where it is used to make a connection between the hepatic vein (the vein running out of the liver taking blood back to the heart) and the portal vein. This connection is then widened, and a plastic tube or stent is inserted to keep it open. The effect of this connection is to relieve the pressure in the portal vein, taking away the driving force for the bleeding. This is a more invasive and risky procedure than endoscopy, so tends to be reserved for situations where the bleeding can't be controlled in any other way. It is, however, literally lifesaving in those situations. TIPSS can cause longer term complications. These include worsening of hepatic encephalopathy (because portal vein blood flow from the bowel is shunted through the liver without the liver having the chance to "clean" it), heart failure (after the TIPSS the amount of blood returning to the heart in the veins is significantly increased because the cirrhotic liver is no longer functioning as a "road-block" to blood flow) and liver failure (the liver normally gets a lot of its oxygen from the portal vein blood and this supply is lost after TIPSS). All these complications are much commoner in older patients and TIPSS should be avoided if at all possible, beyond the age of 65. The complications can, however, arise in younger patients and cannot be easily predicted in advance (and once the TIPSS is in it is in; it can be blocked but that procedure has its own downsides and risks). For all these reasons, the use of TIPSS is better off being avoided unless there is really no alternative.

If bleeding recurs despite the use of these treatments, then, once the patient is stable, the possibility of transplantation should be considered. Transplant would never be considered acutely in the context of an active bleed, however, as it is simply too dangerous.

It is difficult to overstate just how transformative the development of these approaches has been for the safe and effective management of liver disease patients. When DJ started as a liver doctor in the late 1980s it was far from uncommon for people to come into hospital with their 5th (or more) variceal bleed. The bleeding episodes were themselves very unpleasant, and fear of bleeding had an almost paralysing effect on people, preventing normal life. This just doesn't happen anymore. Variceal bleeding as a complication should always be respected (and certainly varices sought in advance of a bleed and managed effectively) but perhaps we have moved to a time when it shouldn't be quite so feared.

**Ascites:** Ascites is, in part at least (low protein levels and hormone changes also play a part), another manifestation of portal hypertension and is, again, a feature of cirrhosis in MASLD. It can cause discomfort, or if very large in volume, problems with breathing because the fluid presses against the diaphragm and stops it moving. The mainstay of initial treatment is with diuretics ("water tablets"). Typically, this is with either spironolactone alone (a useful drug as it has a specific action on the fluid accumulation mechanism in ascites) or spironolactone in combination with furosemide. If the volume of the ascites is very large, and if it is causing problems with breathing, then it is sometimes necessary to drain it through the abdominal wall using a temporary tube. This makes patients more comfortable very quickly but increases the risk of infection getting into the ascites (peritonitis). Over time, patients can become either resistant to the actions of diuretics or, perhaps more commonly, experience kidney complications which mean that the diuretics need to be stopped (essentially diuretics work by working the kidneys hard, and this can have long-term downsides). Many patients with ascites are familiar with the yo-yoing effect of diuretics being started because of ascites then stopped because of kidney problems meaning that the ascites reaccumulates, leading to the diuretics being started again and the whole cycle recurring. In these settings, often the only approach that can control the ascites is repeat draining. Not only does this repeat the risk seen with each drain insertion, but it can lead to a process where the ascites ends up in walled off bubbles of fluid which makes even drainage difficult. In this situation TIPSS can again be effective. The same cautions apply to TIPSS in the setting of ascites control as for bleeding control, and need to be applied even more rigorously as TIPSS for ascites control is rarely a life-saving procedure (unlike TIPSS for bleeding) and patients potentially needing TIPSS for ascites control are frequently older and thus more at risk of complications. This state of resistant ascites is one of the indications for consideration of liver transplantation in MASLD.

Sometimes, bacteria can get from the bowel into the ascites and cause a low-grade infection; a process known as spontaneous bacterial peritonitis (SBP). If SBP is thought to have arisen, a small sample of ascites is taken through the abdominal wall (a small syringe-full with a small needle) for examination in the laboratory. If SBP is found, then the treatment is with antibiotics. SBP development does, however, indicate a higher risk liver disease state and is one of the events that would, again, make us think actively about transplantation. TIPSS should absolutely be avoided in the setting of SBP because of the risk of infection becoming lodged in the TIPSS cannula (a disaster as the infection can't easily be cleared and the TIPSS cannula can't be removed).

**Hepatocellular carcinoma (HCC, "primary liver cancer"):** HCC can complicate cirrhosis of all aetiologies and is commoner in men than in women because of the effects of testosterone. MASLD is one of the types of chronic liver disease where it is commoner as a complication, and it should very much feature in long-term management thinking. Given that the risk is with cirrhosis specifically it is yet another reason why we should do everything we possibly can to stop people with MASLD from developing cirrhosis in the first place. As with liver disease of all aetiologies, disease chronicity (duration of the disease) and level of activity are key risk factors.

The art with HCC is early diagnosis through screening. If identified when small, as a result of the recommended 6 monthly screening with ultrasound and a blood test called alpha-fetoprotein which often, but not always, rises when an HCC is developing, followed by further imaging with CT or MRI if a suspicious lesion is seen, there are several treatment approaches. If it presents late when large, or when the liver function has started to deteriorate, it can rapidly become untreatable. Approaches used for small cancers include:

- TACE (trans-arterial chemoembolization). This is a procedure in which the artery supplying the cancer is identified and chemotherapy is injected into it, followed by a plug to block off the artery to lock the chemotherapy in and take away the tumour blood supply.
- RFA (radiofrequency ablation). In this procedure a microwave probe is inserted through skin into the tumour and the tumour is killed in situ by a pulse of radio-waves.
- Transplant. An effective approach in small cancers and should be considered because once one cancer has developed the rest of the liver is at risk.
- Surgical resection. Actually, rarely possible because of the presence of cirrhosis.

Chemotherapy options are relatively limited and the effectiveness low. Drugs like sorafenib are mainly used where the physical approaches outlined above cannot be used because the cancer is too large. It is likely that all this will change as the new generations of cancer drugs start to be applied to HCC.

Initially used in conditions such as malignant melanoma (where they have been startlingly effective) these drugs bypass the normal switching mechanisms of the immune system that prevent what would be a useful immune response directed against the cancer cells. In simple terms, they harness the body's own systems to effectively fight the cancer. Given that one of the reasons why the body struggles to control liver cancer in cirrhosis is that immune responses in the liver are often functionally switched off, these drugs may in fact be uniquely effective in the setting of liver cancer. Time will tell!

**Hepatic encephalopathy:** Encephalopathy (a state of toxic brain dysfunction) is an important complication in cirrhotic MASLD and suggests the presence of a significant component of hepatocellular failure (in comparison to, say, varices development which can simply reflect the structural changes seen in cirrhosis and can occur in people with good hepatocellular function). As with all complications of cirrhosis, we both treat encephalopathy to reduce its impact on patients and register its development as a sign of how severe the disease is and the need to, if possible, tighten up on treatment. If hepatic encephalopathy occurs as part of an acute liver failure deterioration, then it will typically improve as the event is treated. In our experience, the complication to be certain you look for is variceal bleeding, as most sudden onset encephalopathy occurs as the result of a bleed. If it becomes chronic then we treat encephalopathy with lactulose or rifaximin, both drugs that reduce the bacterial and protein load in the bowel. Most people with encephalopathy have episodes of confusion which then improve. This can have a real impact on quality of life if the episodes are very frequent, severe, or long-lasting. It can, however, be a manageable problem. In a small number of people, it becomes a chronic, unremitting problem where they never return to normal, and where treatments become progressively less effective over time. This can be very distressing both for patients and for their relatives (not least because one of the manifestations of hepatic encephalopathy is personality change). In this situation, transplantation is absolutely an option that should be considered. It is a very effective treatment indeed for encephalopathy and, given the sheer burden of chronic encephalopathy in the first place, is one of the transplant indications that is associated with the greatest patient benefit.

## *HEPATOCELLULAR FAILURE*

Over time, function of a cirrhotic liver can begin to deteriorate. At the end of this process, if left unchecked, patients can enter liver failure (because there is insufficient remaining functioning liver for their needs). There can be acute deteriorations in liver function with other complications such as variceal bleeding or SBP, as well as with intercurrent illnesses unrelated to the liver. Once again, sustained control of the disease is the goal for the future to prevent this complication from arising.

The critical step in managing cirrhotic liver failure is to look for, and manage, any event or complication that has triggered the acute worsening of liver function. This is normally bleeding from varices or an infection. If there is a trigger such as this for deterioration, then it is usually the case that we can return people to the level of liver function they had prior to the deterioration. If liver failure becomes established, and does not reverse with supportive care, then liver transplantation should be actively explored.

One trap to be aware of with liver failure in chronic liver disease is that sometimes the obvious thing to do, which is to increase the level of therapy to control the underlying disease process, can actually sometimes turn out to worsen liver function. The experience of drug therapy in MASLD is not yet advanced enough for the same effect to be seen, but over time this information will be collected, as more people use licensed and trial drugs targeted towards MASLD.

Ultimately, with liver failure in the setting of MASLD, we can support and minimise impacts to a significant degree but very often the law of diminishing returns comes into play, and it becomes more and more difficult to reverse deteriorations. We run out of cards to play. In this setting transplant is the only viable option.

## *CIRRHOTIC SYMPTOMS*

One of the recurring themes in this book is the extent to which symptoms in MASLD impact on patients, and the importance that should be placed on their management at every stage of the disease. Cirrhosis is the form of the disease with the greatest symptom burden. There is a "triple whammy". Patients with cirrhosis are just as prone to getting the general symptoms of MASLD that can be seen at any stage of the disease. Cirrhosis most certainly doesn't protect against them. There are then the symptoms associated with the specific cirrhosis complications outlined above. Hepatic encephalopathy is a pure symptom process. Ascites can cause a lot of functional limitation because of the volume of fluid in the abdomen and can even cause pain because of the stretched abdominal wall. Finally, and importantly, there are the generic symptoms associated with the metabolic state of advanced liver disease with some degree of liver failure. People can lose weight, feel lethargic, feel nauseated and, as a result, struggle to eat. In practice, cirrhosis causes a state of chronic ill health that can have a marked impact on people's lives. Transplant can be very valuable in this setting……. even more valuable would be avoiding the need for it.

## *WHEN TO CONSIDER LIVER TRANSPLANTATION*

Liver transplantation is an effective treatment for end-stage MASLD. The practicalities of transplantation are discussed in **Chapter 10**; however its use should be considered as a normal part of the management pathway for the disease. In other words, it is a completely normal treatment that should be thought about in all MASLD patients, even if it is dismissed very quickly because the disease is too mild or is well controlled. We always set out to "de-mythologise" transplantation for our patients.

In MASLD there is only really one setting for transplantation: to mitigate the impacts of cirrhosis (in their many forms). There is no equivalent of the transplantation for an acute variant of the disease that might be seen occasionally in, for example, hepatitis B infection or autoimmune hepatitis. The most frequent scenario is one of disease which has advanced, over a period, to its very end stages and the likely risk of the complications of advanced disease that would be seen if you did not have a transplant have become greater than the risk of the operation. Occasionally, cirrhotic symptoms (such as hepatic encephalopathy or resistant ascites) can be a significant factor in the decision about transplantation, but they are rarely the only consideration, not least because symptoms typically only arise in patients with complicated cirrhosis which inherently increases the risk to life.

As we have discussed before, the development of cirrhosis is not, in and of itself, a reason to consider transplantation. Most patients with MASLD cirrhosis, in fact, remain well with it (although they need to be watched very carefully). This is because the liver has a lot of reserve capacity. Although cirrhosis reduces the functional capacity of the liver, for many people all that does is reduce the reserve. It is only once the reserve has run out that problems arise, and transplant becomes more relevant. In practice, loss of reserve in MASLD is best indicated by a rising bilirubin level and a falling albumin, especially if accompanied by ascites and/or encephalopathy.

There are no hard and fast rules for degree of abnormality in blood tests, and/or frequency of complications, that would trigger consideration of transplantation. This is because the time scale over which change is occurring is a key additional factor. The more rapid the change the greater potential for things to continue to deteriorate quickly, running the risk that the opportunity to consider transplantation is lost. As a rule of thumb, it takes between three and six months to go from considering transplantation to going onto the list. This is the time taken by the mandatory assessment process. Add to this the time that people may need to wait on the list for a suitable organ (which differs depending on blood group and body weight) and it is seldom less than 12 months from beginning the process to being transplanted. None of us can predict the future so it is essential we build in a comfort margin to our timing. We would much rather know of all patients in the catchment area for our transplant programme with MASLD who are heading towards transplantation so that follow up can be taken in our clinic that links directly to transplantation. "Forewarned is forearmed" is an expression we use frequently.

Occasionally, patients with cirrhosis will develop difficult to manage complications (such as variceal bleeding, ascites not manageable using diuretics, or hepatocellular carcinoma) without a rising bilirubin. Transplant should be considered in these situations as we know that each of these complications suggests that the patient is, either directly or indirectly, at significantly increased risk. Rarely, the albumin can begin to fall without either complications developing, or a bilirubin rise. If this is definitely related to MASLD cirrhosis, then it is an adverse finding. In most cases, however, there is another explanation related to bowel dysfunction or nutritional problems.

The biggest barrier to transplant in MASLD is, as we will discuss in the next chapter, the cardiac and other risks that results from the metabolic syndrome and its constituent conditions. One of the toughest things we ever have to explain to people is that although they "need" a transplant and would undoubtedly benefit from one if it were to be possible, the operation is just too high risk because of other health issues that could have been prevented or treated better. Remember **you have this in your hands.**

# CHAPTER 10: **TREATING MASLD 6:** *LIVER TRANSPLANT*

### *The 2-Minute Version*

- Liver transplantation is an effective treatment for very advanced MASLD, as it is for many forms of end-stage liver disease. The need for it is normally in patients with the MASH form of the disease where risk of progression to cirrhosis is the greatest.
- The aim of our approach to treatment in MASLD these days is, however, to avoid it being needed if possible. The effectiveness of lifestyle modification approaches (if used early enough in the disease and embedded in peoples' lives), and emerging drug therapy approaches mean that, hopefully, the need for it will gradually reduce over time.
- Many MASLD patients who end up needing a liver transplant are first diagnosed late in the disease course (when cirrhosis is already present). This significantly limits the potential effectiveness of therapies and emphasises the importance of early diagnosis and treatment.
- In most cases, liver transplant in MASLD is carried out because of the risks to life of very advanced chronic disease. This could be through the complications of cirrhosis (difficult to control variceal bleeding, ascites with complications, liver cancer etc) or through liver failure (rapidly rising bilirubin is the usual sign).
- A small proportion of liver transplants in MASLD are carried out specifically because of the symptomatic impact of advanced cirrhosis (most often chronic encephalopathy). Transplantation is not appropriate as a treatment for non-cirrhotic symptoms in MASLD (such as fatigue). The risk of the procedure remains, and the benefits are insufficient in practice to justify it.
- Before transplant, patients go through an assessment process to explore the likely benefits and risks to them as an individual. MASLD patients are often higher risk than patients with other forms of chronic liver disease because of the association with metabolic syndrome. Type 2 diabetes, ischaemic heart disease, hypertension, obesity and hypercholesterolaemia are all seen at an increased rate in MASLD patients, and all increase the risk of major surgery (and liver transplantation is a major operation).

- The risk of transplant surgery can be reduced by reducing the severity and impact of associated risk conditions. All of the elements of the metabolic syndrome can be controlled effectively. This takes time and patient motivation. It is therefore important that the potential need for transplantation is recognised early so that everything can be done to reduce the risk of the procedure when it is eventually carried out.
- The only matching between donors and recipients in liver transplantation is for blood group and for organ size (to ensure the new liver will "fit").
- Early complications can include non-function and thrombosis of the hepatic artery. Both are rare but potentially significant. Advances in technique have reduced their frequency and impact.
- Rejection (the attempt by the immune system to "fight" a liver it sees as being foreign) typically first arises as an issue at around seven days after the transplant but can occur at any point after that. Patients typically take lifelong immunosuppression (usually a drug called tacrolimus combined with azathioprine or MMF) to prevent this.
- Recurrence of MASLD after liver transplantation is a real and growing problem. Although the liver is "new" the rest of the person (and their metabolism) remains the same, meaning that fat deposition will occur in the new liver as it did in the old one unless lifestyle change is made. This is important. We have seen recurrent cirrhosis in the new liver within a year of transplantation. Some of the drugs given for immunosuppression such as steroids can increase the risk of MASLD recurrence so treatment choices need to be made carefully.

For all types of liver disease, the ultimate treatment option is to replace the damaged liver with a new one. This is liver transplantation. The good news about liver transplantation for MASLD patients is that it exists as a treatment option. It is a great safety net to have. It is better for everyone, however, if it can be avoided by better earlier management to avoid the development of cirrhosis. For most of the readers of the book, this chapter is for information and interest only as it hopefully will never be directly relevant to you. For the small group who are maybe heading towards, and the larger group of people who have already had, a transplant this is meant to inform and guide you and, hopefully, give you confidence. Transplantation policy and practice is one of the areas that can differ from country to country and inevitably given the authorship, this chapter mainly focuses on policy and practice in the UK. For patients with more advanced disease, understanding the opportunities around transplantation in your own health care system are important and you should discuss these with your clinical team.

## *THE BASICS OF LIVER TRANSPLANTATION*

The term liver transplantation is short for "orthotopic liver transplantation". In this title orthotopic means that the old liver is removed and replaced, in the same place in the body, with a new organ (this contrasts with kidney transplants which are often heterotopic (i.e., the new organ is placed in a different location in the body to the old kidney; usually in the pelvis, leaving the old kidneys in place)). There are four aspects to transplantation for all liver diseases. These are the donor organ, the operation itself, the assessment process before transplant and the follow up after the operation. We will discuss these in general terms first and then, in the next section, discuss the specific issues in relation to transplantation for MASLD.

**Donor livers:** In simple terms, there are two sources of a donor liver. Cadaveric donation (meaning from a person who has died) and living-related donation (a family member giving a portion of their liver). Most liver transplantation historically has used cadaveric donors. This was, until, recently, using what are termed donors by brain death (DBD). This is where the donor has suffered some form of significant brain injury (usually a bleed or head trauma) which means that they cannot survive and will not recover. In lay terms they are "brain dead". They are on a ventilator (without brain function you don't breathe spontaneously) but the heart continues to beat normally, and the other organs of the body are getting their blood supply. Many countries in the world (but not all) have a legal framework by which the organs that are functioning well can be taken in an operation for use in transplantation. In the UK, historically, we used an "opt in" system, meaning that people carried a donor card, or put their name on a registry, to indicate that in the event of brain death they would become a donor (provided their next of kin at the time also agreed). The UK is now moving to an "opt out" system where consent is presumed unless the person has indicated otherwise. DBD livers tend to be good quality because the events around their collection are controlled (the operation to remove them is planned and the body has a good blood pressure). People can sometimes worry about the imagery of an operation with an anaesthetist, with surgeons removing organs. Doesn't this mean the donor is still alive? The answer is **absolutely not**. There are strict laws about ensuring that a person's brain is dead before they become a DBD donor, and that the situation is completely non-recoverable. People often confuse brain death and persistent vegetative state (one from which very occasional people have recovered). A persistent vegetative state is a state of grossly affected brain function, but which falls short of complete brain death (i.e., there is some small neurological function). People in a persistent vegetative state are often breathing spontaneously. It is the existence of some ongoing brain function that makes all the difference.

The issue all transplant programmes face with DBD organs is that fewer and fewer are being donated. This is largely not because of reluctance to donate (although we can always do more on education and awareness), but because the causes of catastrophic brain trauma that lead to the brain death state are getting rarer (fewer intracranial bleeds because of better blood pressure control, fewer massive head traumas in road traffic accidents because of safety legislation etc.). These improvements in population health are, of course, to be applauded. To maintain the numbers of organs available for donation, however, there has been a move towards the second type of cadaveric donor; the donor by cardiac death (DCD). Death in the conventional sense has always been recognised as the point at which the heart has stopped beating (which is why someone who has had a cardiac arrest is technically dead). DCD donors are donors who are dying for reasons that are not recoverable, and from whom the organs are removed immediately after the heart has stopped beating. The use of this approach has increased the number of potential donors significantly. It has, however, significant limitations. The obvious one is that the whole process is less controlled, and is more rushed, meaning that the condition of the organ is often less good. The cause of death can have a much greater impact on organ quality as well.

For all cadaveric donor organs, a detailed assessment of the donor is made in advance of the organ being retrieved. The organ is also assessed at the time of retrieval. Concern at either of these stages means the organ is not used. The pre-donation assessment is around underlying health state and cause of death. Contraindications to donation include disseminated cancer and chronic infection such as hepatitis B or C, HIV or TB. Significant pre-existing liver disease would also be an obvious contraindication. The assessment at the time of retrieval is largely around how much fat is in the liver. As we have been discussing throughout this book, fat deposition in the liver is a significant and growing problem in our society, largely as the levels of obesity grow. Although this is a key part of the disease process in MASLD, this problem can also affect potential liver donors. If a donor liver is too fatty it will not cope with the whole process of removal, transport, and reimplantation, and runs an increased risk of not functioning after reimplantation in the recipient. After removal from the donor, the liver is perfused with a special fluid that is designed to lessen the potential injury that might occur with the organ outside the body. Conventionally, the organ was then stored on ice until the operation to implant it into the recipient. More recently, a new technique of organ perfusion has been developed in which, prior to implantation, the liver is reperfused on a machine, warming it and providing oxygen and nutrients. This approach is becoming routine and may make a significant contribution to increasing the health of organs for transplant in the future.

Living donation is a much newer approach, and one that is growing in its scope. In some countries, the law does not allow cadaveric donation, and this is the only route to organ donation. Predictably, these countries are the ones that have led the way in the surgical approach to living-related transplantation. In simple terms, a donor, usually a family member or spouse, volunteers to donate a section of their liver that is then removed at operation and implanted into the recipient. The technique was originally developed for children, where a parent would donate to a child. In this situation, the approach has proved highly successful. Living related transplantation has key advantages, but also important challenges. The obvious advantage is that both donation and transplant operations can be planned and coordinated. This allows the health of the recipient to be optimised to reduce the risk of the operation, and for the time between removal of the donor organ and its reimplantation in the recipient to be minimised, thereby reducing the impact on the liver.

There are, however, two major challenges. The first is the need for, and impact on, the donor. Clearly, a donor cannot have any of the health issues which would preclude cadaveric donation and can't have liver disease (more of a challenge than you might think given how common fatty liver is in the community). They must also be emotionally able to donate, and to be doing so without any element of obligation or coercion. The whole issue of consent is critically important because the donor faces some degree of risk (resection of a lobe of liver, which is the operation they undergo, is a significant procedure). There have been, thankfully only very occasional, instances where the donor has died after the operation, but the recipient has survived. One of the reasons why the approach is so successful for child recipients is that most parents would regard risk to their life to save the life of their child as being completely acceptable. The ties might not be so strong for a friend or a distant adult relative. The other major challenge is organ size.

Again, adult to child transplant works well as most of the child recipients are under 5 and only need a small amount of liver. This leaves plenty behind in the donor. At the other extreme, if a small wife is to donate liver for a large husband her liver may not be large enough to provide sufficient tissue for both. The challenges mean that, outside adult to child donation, living related transplantation is something that tends to be considered as an option vastly more frequently than being performed.

One thing that often surprises people about liver transplantation is that there is no need to match the donor and recipient by tissue type, as would be the case for all other types of organ transplantation. The only matching done between recipient and donor is by blood group and body mass. Body mass matching is important as a donor liver that is too large for the recipient can become compressed, pressurising it and making closure of the wound difficult. Too small a liver has the potential to twist around its blood supply, putting it, in theory at least, at risk of blocking off its blood supply. In non-liver transplant settings, if tissue type matching isn't carried out the organ is at a much greater risk of rejection. This is not the case for livers for reasons that aren't entirely clear. It may be that the liver is just so large that the immune system does not attempt to reject it. Alternatively, the complex mechanisms that exist in the liver to allow us to tolerate protein from the diet without mounting an immune response may come into play.

**Liver transplant surgery:** The transplant operation itself is a significant one, taking between 4 and 12 hours. It has two symmetrical elements to it, the removal of the old liver and the implantation of the new. Removal of the old liver may, of course, be complicated by its diseased state and by the presence of portal hypertension, which can increase the risk of bleeding significantly. Previous spontaneous bacterial peritonitis (SBP) can also make the removal of the old liver difficult. It is now standard practice to use bypass to maintain the blood drainage from the bowel and lower half of the body. The portal vein and the inferior vena cava (the large vein carrying blood from the lower half of the body back to the heart (the counterpoint to the aorta) and which passes through the liver) are both removed as part of the transplant operation and therefore must be clamped off. Without bypass, venous blood would not be able to drain from the lower body and the bowel, potentially causing damage to the more delicate tissues such as the kidney and the bowel. Implantation and anastomosis (the reconnection of the hepatic artery, vena cava, portal vein and bile duct) are normally technically straightforward, although there can be issues with size disparity between the donor and recipient blood vessels. This is particularly the case for the portal vein, which contributes a different proportion of the total liver blood flow in different people (ranging from 50 to 80%). Where there are likely to be issues with anastomoses these are avoided by changes in the operation. The details of the surgical technique are, however, beyond the scope of this book. The time of the greatest potential risk in the operation is when the new liver is perfused for the first time (the bypass is switched off and the arterial and portal venous blood flow allowed into the new liver). This is a time of great potential stress for the body as it washes out any remnants of the preservation fluid used for the liver in transport from the donor site, as well as any toxins that have built up in the liver during its storage. Blood pressure can fall and may need to be supported by the anaesthetist. This stress point is the main reason for the detailed assessment of cardiac function undertaken as part of the assessment process pre-transplant. Significant obesity can really make transplant surgery complex because of the simple challenge of access to the abdominal cavity.

**Liver transplant assessment:** Before a patient ever comes to a transplant operation (for chronic disease; the rules are different for acute liver failure, but this scenario is, in essence, never seen in MASLD) they need to have gone through the process of transplant assessment. This is a formal process that needs to have been undertaken before people can have access to the national organ allocation programme. Similar models are in place for all countries. The terminology "waiting list" is widely used for organ transplantation but in practice there is no such thing; a patient will be transplanted at the time an organ best suited to them becomes available, which means there is no strict ordering of recipients.

The format of transplant assessment will vary from centre to centre, but the aim is the same. The goal is to understand the benefit that someone might get from transplantation (the risk posed to them by their liver disease, which might be reduced by transplantation), counter-balanced by the risk of the procedure to them, in particular in relation to their cardiac and lung status. Most centres also use the assessment process as an opportunity for potential recipients to get to know the transplant team, and to understand more about the procedure. In our centre we undertake imaging of the liver to map the blood vessels and assess heart and lung function in dynamic tests as a baseline. Other investigations are then added based on someone's individual disease and risk profile. Once the risk and benefit data are collected, all the potential transplant recipients are discussed in a formal assessment meeting with all the team members present (including the transplant coordinator, one of whose roles is to express the views of the patient). Our assessment process is very successful at avoiding "getting it wrong" (i.e., transplanting someone who goes on to have avoidable complications during the operation or who struggles to cope with the emotional side of the procedure). Once someone is accepted onto the list, they continue to undergo close follow-up to make sure there is no material deterioration of their condition that might impact upon successful transplantation.

**Post-transplant management:** Whereas patients often think of liver transplantation as being the end of the part of their life with liver disease, the reality is that it is the beginning of a new life as a post-transplant patient. Transplantation should not, therefore, be thought of as a cure, rather a procedure that prevents the complications of chronic liver disease but is subject to its own long-term problems. An integral part of post-transplant management is to use drugs to reduce the risk of organ rejection. Organ rejection is the process by which the immune system recognises the new organ as being "foreign" and mounts an immune response against it. Think of this as a potentially much more aggressive form of an autoimmune disease process. The good news is that, unlike autoimmune disease, the point of first "recognition" of the new organ by the immune system is known in advance, meaning that treatment can be given to prevent the onset of the immune response. This is what is known as "immunosuppression", a blanket term for several different drugs.

Immunosuppression will be started the day after theatre and will essentially continue for life thereafter. Different units have different approaches to drug combinations, which will also be tailored according to the health of the recipient (if they have kidney problems for example) and the underlying liver disease. In most centres, a drug called tacrolimus (previously known as FK506) is the mainstay of treatment, usually accompanied by steroids (initially hydrocortisone injections replaced by prednisolone tablets when patients can eat and drink) and azathioprine or mycophenolate mofetil (MMF). The tacrolimus dose is adjusted up or down according to blood levels, whilst the other drugs are given either at fixed doses or adjusted for dose according to patient body weight.

Post-transplant management begins immediately after surgery when patients are managed on the critical care unit. In the first 24 to 48 hours after a transplant operation the potential complications and problems are largely related to the operation itself (anaesthetic issues and bleeding from vessels around the operation site). The two specific complications that can happen in liver transplantation are hepatic artery thrombosis and primary non-function. The hepatic artery is, despite supplying a large organ, often a very small vessel (remember that a significant proportion of the blood coming into the liver comes via the portal vein), with a difficult anastomosis (the joining up of the donor and recipient arteries). For this reason, it is at risk of clotting off, typically in the first 24-48 hours after the operation when there is swelling in the artery wall that narrows it further. If the surgeons are concerned about the risk to the artery, they will fashion what is called an arterial conduit, which is a linker between the donor and recipient arteries and which significantly reduces the hepatic artery thrombosis risk (but does slightly lengthen the transplant operation and make it more complex). Blood flow will usually be assessed in the hepatic artery on the day after surgery using ultrasound, with a more detailed CT or angiogram study carried out if there are any doubts about the flow. If the hepatic artery does thrombose, the effect is much less dramatic (in the short term at least) than people think it will be. Because of the portal vein blood supply, the liver will only lose a relatively small percentage of its total blood flow. The slight blood supply shortage will show up as a deterioration in liver function tests.

Hepatic artery thrombosis is not, however, a benign process. The artery may only supply a fraction of the blood needed by the liver, but it supplies most of the blood needed by the bile duct. Thrombosis of the artery can, therefore, cause ischaemia (oxygen starvation from lack of blood flow) of the bile duct, which can lead to it necrosing (dying) and beginning to leak bile into the abdominal cavity, where it is highly irritant. Longer term, ischaemia of the bile duct can lead to stricturing or narrowing in the duct, which reduces bile flow and can replicate many of the clinical features of PBC or PSC, the bile duct liver diseases. The other complication of hepatic artery thrombosis is that it can leave areas of the liver with relative ischaemia. The loss of arterial flow is not enough to cause the liver to infarct (die) but it can become isolated from the immune system. The ischaemic zones can thus become areas where bacteria in the circulation can lodge and thrive, protected from the immune system. This leads to the formation of liver abscesses that can be very difficult indeed to manage. The risks associated with hepatic artery thrombosis mean that it is an emergency, and there is only a relatively short time period to restore flow before damage becomes permanent. In the first instance, the approach is radiological - insertion of a tube or catheter into an artery which is manoeuvred to the hepatic artery. The artery is opened and a stent (a liner tube left in place to keep the artery open) is inserted. If this is not possible technically then an operation to replace the thrombosed artery with a conduit is likely to be needed. Occasionally, none of these approaches work, or it is not possible to restore blood flow, and, in these situations, repeat transplant may be needed.

The other early complication is primary non-function (a state in which the liver simply does not start working in the recipient) or delayed function (a milder process where function is impaired for a while). Both of these processes are thought to be a consequence of preservation injury (damage caused to the liver in the removal and transport process). A major contributor to this is fat in the donor liver (an increasingly common problem in society as a whole and therefore in organ donors as well). In simple terms, livers with a lot of fat in them do not cope well with being ischaemic (losing their blood supply). The fat in the liver exacerbates the ischaemic injury. High fat level in the donor liver is the commonest reason for a liver to be deemed non-transplantable. Improvements in the science of organ retrieval and preservation, including with the preservation fluid, have reduced the risks. It is likely that the new organ perfusion techniques, which are now entering into routine practice, will make a further major difference in the future.

The aspect of post-transplant management that everyone thinks about is, of course, rejection and its prevention using immunosuppression. As introduced above, rejection is the process by which the immune system recognises a transplanted organ as being foreign and attempts to mount an immune response against it. This injury can cause damage to the liver and, over time and without treatment, its loss. The term rejection is not helpful as it conjures up images of dying organs. In reality, rejection is a process which, if it happens at all, is identified early when the changes in the liver are minor, and which is reversed, in most cases, by a short burst of additional treatment followed by a slight increase in the long-term immunosuppression. The net result is that rejection, once feared, is now more of an inconvenience for most people. It could be completely prevented by using higher levels of immunosuppression, but that would open patients to significant risk of drug side-effects. The optimal approach is to find, for each patient, their "sweet spot" where rejection risk is minimised whilst maintaining immunosuppression at an acceptable dose. The typical pattern of rejection, where it occurs (at least 50% of patients never get an episode), is a slight worsening of liver blood tests at around 7 to 10 days after transplant. This is sometimes, but not usually, accompanied by a fever and aches and pains which can make the unwary think it is an infection. Rejection should always be confirmed using a liver biopsy, which reveals a typical pattern of immune-mediated injury to the bile ducts. If significant rejection is seen on liver biopsy (determined by the nature of the injury and the extent of involvement) then standard therapy is pulsed intravenous methylprednisolone (a very powerful form of steroid given as two doses a day for three days via a drip). After this, it is normal to go on to a reducing dose of oral prednisolone. At the same time, it is appropriate to review all the immunosuppression being used to try and identify a treatable reason for rejection (there usually isn't one). For most people, getting rejection is a case of a single episode that responds well to treatment and does not recur. Occasionally, a first pulse of enhanced immunosuppression is not sufficient and the three-day course must be repeated. On the rare occasions when this does not work then an alternative therapy, usually with one of the biological agents such as anti-thymocyte globulin (ATG), is appropriate.

There are two further forms of rejection which bring their own issues. The first is antibody-mediated rejection that typically arises very early and is driven by antibodies in the recipient that are specific for donor proteins (it can also be one of the explanations for a later episode of acute rejection that fails to settle with methylprednisolone). This doesn't mean that the recipient has previously been exposed to the donor, rather it is sometimes a consequence of a previous blood transfusion where the blood donor was coincidentally a partial match to the liver donor. Alternatively, it can be just bad luck (the immune system works on the basis of making any immune response possible unless it is negatively selected because it is too close in sequence to one of the body's own proteins). Antibody-mediated rejection can be a very severe form of rejection (although thankfully it is rare) and typically needs action to be taken to remove the antibodies (antibodies are long-lasting in the blood and aren't removed by steroids or other conventional forms of immunosuppression). Approaches can include the use of plasmapheresis (a form of dialysis that removes antibodies from the circulation) and of rituximab, a biological drug that removes B-cells (the cells that will go on to produce antibody) from the circulation, often in combination.

The second additional form of rejection used to be called chronic rejection, to contrast it with the acute cellular rejection (i.e., mediated by the T-lymphocytes in the circulation) which is the typical early form of rejection. The term now used for the more chronic process is ductopenic rejection. This is partly because it more accurately describes the process, and partly because the terms acute and chronic imply a sequencing that isn't in fact the case (ductopenic rejection can occur early and in patients who have not had acute rejection). Ductopenic rejection is a rare but very difficult complication of liver transplantation that is very hard to treat. The first step in management is normally to optimise standard immunosuppression in case the process has been driven by under-treated acute rejection. The issue is probably, however, that the injured bile ducts enter into a cycle of ongoing damage where an initial rejection injury has given rise to bile acid retention which causes further injury. Intriguingly, this is the same concept that is currently very much in vogue for how PBC develops, and where ductopenic rejection occurs the clinical features are, perhaps unsurprisingly, very similar to those encountered in PBC, with cholestatic itch being particularly prominent. The approach to treating ductopenic rejection is, first and foremost, to try and avoid the cycle ever starting by getting effective long term immunosuppression regimes in place. Once established, there is no recognised treatment, however we use, again unsurprisingly, UDCA, the standard first line therapy for PBC.

Immunosuppression in essence "does what it says on the tin" which can bring its own long-term problems. In fact, in many ways the complications of immunosuppression are, these days, more of an issue for patients than rejection. This is the reason why we always try and find the treatment "sweet spot" of just enough, but not too much. The first obvious potential problem is infection. Given that the immune system evolved to protect us against infection, limiting the function of the immune system naturally increases infection risk. A bit like rejection, however, this is a manageable risk, and not quite the problem people think it is. There are certain very specific infections transplant patients can be at risk of. These include fungal infections such as pneumocystis and aspergillus. Both are important and dangerous infections which are avoided by prophylactic drugs (typically a weekly dose of specific antibiotic) and risk avoidance respectively. Aspergillus tends to hide in spore form in dust in old buildings so we always recommend transplant patients stay well away when building work is being carried out! There is also an increased risk of certain viruses such as cytomegalovirus (CMV) and human papilloma virus (HPV). We make sure people's vaccinations are up to date before the transplant to reduce risk and recommend normal vaccinations after the transplant BUT ONLY IF THE VACCINE IS NOT A LIVE ONE. In our experience, however, patients are not troubled by increased numbers of "ordinary infections". Sometimes, people worry about infection and avoid crowded places such as cinemas. Our advice is to use common sense. Avoid people with known active infection if you are not immune to it, otherwise live your life!

The second immunosuppression risk is of cancer. In large part, this is in relation to those cancers that are driven by viral infection such as cervical cancer and squamous cell carcinoma of the skin, both of which can be driven by human papilloma virus (HPV) infection. It is important that all transplant patients (and indeed anyone on long-term immunosuppressive therapy) gets all relevant cancer screening (especially cervical) and is aware of the potential skin cancer risk, checking for unusual skin lesions and getting them checked quickly if they arise. The other main cancer risk is for lymphoma, a cancer of the lymph glands. This can be a particular issue if people have had one of the powerful biological drugs such as ATG, which, by their very nature, disrupt the immune systems checks and balances (that's how they work!). The commonest version of this is a condition called post-transplant lymphoproliferative disease (PTLD). This starts out as overgrowth of the B-cells that is not cancerous but has the potential to turn rapidly into a lymphoma. It appears to be, as with the other transplant-associated cancers, driven by a virus; in this case Epstein-Barr virus (the glandular fever virus). Treatment is, in the early stages, to reduce or stop immunosuppression to allow the immune system to be able to clear the virally infected B-cells. If necessary, rituximab can be used effectively to clear the B-cells. If PTLD evolves into an active lymphoma, then the treatment is chemotherapy. The message that PTLD sends is to be cautious about the immunosuppression you use. Hitting the immune system hard to avoid any chance of rejection may feel like a good idea as a clinician when you are focusing on rejection as an issue. Be careful, however, to ensure that the treatment is really needed as it can store up major problems down the line.

The final major complication of immunosuppression is one that people often don't think of, and one that is important in people having liver transplantation for MASLD. It is the metabolic effects of the drugs. The issues with prednisolone (weight gain and risk of type 2 diabetes) are well known and are one of the reasons why these drugs are weaned down and stopped whenever possible. What is less well known is that tacrolimus and cyclosporine, the mainstays of immunosuppression, have their own metabolic impacts. Tacrolimus can, itself, cause type 2 diabetes mellitus and an increased risk of ischaemic heart disease. Both tacrolimus and cyclosporine can cause kidney damage if their levels are too high, and can, over time, lead to kidney failure. Finally, both can cause neurological symptoms. These include a fine tremor (DJ once met a watchmaker taking tacrolimus who knew his blood level by the degree of hand tremor he had, and who would stop the drug when he was working on a very expensive watch!). Other problems can include headaches, confusion and even fitting on occasions. It is very important when taking tacrolimus or cyclosporine that the blood levels of the drug are monitored carefully, and the drug dose adjusted accordingly.

## *LIVER TRANSPLANTATION IN MASLD*

There is no doubt that liver transplant in MASLD is a significant undertaking with challenges and, perhaps more so than in any other type of liver disease, risks. It is also, however, frequently life changing. Transplantation is, therefore, a treatment to be valued if it is needed and avoided if possible. My (DJ) personal goal as a liver disease doctor is to, eventually, consign transplantation for patients to the history books because diagnosis and treatment will have improved to the point where it is no longer ever needed! In this section we will look again at the 4 aspects to liver transplantation, but this time specifically in relation to MASLD.

**Donor Livers:** This is the one aspect of transplantation that has few MASLD-specific features, as the nature of the donor organ is beyond the control of patients (other than, of course, if living-related transplantation is being considered). Living-related transplantation has not, in the UK at least, become a routine procedure other than in the case of children and the systems aren't really in place in adults to change this. One issue that we will need to be aware of (in addition to the general practical and ethical issues associated with living related liver transplantation) if this is to change is the demographics of potential recipients and donors. Advanced MASLD is commoner in men than women, and, in practice, most live-related donors are spouses. The commonest potential pairing is therefore a female donor to a male recipient. The issue that this gives rise to is organ size limitations. Women tend, naturally, to be smaller than men and the amount of liver that would need to be donated to be sufficient to support a larger man would be problematic (in essence one smaller liver is split between two people). The reverse spousal pairing (larger man donating liver tissue split between two people) is, in contrast, rarely an issue. As is always the case with living-related donation, where the lives of two people are impacted, the issues need to be thought about very carefully indeed.

**Liver transplant surgery:** Liver transplantation surgery in MASLD is usually mostly impacted by obesity (in simple terms access to the liver is made more difficult by adipose tissue) and the anaesthetic risks associated with diabetes, heart disease and kidney disease related to diabetes. This is why transplant assessment is so very important in MASLD. It allows the anaesthetists to understand the risk of the operation, and to reduce that risk as much as is possible before the operation.

The aspects of previous liver history that can cause issues are portal hypertension and its complications, and a history of spontaneous bacterial peritonitis. When people think of portal hypertension they instantly think of oesophageal varices, the blood vessels at the base of the gullet, as being the primary complication. In terms of overall complication risk this is indeed the case. In the context of transplant surgery (and indeed any other form of surgery involving the abdomen) it is important to realise that varices can also develop anywhere throughout the abdominal cavity, including on the inside wall of the abdomen, where they can be damaged by the surgeon opening the abdomen. This can mean that bleeding issues are encountered right from the point at which the abdomen is opened, and long before the liver is reached. For this reason, it is really important to be aware of the degree of portal hypertension prior to transplant surgery, and to undertake whatever steps are possible, up to and including TIPSS, to reduce portal hypertension. In terms of the other complications of portal hypertension, ascites in isolation isn't an issue (indeed it can sometimes "stretch" the abdominal wall making the insertion of the donor liver easier). There is, however, a rare feature, called porto-pulmonary hypertension in which the pressure in the artery leading from the right side of the heart to the lungs has a significantly higher than normal pressure. This can lead to complications during the anaesthetic because of increased burden on the heart. This is a process associated with portal hypertension and should be screened for at transplant assessment.

The one aspect of ascites that can cause real problems in transplant surgery is if that ascites has been infected: spontaneous bacterial peritonitis or SBP. If such infection is present at the time of the transplant it can cause major issues with infection risk in and around the new graft, as well as bleeding problems because the tissue surfaces become very inflamed and friable, bleeding at the slightest touch. Where there has been ascites infection in the past, scar formation can occur with loops of bowel stuck to each other and to the abdominal wall. This can make it a real challenge to take the old liver out, often leading to a prolonged operation. As with all complications of cirrhosis in MASLD, avoiding the problem in the first place is the best option!

**Liver transplant assessment:** This is probably the most critical aspect of safe liver transplantation in MASLD. All operations place stress on the body through the effects of anaesthetics, the stress of the surgery itself and changes in blood pressure (which can occur because of blood loss, the body response to pain and the effects of the anaesthetics). As we have discussed earlier, to this is added the impact of liver transplantation itself. As well as being a long and significant procedure in general terms, liver transplant has uniquely stressful aspects to it (in terms of the patient's physiology). These are to do with the significant changes in blood pressure that can be associated with going onto bypass and then the perfusion of the new liver. This can result in quite rapid, and significant, changes in blood pressure. This is typically temporary, but the stress on the body can be marked. Two organs can be particularly affected. These are the heart and the kidneys; organs that are often abnormal in MASLD anyway because of the effects of the metabolic syndrome. If there is significant abnormality in heart function then the rapid changes in blood pressure can overwhelm it, causing heart failure. Furthermore, heart failure adds to the tendency to drop blood pressure (the heart's "pumping" capacity is reduced) and the net effect of all the blood pressure issues is that the coronary arteries, the arteries that supply the heart muscle with blood, don't have enough blood supply. This can cause shortage of oxygen to the heart muscle and a form of heart attack, all of this happening in coronary arteries that may already be narrowed by the atherosclerosis. If kidney function is abnormal then, again, blood pressure changes can send people into full kidney failure.

It is easy to see that a spiral of problems could arise in the middle of a liver transplant operation in MASLD, and that things could continue to deteriorate rapidly once the spiral starts. At this point it is typically far too late to back out of the operation. This can be a very difficult situation indeed. One final challenge is that people with fatty liver and metabolic syndrome can often reach a state of stable abnormality regarding heart and kidneys (we call this "compensation"). What this means is that heart function isn't normal but is normal enough to allow day to day life to go on okay. People may have no symptoms (although in the case of heart disease this is often because they adapt their lifestyle (often subconsciously) to avoid stressing their heart). This stable abnormality is fine until a real stress event, such as a liver transplant operation, comes along.......

All this may sound negative. It isn't meant to. It is meant to help you understand why transplant assessment is so important (and why, in an ideal world, we would avoid the need for liver transplantation in MASLD in the first place!). In reality, MASLD is now an important and common indication for liver transplantation and many patients undergo it very successfully. It is essential, however, to be prepared.

Given the importance of the heart in terms of risk reduction for liver transplant in MASLD (because of the heart disease risk of metabolic syndrome) assessing the functional status of the heart and circulation is key. This can be done in two ways, static tests and dynamic tests. The static tests are an ECG and an echocardiogram (a type of ultrasound that looks at the heart moving). These assess the electrical function of the heart (the trigger for the heartbeat) and the function of the heart respectively, and are very standard tests. The problem with these tests is that they are done at rest and although any abnormalities found using them are likely to be important, they don't really look at the key issue, which is the likely response of the heart to the stress of the operation. This is where the dynamic tests come in. In the past these included exercise testing. This is a test where the ECG is recorded, not with someone sitting down but whilst they are walking on a treadmill. The treadmill speeds up, and the slope increases progressively, to test the response to stress. This is a very long-standing approach, usually used to investigate people with angina. It is still useful in transplant assessment but still doesn't quite address the key question which is whether the heart and circulation as a "unit", linked to the lungs, are able to deliver the oxygen needed to the cells as the body becomes stressed. This is where cardiopulmonary exercise testing or CPEX comes in. In this test people (usually) ride an exercise bike where, again, the amount of resistance increases progressively, making them work harder and harder. In addition to an ECG, what is recorded is the amount of oxygen that people can absorb, and the amount of carbon dioxide they are able to breathe out. This is an effective way of assessing how well the heart/lungs/circulation are working in practice. The values that come from this test are really accurate at predicting risk, and if the test result is good, it really allows people to go into a transplant operation with confidence. One thing to always remember if you are doing a CPEX test is that there is no pass/fail element to it. The amount of exercise will increase progressively until you can't manage any more, or until the person supervising the test decides, based on the values that they observe, that you have reached the maximum level of exercise that you will be able to do.

If the cardiac and lung assessment suggests that your transplant risk is higher than we want this doesn't necessarily mean that transplant isn't possible. It just means that there is work to do before you can go onto the list. If the lungs are an issue, then it is a case of treating the problem appropriately. If the coronary arteries are an issue, then the modern interventions like stenting (where an artery is opened up and kept open by insertion of a tube) are safe to be done before a transplant operation, and effective. Perhaps the commonest issue that we see is less about specific problems like coronary artery narrowing and more in relation to a lack of fitness. Many patients with advanced MASLD struggle to exercise, and this can have a real knock on effect on physical fitness. This is where an approach that has been christened "pre-habilitation" comes in. You wouldn't expect to be able to run a marathon without doing any training so, by the same token, unless you are reasonably fit to start with, you shouldn't expect to be able to go through a big operation without also training. We can, and do, devise fitness programmes for people to help them become transplantable, and we monitor their improvement through repeat CPEX. One of the recurring themes in this book is "own the problem, own the solution". So much of MASLD is controllable if people have the desire to control it, and guidance as to what to do (the very essence of this book). This absolutely applies to physical fitness before liver transplant.

**Post-transplant management:** The early post-transplant management of MASLD patients is usually straightforward, with no specific risks over and above those seen in all post-transplant patients. None of the early surgical complications are seen at an increased rate in MASLD, other than, perhaps, some knock-on effects from the operation being a little slower because of the difficulty of access in the context of obesity.

One aspect of post-transplant management where thought needs to be applied is around anticoagulation ("thinning the blood" to prevent clot formation). This is relevant in MASLD patients for two reasons. The first is that obesity can, rather like being a pro-inflammatory state, be procoagulant. This means that MASLD patients are rather more prone than others to develop blood clots. Add to this mobility limitations because of body weight and the risk of blood clots in the leg (deep vein thrombosis or DVT) and those clots going to the lung (pulmonary embolism) is real. This risk can be managed by the use of anticoagulant drugs (heparin injections under the skin), the use of compression stockings on the legs to aid blood flow out, careful attention to keeping well hydrated (if people become dehydrated the blood can become "gloopier" and thus be more likely to clot) and early mobilisation. The other risk that is more specific to liver transplantation is that of hepatic artery thrombosis, clotting off the main artery to the liver, which is a specific complication of liver transplantation. The same approaches that prevent DVT (other than stockings) are applicable to this. Despite the most effective prevention approaches the risk remains (small but present) and this needs to be factored into all decision making about the appropriateness of liver transplantation in any individual.

Perhaps the thing that people most frequently think about and discuss in liver transplantation in all patient groups is immunosuppression to prevent rejection. Most first rejection episodes occur around 7-10 days after transplantation; typically, at the point where the risk of primary function issues is reducing. Immunosuppression is, of course, an important issue in MASLD transplantation as it is in transplant for all other conditions. A

MASLD background does, however, give rise to some specific issues relating to the optimal drug regime. The earliest decision to be taken is whether to use one of the newer "biological" drugs such as basiliximab. These act to make a newly transplanted organ "invisible" to the immune system. The logic is that if the new organ is "invisible" then the immune system won't mount a response. A critical aspect of their function is that they don't eliminate the capacity to reactivate pre-existing immune responses (immune memory after past infections); something which older and cruder biologicals such as ATG do. This means that patients retain protection against many infections. Use of basiliximab (and related drugs) needs to be at the time of the transplant, before the blood flows into and out of the new liver as, once seen, the immune system can't "un-see" the liver. This means that the use of basiliximab needs to be thought about in advance and planned for if it is going to work. Why therefore consider it? The key reason in MASLD is that it means that starting tacrolimus can be delayed for up to around a week. This allows the kidneys to be protected from a "double hit" of the operation itself combined with tacrolimus (which can itself cause kidney toxicity). Given that many MASLD patients have diabetes that can cause kidney issues this is an important option to consider.

As alluded to in the previous paragraph, conventional immunosuppressive drugs can cause their own significant issues in MASLD patients. In addition to the kidney risk in diabetic patients, both tacrolimus and steroids can significantly worsen type 2 diabetes; an important issue in patients already at risk of both type 2 diabetes and its consequences. In many ways, the choice of immunosuppression in MASLD patients post-transplant is about choosing the "least bad" regime, monitoring really carefully for complications and intervening early and rapidly when they start to arise.

Slightly further down the line, the possibility of complications of three types is particularly important to remember. These are: late acute cellular rejection (a form of rejection arising outside the normal window where the process is typically seen), infection and, of the greatest relevance in MASLD, disease recurrence. In most liver transplant settings, a "modus vivendi" seems to arise between the liver and the immune system. In simple terms an "uneasy truce" is brought about by the effects of immunosuppression that can even evolve into a state of tolerance where immunosuppression is no longer needed (although practice in the UK is very much to not stop immunosuppression). In some patients this doesn't really seem to happen and for this reason life-long immunosuppression is the norm.

Infection is an ever-present concern after liver transplantation. There are specific infections that arise almost exclusively in immunosuppressed patients (for example pneumocystis pneumonia) and some infection types that can occur in all populations but are a specific risk after transplant (for example cytomegalovirus (CMV) infection and human papilloma virus (HPV), which can contribute to several types of cancer). In practice, however, most infections that people have are simple bacterial and viral infections (such as urinary tract infections) that have a greater impact because the body's capacity to fight them is reduced. They may be a little worse than in non-transplant patients, and go on a little longer, but they are fundamentally the same.

Perhaps the greatest emerging problem in patients having liver transplantation for MASLD is disease recurrence. As we have discussed in earlier chapters, MASLD is, to a significant degree, something that happens to the liver as a result of changes occurring elsewhere in the body (diet, metabolism, type 2 diabetes, obesity etc). Crucially, although the liver is new after a liver transplant, none of these other problems is addressed by the operation. In fact, it is worse than that. Patients are frequently immobile, or at least have reduced mobility, for a sustained period after transplant (and exercise is one of the most effective ways of controlling fatty liver). Furthermore, we give drugs such as steroids that actively make the problem worse. The scene is therefore set for MASLD recurrence (often rapidly). One of oddities about liver transplantation in MASLD is that we do very little to address risk factors either before or after transplant. We work intensively with people with alcohol-related liver disease to address harmful drinking but do nothing systematically in MASLD to address harmful eating, an interesting paradox. The important thing to say is that absolutely everything we have discussed in the chapters on diet and weight loss in MASLD apply in the post-transplant setting many times over.

# CHAPTER 11: **SYMPTOMS IN MASLD**

## *The 2-Minute Version*

- Historically, the focus of doctors in MASLD, as with all other liver diseases, has been on treating the disease to prevent progression to cirrhosis. The question of the symptoms of MASLD has been much less extensively addressed and there are important gaps in our understanding. There is a particular potential for symptoms to impact on important aspects of disease management such as lifestyle modification.
- The way diseases are thought about now has changed and a more balanced approach is increasingly being taken, focusing more on the needs of patients. It is time, therefore, to put more of a focus on symptoms in MASLD, their impact on people lives and, crucially, how we can prevent them from developing and treating them when they occur.
- Symptoms in MASLD patients fall into three groups, although in any individual patients none, one, two or three can be present, so a holistic view must be taken.
- The first symptom group are the ones that doctors always think about, which are the symptoms associated with the development of cirrhosis and its complications. These include abdominal swelling because of ascites and impaired conscious level because of hepatic encephalopathy. It is also clear that simply being cirrhotic is associated with fatigue with an often significant impact on life quality and function. There are treatments, but avoidance of their development in the first place is the key to better treatment. Transplantation can also be an effective treatment.
- The second type of symptoms are less frequently thought of, but in overall population impact terms more important. These are the symptoms that result from the chronic inflammation and metabolic derangement that characterises MASLD. These are not direct cirrhosis features (they can occur throughout the disease course and certainly long before cirrhosis develops) and include fatigue, cognitive symptoms (memory and concentration issues) and itch. These are, again, a major issue and a neglected one. It may be that current approaches to better control of MASLD will mean that they don't arise in the future (although the potential for them simply to be swapped for treatment-related symptoms is there).

- The final symptom type is the symptoms associated with the metabolic syndrome (i.e., the conditions that are associated with MASLD). There is probably a very significant overlap between these and the second type. Most clinicians "know" that type 2 diabetes is associated with significant fatigue. It is almost completely unknown, however, why this is the case. People naturally think that it is a direct effect of elevated blood glucose values. The same degree of elevation is not, however, typically associated with the same degree of fatigue in type 1 diabetes. It is, therefore, something much more linked to the type 2 process. Could this, in fact, be the impact of latent MASLD? The key point is that effective control of symptoms in MASLD requires effective control of all the potential associated conditions.
- The good news about symptoms in MASLD is that many patients have none whatsoever and have a completely normal quality of life over many years. Complete symptom control is therefore an achievable goal. Every patient with MASLD should be asked about their symptoms on every clinic visit and where issues are arising, early treatment should be started. Attention to detail is key.

One of the major steps forward in the management of the autoimmune liver diseases, the subject of the first three books in this series, has been the appreciation, by clinicians, of the extent to which symptoms can occur and can impact on peoples' quality of life, and the importance of treating them (patients, of course, have always known about them!). In our experience, although symptoms can be just as big an issue in MASLD they are much more likely to be ignored by clinicians, or their significance underplayed. Why this happens is an interesting question and one that goes to the mindset of liver doctors. All hepatologists are brought up to regard cirrhosis development as the critical issue in liver disease, and the management of its complications the main aspect of treatment. The perception of MASLD for many clinicians is, therefore, all about preventing the disease from killing people. This clearly should remain a priority, but we do need to balance it with an awareness of the broader impact of the disease on people and their day to day lives. A patient with no cirrhosis, and good control of their liver blood tests, but who is still symptomatic, still has a problem and it is not helpful to them to tell them that they don't! We need to take a step back and take a broader view of the disease and its impact, a holistic view. We have two goals in treatment -the longest lifespan we can possibly get and the best quality of life we can get. One without the other is a failure. In the next chapter we will talk about the important role that patients can play in raising the issue of symptoms and their impact on life quality with their doctors.

In thinking about symptoms in MASLD it is useful to break them down into the settings in which they occur. The reason for this is that this helps us think about the causes and then the treatments (the thing that, of course, matters most of all). A final important point is that none of the symptoms seen in patients with MASLD are unique or specific for this disease. This is one of the problems with symptoms in liver disease. There is often nothing that should specifically make doctors suspect the presence of liver disease. This can have the important effect of delay in diagnosis.

## ***SYMPTOMS RESULTING FROM CIRRHOSIS***

Perhaps the simplest symptom set to understand are those that do arise because of cirrhosis. These are generic in nature and are similar in cirrhosis of all causes. This has the important implication that the development of these symptoms indicates the presence of cirrhosis rather than implying any individual liver disease aetiology.

Self-evidently, these symptoms only develop in people whose disease has progressed to cirrhosis. Our goal for the future must be effective management through diet, exercise and medication (if available and indicated) given early in the disease to prevent progression. It is also important to say that many people with cirrhosis will not have any symptoms from it, meaning that absence of cirrhosis symptoms should not falsely reassure someone. The complications of cirrhosis (and it is the complications that give rise to symptoms) have been discussed in **Chapter 9.**

The complication most likely to give rise to symptoms, and to reduce patient quality of life, is *hepatic encephalopathy*, a state of reversible brain dysfunction that arises because of the retention of toxins in the blood that the liver is unable to effectively clear. In its mildest form this can be a change in personality, noticeable only to close acquaintances. This is sometimes accompanied by a reversal of day and night sleep patterns (a tendency to sleep during the day and be awake during the night) and poor concentration and memory. In more severe forms there can be impaired conscious levels (initially a tendency to fall asleep at unusual times) with, in its ultimate form, unconsciousness and coma. Where hepatic encephalopathy arises, it can be very distressing for both the patient and for family members (we have often heard it said that it feels like people don't know their loved one anymore). Initially, the process is typically subtle and episodic, with periods of abnormality that resolve, returning people to normal. The episodes usually arise when an event occurs either temporarily reducing liver function further or increasing the level of function needed. Examples include an intercurrent illness (often just a mild viral infection), taking sedative drugs or even just constipation. Encephalopathy can also occur when someone with advanced cirrhosis has a bleed into their bowel for any reason (the liver can't cope with the increased workload processing the broken down and reabsorbed blood in the bowel). The obvious concern in this setting is a variceal bleed. It often surprises people how minor the triggers for encephalopathy can be. The point is that they are "tipping point" events occurring in people whose liver is only just coping, and who need only the tiniest thing to push them over the edge into liver dysfunction.

Early encephalopathy is usually very straightforward to manage. We try and identify the event or events that tipped the balance and treat them, thereby restoring the balance. If it is an infection, treat it (or at least wait for it to settle of its own accord), if it is a sedative drug, stop it, if it is a bleed find out why and treat it and if it is constipation get the bowels moving. In practice, the workload given to the liver from the bowel is always a factor and we optimise this aspect in everyone. The first-line treatment for encephalopathy is the laxative lactulose, given at a level to get the bowels opening two to three times a day. We also use the non-absorbed antibiotic rifaximin that reduces the workload resulting from the bacteria in the gut.

In most people, a single episode develops and resolves. The risk of it recurring is always there (getting a liver at the tipping-point back into balance is fine but unless we do anything to improve residual liver function, the risk of future imbalance will always remain). The most important prevention step is to make sure control of liver function is as good as possible, and to avoid situations with a high risk of triggering an episode (constipation and taking sedative drugs are the most easily avoidable). There can come a point when the episodes never return to normal, and a state of chronic hepatic encephalopathy arises. This can really impact on quality of life and is particularly distressing for relatives and carers.

Ultimately, hepatic encephalopathy can be a reason to consider liver transplantation. It is important to say that transplant is a highly effective treatment for encephalopathy, and the quality-of-life gains seen after liver transplant are probably higher in people with encephalopathy than any other group. In practice, a first episode of encephalopathy should ring alarm bells as it tells us something about the state of underlying liver damage and function. Unless there was an obvious, and reversible, trigger for encephalopathy clinicians should have transplant in mind from that point onward and begin to talk to patients about it as a possible future option. That way, if it becomes necessary, people are prepared.

The second main symptom of cirrhosis is ***abdominal swelling from ascites***. This arises because of increased pressure in the portal vein, combined with low albumin level and retention of a hormone called aldosterone. The pressure rises in the portal vein occur because of the impediment to normal blood flow through the liver, which results from liver scarring in cirrhosis (compounded by the attempt of the liver to regenerate within the scars leading to the liver cells being "squeezed"). Albumin in the blood acts to keep fluid in the circulation through the effect of oncotic pressure. It is normal for fluid to leak from the blood vessels under pressure (even the low level of pressure seen in veins). The effect of high protein levels in the blood is to draw the fluid back into the vessel. Without this drawback effect the fluid remains in the tissues. The abdomen cavity is particularly vulnerable to this effect because it acts as de facto "free space". Aldosterone is a hormone naturally produced by the body to help regulate fluid and salt levels. It is normally broken down by the liver, meaning that if the liver isn't functioning it builds up, causing both fluid and salt retention. This all adds to the effects of portal hypertension and low albumin levels.

The presence of significant ascites can cause symptoms in several ways. First it is cosmetic, giving an appearance that people don't like. It can also feel like a "heavy weight" in the tummy, reducing mobility (remember, each litre of ascites fluid weighs over 1kilogramme and someone with a lot of ascites may have 20+ litres present). Large volumes of ascites can also lead to breathing problems when people lie down (it presses against the diaphragm, restricting its movement). This can cause significant shortness of breath and also interfere with sleep, leading to knock-on effects in terms of fatigue.

Treatment of ascites is, in the first instance, by reducing fluid intake and by using water tablets (especially spironolactone which is particularly useful because it blocks the actions of aldosterone).

## *CHRONIC INLAMMATORY DISEASE SYMPTOMS*

It used to be commonly thought in liver disease that symptoms were a feature of advanced disease alone. In other words, symptoms developed only when people progressed to cirrhosis. We have discussed, in the previous section, one setting in which this doesn't hold true; the fact that many people with cirrhosis don't develop any symptoms at all. The reverse is also true. Many people with symptoms in MASLD don't have cirrhosis. The explanation for this is that the chronic inflammation and metabolic abnormalities that underpin MASLD can themselves be symptomatic. The most characteristic of these are fatigue and cognitive symptoms (memory or concentration problems). Fatigue in MASLD gives rise to an important "double whammy". It both impairs quality of life, with a particular impact in children, and reduces peoples' capacity to undertake lifestyle modification interventions as a route to disease control.

**Fatigue:** In our experience, the most challenging symptom in non-cirrhotic MASLD is, as with most other types of liver disease, chronic *fatigue*. This is partly because of its all-pervasive nature, and partly because of the lack of effective drug treatments. At present, there is no evidence to suggest that emerging drug treatments for MASLD are effective at reducing fatigue, and there are no specific drug therapies for fatigue as a symptom (akin to, for example, paracetamol for pain). Our comment about the effectiveness of drug therapies for MASLD is very carefully worded. Part of the issue is probably lack of effect, but this is probably added to by a lack of evidence because this important aspect of the patient experience has often not been well studied in clinical trials of novel therapies. Despite all this, the most effective treatment approaches that we have should be used in the setting of fatigue in MASLD. This is for two reasons. The first is that if disease progresses to cirrhosis, it is likely (although not inevitable) that additional symptoms will develop. Developing cirrhosis never improved anyone's symptoms and quality of life so preventing cirrhosis must be an important part of long-term symptom management. The second reason why we should still focus on disease control is long-term disease trajectory. Ultimately, we suspect that it is the inflammation component of MASLD that drives chronic fatigue (the pro-fatigue effects of cytokines such as TNF and IL-6, both know to be produced at elevated levels in MASLD patients, are well known). As we have discussed throughout the book it is fat itself that drives the inflammation. Intuitively, therefore, fat reduction must over time reduce inflammation and thus fatigue. The key thing is that it is likely to take time to achieve, and this rather goes against the (entirely reasonable) desire of both patients and doctors for rapid symptom improvement. In simple terms, MASLD therapy may "not work for fatigue" for the simple reason that it hasn't been given early enough in the disease and for long enough. If regulators move to target therapy exclusively towards patients with evidence of established fibrosis falling short of cirrhosis (as they may well do) this may target the benefit in terms of risk to life at the highest risk patients but do so at the cost of potential symptomatic benefit.

The lack of specific drugs does not mean, however, that we can't improve patients' quality of life. Our approach to managing fatigue in chronic liver disease is constructive, positive and, most of all, supportive. This can make an important difference to people, although ideally, we would be able to go further into the territory of active treatment. One of the reasons why a supportive approach is so important is the negativity around chronic fatigue that patients can encounter from families, the public and, all too frequently, health care professionals. One reason for this is what we call the "normality" of fatigue. What do we mean? Other symptoms people encounter in their day-to-day life are black and white. It is normal not to have them, meaning that their presence clearly indicates abnormality. Pain would be a classic example of this. We don't normally have pain other than, perhaps, as a fleeting sensation. It is, therefore, easy to compartmentalise as something that is abnormal and present as part of a disease. This does not reduce its impact, of course. It does, however, make it easier for patients to understand and accept it. Fatigue is very different. It is something that many of us feel as part of ordinary life (working too hard, too many late nights etc). This leads many patients to struggle with understanding whether their fatigue is part of the disease or not. Is what they perceive real? It is no coincidence that one of the important steps in managing fatigue in the clinic is to explain it in the context of MASLD, and to describe the experiences of other patients. Patient groups facilitating meeting with other patients with similar experiences are also very helpful in this regard. This, again, does not reduce the fatigue but it does make it easier for patients to accept it.

The attitude of the medical and nursing professions to fatigue can, unfortunately, be negative. Far too many patients describe doctors tutting, rolling their eyes, saying that they "only treat proper problems" and saying how tired they are because they were "on-call" last night. One of the things we find most puzzling in chronic liver disease is why doctors find it so easy to accept that itch in PBC (along with fatigue one of the classic symptoms of PBC) is "real", whilst at the same time believing adamantly that fatigue is not. We suspect that the fact that the former is easy to treat whilst the latter is not has a lot to do with it.

One of the main challenges with fatigue is that the concept itself is difficult to explain. Whereas pain or itch are quite easy to explain and understand, and the terms largely mean the same thing to different people, the term fatigue is challenging. DJ once met a patient after a lecture who told him that some days it was her fatigue that was bad and some days her tiredness. The terms had been used interchangeably in the lecture, but to her each had a distinctive meaning. The problem is that the same words may well have meant different things to another patient. When using patient descriptions of their own experience, fatigue appears to be present in approximately 60% of patients, with around 25% of all patients having significant fatigue. Tools such as the Fatigue Impact Scale (FIS) are very useful for allowing us to quantify fatigue; something which is an important step if we are going to understand it and treat it. As with itch, one of the important groups of patients is that of people who are clearly not affected. It is the comparison of these people with patients with fatigue that has been most informative in understanding the problem.

There appear to be two main variants of fatigue in MASLD (although we would reiterate the point that this area hasn't been well studied). The first type is a very peripheral form, which patients often describe as feeling like their "batteries running down". This type of fatigue is associated with real struggles doing day to day things (people often describe planning shopping trips to shopping centres where they know they can sit down halfway round). There can often be a sense of a finite amount of energy that, once used up, means that the rest of the day is a struggle (mornings are often much better than afternoons for this reason; something which is an important part of the approach to coping with fatigue that we work with patients on). Resting restocks energy to a degree, but it is normally only the next day that people can get going again. Another common phenomenon is that of "good days and bad days". A few years ago a patient who, earlier in life, had been a keen runner said to DJ that her fatigue felt just like she had "finished a half marathon" with her legs turning to jelly. This form of fatigue may well be a result of what is called deconditioning; a process where underuse of muscles, and the body processes needed to supply them with energy, leads to their becoming less efficient. A medical form of being "unfit" if you like. A good example of this is someone who has their leg in plaster following a fracture. When the plaster is eventually taken off, the muscle of the leg is often smaller, and certainly less strong. The way to prevent and reverse this effect is through increased activity which improves the levels of muscle function. Athletes get to be able to perform at a higher level by training. My person with a leg fracture returns the leg muscle to normal by going to the gym and weight training. The challenge, of course, for people who are fatigued is that it is difficult to start and then maintain an exercise programme (our own research in this area indicates it is a particular problem in MASLD). This is, however, important and is a key part of the "owning the solution" aspect to living with MASLD that we will discuss in **Chapter 12**.

The second type of fatigue is what we call central fatigue. As its name suggests, this is more about brain function than peripheral muscle capacity and is thought to be a direct result of low-grade inflammation impacting on the brain. In this sense, central fatigue is a phenomenon that can be seen in many different inflammatory and immune disease (arthritis, colitis, multiple sclerosis etc). It is certainly not unique to MASLD. Patients often use terms other than fatigue to describe this problem, and a term frequently used is "brain fog"; a term that has been used for many years in the setting of chronic liver disease symptoms but which, intriguingly, has made a recent reappearance in the context of "long COVID". Furthermore, problems such as disturbance of sleep are common. Concentrating can be hard, and short-term memory can be a real problem. People feel like they must make a huge effort to concentrate enough to do things. In its purest form this is very distinct from the peripheral type of fatigue although, of course, the two can co-exist in the same person. One potential mechanism for the co-existence is that in some people central fatigue is the initial problem. This leads to people wanting to, and being able to, do less. This means that they lose physical fitness, which means that their muscles work less well and are more inefficient, reverting to anaerobic metabolism too quickly. The process of deconditioning that we introduced earlier. This dual process to fatigue is of much more than academic interest. The impact of deconditioning is such that even if we found a "cure" for central fatigue it, on its own, would not really help people because although the motivation and capacity to initiate activity will be increased, the muscles will need to readjust to be able to do that. This will take time and rehabilitation. The athlete with the broken leg needs to rehabilitate and so, we suspect, will MASLD patients recovering from central fatigue.

Central fatigue rarely exists on its own. It appears to be linked to two other processes which are important in terms of its clinical impact. The link to a third is very controversial. The first clear link is with dysfunction of the autonomic nervous system, the part of the brain and nervous system that controls the most fundamental automatic functions such as heartbeat and blood pressure, sweating and the function of the bowel. One of the key roles of the autonomic nervous system is to adjust the blood pressure up and down in response to changes in the body position and function. A simple example is standing up in the middle of the night. Blood pressure falls at night in general as the blood vessels dilate up. On top of that, if you suddenly stand up the blood literally rushes to your feet as gravity takes over. If there were to be no response to this, you would feel dizzy and then black out as the blood supply to the brain was compromised. This is a protective mechanism as blacking out makes you lie down again, removing the gravity problem! Normally, of course, this doesn't happen. The instant the blood pressure begins to fall the drop is sensed by receptors in the veins in the neck (the baroreceptors). They signal to the brain, which, in response, activates the autonomic nervous system to tighten the blood vessels in the leg, returning the blood pressure to normal. This all normally happens in an instant without you ever being aware of it. In MASLD patients (and patients with many other types of chronic disease with fatigue) this "reflex" can either function poorly or fail completely; a risk that is increased by the presence of type 2 diabetes. This means that the blood pressure continues to fall when you stand up. A fail-safe then kicks in which is the release of adrenaline to speed up the heart. This is not the most effective way of increasing blood pressure if the problem is dilation of the blood vessels in the leg (it is a bit like stamping on the brake pedal in your car very hard when the fault is a leak of brake fluid), but it is enough to stop blacking-out. The adrenaline release can lead to sweating and palpitations (fast heart rate). Ultimately, if this failsafe doesn't work you will get dizzy and eventually black out. This is fortunately rare in MASLD patients (although it does happen). What is common is a sense of dizziness when standing up, accompanied by palpitations. All of this is particularly common in patients with fatigue. What is the link to fatigue? We do know that autonomic dysfunction is a feature of many chronic conditions with fatigue as part of their clinical picture, suggesting that the link is real. It may be that it is at the level of blood pressure regulation in the muscle with poor blood flow into the limbs (necessary to supply nutrients and oxygen). Perhaps more likely is a dysfunction of the muscle draining blood flow. Pooling of venous blood may lead to poor runoff of lactic acid, contributing to the muscle acidosis and dysfunction discussed previously. Given that increasing venous drainage of lactic acid is part of how we adapt in exercise training this would fit with the finding that exercise training helps in fatigue, representing another rationale for the benefits of exercise in MASLD.

The second key association is with sleep disturbance. Fatigued liver disease patients very frequently have abnormal sleep patterns. The commonest pattern is daytime sleepiness. This can sometimes be severe enough to get in the way of work or family life. People tend not to have the extreme sleep patterns seen in the condition narcolepsy (where people can even fall asleep driving a car) but on occasion it can fall not far short. Obviously, disturbed sleep can occur in lots of conditions (and, of course, can be just the way people are). It can be very difficult to "unravel" abnormal sleep because we are not good at sensing our own sleep patterns. Many of our patients, therefore, go to the sleep clinic to have a formal sleep study where the stages of sleep are assessed. This can be done in a hospital sleep lab during an overnight stay or, more commonly these days, at home using portable equipment. One of the recent revolutions in healthcare has been the rapid development of digital health monitoring technology. These days a "Fitbit" or similar device can give quite accurate sleep data at relatively low cost. It may be, therefore, that we will be able, soon, to introduce sleep assessment into everyday practice. One simple step which may help with sleep is ensuring that vitamin D levels are normal.

The controversial question is around depression. Fatigue is a common feature of depression. It is also, however, a common feature seen in people with several chronic illnesses who are not depressed. To put MASLD fatigue down to depression is, therefore, a rather casual, even lazy, assumption. Some people do get down, and occasionally people get depressed, but this seems to be more a response to the frustration they feel about their fatigue, and worry about the future, than a primary problem. Treating depression with antidepressant drugs such as sertraline is not effective for improving fatigue in our experience.

**Treating fatigue in MASLD:** Our approach to managing fatigue in MASLD is, in many ways, a complete contrast to, say, itch in PBC. Whereas there are several effective drug treatments for itch, and the issue is finding the right agent for an individual, there are, regrettably at present, no drugs effective for treating fatigue. Hopefully this will change soon, but at present our approach is to minimise the effects of fatigue on people and to help them to find a way to live with the symptom. We have developed a 4-step approach which we teach to doctors and nurses. It will only work, however, if the doctors and nurses start from the point of view that fatigue is an important problem that needs a solution. Negative attitudes are highly counter-productive. We have a saying when training people in the approach which is "don't fail before you start". We have christened our approach TrACE after the 4 steps.

STEP 1: TREAT THE TREATABLE
A key first step in managing fatigue in fatty liver is to manage those other conditions that may coexist and which themselves cause fatigue. These include directly associated conditions (those that are frequently seen alongside MASLD), age associated conditions (things which tend to occur more commonly in people who are the typical age of MASLD patients, such as anaemia) and completely non-associated conditions that a MASLD patient may just happen to have. The point is that no matter how much effort we put into the management of MASLD fatigue, if the true cause is anaemia, we will get nowhere at all!

The most important associated condition, by a long way, is *type 2 diabetes* which is inextricably linked to MASLD and has featured in our discussions throughout this book. In simple terms in this context, type 2 diabetes is associated with fatigue, and the better the diabetes control the lower the fatigue levels. The main rationale for better type 2 diabetes control in MASLD is to reduce the complications of diabetes, however fatigue improvement is an important secondary gain and one that, as we have discussed in **Chapter 7**, can really help patients to take up and stick to the lifestyle modification approaches that are so important for both MASLD and diabetes management.

Another potentially important directly associated condition is ***heart failure***, a state where the pumping function of the heart is reduced because of either acute damage (a previous heart attack) or chronic dysfunction (ischaemia (reduced oxygen supply to the heart muscle) affecting the ability of the heart to pump). If the heart is not pumping as well as it should, then it will reduce blood supply to the muscles, with knock-on effects on venous outflow, contributing to the lactic acid build-up in muscle that is a key part of fatigue. Heart failure also worsens autonomic dysfunction. Strictly speaking, heart failure is a cardiac complication of diabetes and thus is rather indirect as a MASLD association, but it is important for doctors to think about it and then to diagnose and treat it. The most useful first-line test to screen for heart failure is a blood test called NT-pro-BNP, often shortened to pro-BNP. A level of less than 400 ng/L (47 pmol/L) is reassuring and means heart failure is unlikely. If the NT-pro-BNP level is between 400-2000 ng/L (47-236 pmol/L) you should be referred for specialist assessment and an echocardiogram, an ultrasound of the heart, which can assess the pumping ability of the heart. If the level is above 2000 ng/L (236 pmol/L) you should be referred urgently for specialist assessment and echocardiography, to be seen within two weeks. The classical ECG or electrocardiograph measures the electrical activity of the heart (the heart rhythm) rather than the pumping function and so is less useful in looking for heart failure.

An important thing to consider, if you have heart failure, is what treatment you are on, and any overlap this may have with treatment for liver disease, particularly if you have complications of cirrhosis. There are four 'pillars' of treatment for heart failure. Not everyone with heart failure will need treatment from each group, and some 'pillars' will be contraindicated in some people. The first pillar is an ACE inhibitor or similar type of drug that reduces blood pressure and takes the strain off the heart. The second pillar is beta blockers. Not all beta blockers are beneficial for heart failure, and not all are beneficial for portal hypertension. It's important that the doctors treating these conditions (if both are present) consider one drug that treats both conditions. Carvedilol is licensed for both, so a good choice. The third pillar is a group of diuretics that block aldosterone. Spironolactone is one of this group, so is a good choice if people have both heart failure and ascites. It can actually be quite hard to know, in people with MASLD and heart failure, how much of the ascites is due to the heart and how much to the liver, but at least the treatment is the same in terms of using spironolactone. The fourth pillar is a group of type 2 diabetes medicines called the SGLT2 inhibitors. Examples include dapagliflozin and empagliflozin, and they are licensed for heart failure treatment even in people without diabetes. Like many of the other diabetes medicines, there is some evidence that they may be associated with some improvement in MASLD, but much more research is needed.

A final association is with *renal failure* (abnormality in the function of the kidneys). As with heart failure this is a type 2 diabetes association rather than MASLD per se. Preventing kidney damage in diabetes is a critical goal of management. Once significant kidney damage has occurred significant fatigue is almost inevitable and difficult to treat. Far better to prevent it in the first place through good diabetes control.

The two commonest age linked problems which can be seen in MASLD, not because people have MASLD but because they are common in people who are the "right age to get MASLD" are *thyroid disease* and *anaemia*. An underactive thyroid is common in the population with a typical age of onset that is like MASLD. This means that it is also common in MASLD patients. It is caused by autoimmune injury to the gland and is therefore not a direct MASLD association. Its classic symptom is fatigue, often accompanied by weight gain (which can, of course, worsen MASLD) and constipation. These effects are all caused by a "slowing down" of the metabolism because of the reduced levels of thyroxine being released by the damaged gland. It is easy to test for using blood tests, and easy to treat using thyroxine tablets. Anyone with MASLD and fatigue should have their thyroid function tested.

Anaemia is the second common issue. Again, this is not directly linked to MASLD but is common in the population. There are many causes of anaemia, and a full discussion is beyond the scope of this book. Anaemia directly causes fatigue (reduced oxygen delivery to the heart and skeletal muscle) and treating it will improve fatigue. The approach to treating it, however, will very much depend on the cause. People tend to naturally assume that the treatment is with iron, however this is only the treatment if iron loss or reduced absorption is the cause. It therefore needs to be investigated before it is treated. There is, however, another important reason to investigate it which is the fact that it can be a signal of another disease which can give rise to real risk. Anaemia because of blood loss into the bowel or the urinary tract can be a feature of cancer, and early diagnosis of these conditions can make a massive difference to the outcome. This type of blood loss can therefore be a "red flag" symptom and mandates investigation. One important thing to know about this type of blood loss is that it can frequently not be directly visible. It is the drip drip drip of blood loss at a low level over a long time rather than a very visible bleed. The absence of an obvious bleed doesn't, therefore, rule out low level blood loss. It is important to say that we are NOT saying that anaemia suggests the presence of a cancer. It is just that it is a possibility, and it needs to be investigated if it is there. Anaemia can also be a consequence of dietary lack of vitamins, and taking a daily multivitamin can be helpful to ensure this is avoided.

It is also important to consider the possibility of *menopausal symptoms* where relevant. Menopausal symptoms include fatigue and "brain fog", and these can clearly be additive to MASLD symptoms. What makes the association particularly important is the fact that menopausal symptoms can be treated using hormone replacement therapy (HRT). The menopause does not completely explain fatigue and brain fog in MASLD, especially as at least half of people with MASLD will never undergo the menopause! However, to not use HRT in relevant patients may represent an important missed opportunity to reduce overall symptom burden. One reason for under use of HRT has been past concern about safety, and in particular blood clot and cancer risk. It is likely, however, that these concerns have been a little overstated, and we have many patients who have now been treated with HRT both safely and effectively for a number of years. One precautionary step that a number of liver clinicians recommend is to use patch-based medication rather than tablet, to reduce the high levels of liver exposure to the drug if it is taken up from the gut after being ingested in tablet form.

*Vitamin D deficiency* can also cause fatigue. Deficiency is common in the UK, and the NHS guidance is to take a supplement throughout the winter months, from October to March, and all year for people with reduced sun exposure.

One condition that, perhaps paradoxically, cannot coexist with MASLD is chronic fatigue syndrome (CFS). CFS is a diagnosis of exclusion, meaning that it is a diagnosis that is only reached by excluding all other potential conditions that could be causing fatigue. As MASLD is a condition that causes fatigue, its presence alone prevents a diagnosis of CFS from being possible.

STEP 2: AMELIORATE THE AMELIORATABLE
This step is about addressing those problems that are clearly part of the fatigue process and which make it worse. These include, as we have discussed, sleep disturbance, autonomic dysfunction, and depression.

The potential for sleep disturbance to make fatigue worse is obvious. We therefore explore to see if there is significant sleep disturbance and then look for ways to reduce it. The first and obvious question in the clinic is about night-time itch because of the clear link. Assuming that there isn't significant night-time itch what do we do next? The first step is to understand the type of sleep disturbance (is it difficulty in getting to sleep, a tendency to wake during the night, early morning waking or a tendency to fall asleep (or want to sleep) during the daytime). Each has its own causes and treatments. Difficulty in getting to sleep can be a result of taking stimulants (tea, coffee, energy drinks etc) too late in the day.

Waking during the night is often a consequence of sleep apnoea (a process of airway collapse that leads to a temporary cessation of breathing which results in the patient waking up). A useful suggestion that this might be the case is snoring; something we ask partners about in the clinic. Sleep apnoea is an important diagnosis to make as there are effective treatments that can be delivered by sleep clinics. It is also important to consider sleep apnoea, and treat it where it is present, because there is some evidence that it is pro-inflammatory and can be one of the drivers for inflammation development in the context of fatty liver.

Waking early is a classic feature of depression, although this phenomenon seems relatively uncommon in MASLD (and certainly less common than doctors sometimes think as a cause of fatigue). The commonest manifestation of sleep disturbance in MASLD is daytime sleepiness, which can often be very prominent. Its impact depends on the lifestyle, and obligations, of the individual. For people who are retired it can be an irritation (perhaps having to cancel a social event at short notice), but people adapt to "go with the flow". At the other end of the spectrum are people who have tight and inflexible timetables in their work (teachers are the classic example) where worry about being overcome by sleepiness can be as big a problem as the sleep itself. In our experience, the sleep pattern is rarely dangerous (people do not fall asleep when the car has stopped at traffic lights as people with narcolepsy do), but it is difficult to address. Our approach is to explore all aspects of sleep with the sleep clinic to attempt to "push-back" sleep into the night-time. There is often an element of poor night-time sleep that contributes. Very occasionally we use stimulant drugs such as modafinil. Developed as sleep suppressants they have got a bad name through their abuse as "cognitive enhancers" and study aids to help students stay awake to revise for exams. Many of our patients who have benefitted from modafinil have never actually taken it! The thought that there is a treatment option available if needed, and if things ever get bad, can itself be highly beneficial. If you are going to use it, blood pressure needs to be carefully monitored and some experimentation is useful to work out the optimal time in the day to take it.

The second modifiable process is autonomic dysfunction and the resulting problems with dynamic control of blood pressure. This is really common in MASLD, and the tell-tale feature is dizziness or light-headedness on standing up. Most hospitals now have a clinical service dedicated to autonomic function (usually called a falls clinic or something similar because autonomic dysfunction is a common cause of falls and injuries). Their testing approach can also be very helpful in MASLD, however. If autonomic dysfunction is present (and it is seen to some degree in most fatigued patients) then the treatment approach is to try and restore effective muscle perfusion and venous flow control. There are several ways to do this. One important area to look at is blood pressure lowering treatments. These are widely used in patients with MASLD because of the associated metabolic syndrome. They lower blood pressure, and typically do so in a rather "blunt-edged sword" way. There is also the issue that as liver disease develops and/or progresses, blood pressure can naturally fall. If blood pressure treatment isn't adjusted to take account of this natural drop, then people can end up overshooting, with low blood pressure. The "lower the better" mindset for blood pressure that many doctors have doesn't help (very low blood pressure can be as risky as high; blacking out because of low blood pressure as you are crossing the road in front of a bus is not good for you!). MASLD patients with fatigue, blood pressure treatment and features of autonomic dysfunction should have their blood pressure reviewed by their doctor. You **must not adjust blood pressure treatment without discussing it with your doctor**. If blood pressure treatment is not the culprit, then there are some simple steps you can take. The first is to increase your fluid intake (our mantra is "two litres before lunch"). This will increase the intravascular volume. Make sure this isn't sugary drinks (diabetes risk) or tea or coffee (they will add to sleep disturbance and are fluid depleting as they have a mild diuretic or water tablet effect). Another simple measure is graded pressure stockings that squeeze the lower limb and increase venous return (these are available in pharmacies). Beyond these simple measures, there are drugs such as fludrocortisone and midodrine which directly increase blood pressure. Given the risks associated with very high blood pressure these are, as you might expect, very specialised drugs that should only be used in expert clinics. You might also be advised to increase the amount of salt in your diet, which goes against much of the advice people have been given over the years, but should only be advised based on individual circumstances, where the healthcare team know what a person's blood pressure, kidney and liver function is like.

The final associated problem is the challenging one of depression. In our experience, the role of depression in MASLD fatigue tends to be overstated, with true depression being uncommon. Clearly, if present, it needs to be managed through talking therapy and antidepressant treatments as appropriate. Lower levels of depression can be seen and can contribute to the overall perception of reduced wellbeing. This tends to be a consequence of the problems that people perceive; the limitations to life that people feel, accompanied by worry about the future. This is one of the reasons why self-management is so important. Taking as much control as you can is a natural way to reverse these feelings. Sometimes drugs (for example the SSRI drugs such as sertraline) can help, and counselling and psychological support are often needed. Patient groups have an important role to play to bring people with similar problems together and to offer mutual support.

STEP 3: COPE
Coping strategies are fundamental to living well with MASLD fatigue (and indeed MASLD in general). These are explained in detail in **Chapter 12**. The key issue is owning the problem so that you can own the solution. Understand what is going on and why, and how you can plan and live your

life to minimise the impacts. This can improve symptoms and, especially, improve wellbeing.

STEP 4: EMPATHISE (& EXERCISE)
This step is mainly for doctors and other clinicians but is a useful thing to think about for partners and family members. It is about understanding and caring for your patients/loved ones. In our experience, liver disease patients with fatigue don't want their doctors to sympathise; to feel sorry for them. They want them to understand and appreciate how horrible it can be. They want someone who will help them to come to terms with it and make it as good as it can be. If you as a doctor do not think fatigue is "real" or a "proper problem" then you will be unable to work effectively with your patients and you shouldn't be managing these patients.

The other E in step 4 is a reminder that exercise, even if a gentle walk outside, is both good for fatigue and for wellbeing.

**The Newcastle approach to managing fatigue in chronic liver disease is outlined in the appendix.**

## *COGNITIVE SYMPTOMS*

These are the symptoms of poor memory and concentration which are experienced by many patients with MASLD. Clinicians tend to think of hepatic encephalopathy in cirrhosis as the cause of this type of symptoms and it is clearly the case that people with encephalopathy complicating cirrhosis will have memory and concentration problems. These symptoms can and do, however, develop in people who don't have cirrhosis, as part of the inflammatory/metabolic disease process. The distinction between these and the symptoms of central fatigue (fatigue with "brain fog") is probably arbitrary, and these are best thought of as part of the central fatigue process. It is likely that treatments in the future that benefit central fatigue will also benefit these symptoms. They can, in practice, be troublesome for people, particularly if they have jobs that require a lot of concentration or information processing. They can also be a real concern to people who worry that they are developing dementia. It is interesting that in the clinic people will often talk about fatigue but rarely about memory problems (unless we ask them). We suspect that this is because of the deep-down worry about dementia. The important thing for patients to realise is that dementia is no more common in MASLD than in the non-MASLD population, and that although these symptoms can be a real nuisance they do not progress to dementia. In the absence of a specific treatment, the approach is to find ways to cope with the problem. Writing list, using apps and trying to finish one thing before starting another are the sorts of things that patients do which help.

## *ITCH*

Many doctors managing patients with MASLD would be surprised to see a discussion of itch in a section on typical symptoms. Itch is a symptom that can often be seen in liver disease patients. It is, however, a typical feature of cholestatic diseases (diseases of impaired bile flow) rather than hepatocellular (diseases of the liver cells themselves). Given that MASLD is conventionally thought of as hepatocellular it "shouldn't" be characterised by itch. However, like so much in this enigmatic disease, it isn't quite as simple as that. In fact, a proportion of MASLD patients do show some injury to their bile ducts and, in some patients, this can be associated with typical cholestatic blood tests (elevation of alkaline phosphatase) and symptoms such as itch. It isn't clear whether having a cholestatic element to MASLD increases the risk of progression (probably not) and changes disease treatment (again probably not) but if cholestatic symptoms such as itch are there then they are an important aspect to quality of life. This importance comes partly from the nature of the symptoms and partly from the fact that itch both has a knock-on effect for other symptoms (interfering with sleep and contributing to fatigue, making people feel self-conscious and interfering with social activity etc) and is relatively straightforward to treat. It is, in essence, a symptom "quick win". We will discuss treatment options in the next few paragraphs, but the "short version" is that treatments that are effective for cholestatic itch in conditions such as PBC are also effective in cholestatic itch in MASLD.

The itch in PBC and MASLD patients is different in character to that seen in settings such as allergy or eczema. It also, importantly, needs to be treated using specific approaches rather than with the antihistamines typically used in allergy. Cholestatic itch is often described by patients as being "deep under the skin" with "creepy crawlies" there and is often made worse by a hot bath. Its characteristics are, therefore, very different to allergic itch which tends to affect the surface of the skin. The body distribution is also characteristic, with affected areas including the soles of the feet and the palms of the hands, as well as the scalp. Perhaps inevitably, the first thought of clinicians is that itch has a skin cause rather than being a feature of a distant disease process. Cholestatic liver disease patients do not, however, have any rash or skin abnormality (other than where they cause skin damage through scratching) and the absence of rash should always make clinicians think of another cause. The severity of cholestatic itch ranges from a mild sensation which is present, but which does not warrant treatment, all the way through to a life-altering, very severe symptom. Fortunately, the former is far commoner than the latter in MASLD.

The actual cause of itch in cholestasis remains unclear. The response to treatment, however, gives us some clues. The most striking response to treatment is that seen following liver transplantation. Itch disappears immediately (patients tell us it has gone by the time that they wake up after the operation) and, in our experience, rarely, if ever, comes back. This suggests that a fully functioning liver clears whatever it is that causes itch (or at least sets off the chain of events that leads to itch) very quickly. We also know that an approach called naso-biliary drainage, in which a tube is used to drain the bile from the bile duct out of the body, is also highly effective. These two observations point to something which is present in the bile contributing directly to itch. Furthermore, the first-line treatment for itch is a drug called cholestyramine which acts, within the bowel, to bind bile acids and prevent them from being taken back up at the end of the small bowel (the ileum) and recycled to the liver. To take the bile link further, one of the new classes of itch treatment which has been successful in trials in PBC is a drug which specifically blocks the uptake of bile acids within the ileum. These observations all point to bile acids either being directly responsible for itch or acting as triggers for the itch pathway. Whatever the underlying cause of the stimulation, the actual sensation of itch is mediated by activation of nerve receptors in the skin which then signal to the brain. Interestingly, drugs that block the actions of opiates (the morphine family of pain killers which are also present in the natural state in the body to act as an internal pain control system) are effective for PBC itch, suggesting that the activation of nerve sensors in the skin may be via natural opiates.

We take a stepwise approach to itch management in liver disease. The first step in managing itch is to understand whether treatment is needed at all! For many people, understanding that itch is part of the disease, and is treatable if needs be, is enough. The art with controlling itch is to be able to forget about it or block it out. The brain has highly developed pathways to prevent sensory overload by information coming from the skin; none of us normally thinks about being able to feel our clothes on our skin, yet once you do think about it you can indeed feel them. This continues for a few minutes until you "forget" about the sensation again. The art with itch treatment is therefore to help people to get to the point where they can forget about the sensation. Awareness of itch during normal activities, the need to scratch and significant itch at night are the features that suggest treatment may be necessary. Sleep disturbance from itch can be a particular issue as it can have knock on effects in terms of fatigue and cognitive symptoms. The issue of night itch is partly a result of the symptom being worse at night, and partly the lack of other daytime distractions at night, meaning that the brain has less in the way of other stimuli to focus on.

Before moving to drug-based therapy many patients try moisturising creams and vitamin E cream. These have never been formally tested in clinical trials, but they are very safe and as this is a purely symptom issue (the only goal is symptom control as disease risk is managed via different routes) if they work for a patient then they are effective. One preventative step that patients can take is to avoid opiate painkillers (e.g., codeine phosphate, dihydrocodeine, morphine etc). These can add to the level of activation of the body's own opiate signalling system, which, as we have discussed, probably signals itch in the skin.

First-line treatment for itch, once a decision has been taken to go down the medicine route, is cholestyramine. This is the only licensed drug for itch related to liver disease and has the advantage of being very safe (it stays in the bowel and has its actions there). It is, however, limited in its actions and can be unpleasant to take (it has a bitter taste and an odd texture). We suggest to people to try adding fruit juice to it (it comes as sachets that are mixed into a drink) or chill it in the fridge before use; both of which patients describe as making it more palatable. The use of cholestyramine as first line treatment for liver itch, rather than antihistamines (the type of medicines and skin creams easily available for itch due to allergy and inflammation), often comes as a surprise to doctors. In fact, antihistamines are to be avoided in patients with liver disease for two reasons. The first is that they do not particularly work in this setting. The second is that they are even more sedating in liver patients than is normally the case (and sedation is their commonest side-effect). The one time we use antihistamines in liver patients with itch is in people with real difficulty in getting to sleep because of the itch. In this situation the sedating property is quite useful! When they are used, people need to be careful about hangover effects. They can be slow to clear from the circulation in people with cholestasis, meaning that if they are taken late at night they can still be acting in the morning. Something to be very cautious about if you are driving to work….

If cholestyramine is not effective, or people simply can't tolerate it, and itch is severe enough, then consideration should be given to second-line itch therapy. It is important for patients to understand, though, that although none of the second-line drugs are particularly risky as such, they do have more in the way of side-effects than cholestyramine. Using them means that the stakes are rising. Practice differs from centre to centre, but our preferred second-line therapy is a drug called rifampicin. This is an old antibiotic, originally used for the treatment of TB and still used for preventing disease in the contacts of people with bacterial meningitis. Its actions in the liver are unrelated to its antibiotic actions. Rifampicin represents a clear step up in both potency and potential side effects compared to cholestyramine. It is, therefore, important to be certain that cholestyramine is not effective before moving on. All too often, we see patients with "intractable itch" who, in practice, have only had a couple of days or weeks here and there with treatments. In almost all these cases, going back to the beginning and using the earlier therapies again, but properly this time, results in good itch control. The issue with rifampicin is that it can (rarely) cause liver injury. This is not particularly worse in liver patients than it is in patients getting the drug for other reasons, but the concern about additive injury is obvious. The good news is that the injury, if it happens, settles down very quickly if rifampicin is stopped. We start people on a low dose (150mg (1 tablet) daily) and check liver blood tests at 2-4 weeks. If there has been a deterioration, in particular a rise in ALT or bilirubin, the rifampicin should be stopped, and the blood tests watched until they return to the levels they were before it was started. If the blood tests are fine (as they usually are) then we monitor the effect on itch. If it isn't controlled completely, we slowly increase the dose as far as 600mg daily (4 tablets). If we get good control of the itch at a lower dose, then there is no need to keep increasing the dose. In our experience, about half of patients get good control just on the lowest "test" dose of 150mg. One thing we always warn people about with rifampicin is that it can colour urine, sweat and even tears pinky-orange; a real surprise to people who are not expecting it. Although this discussion of side-effects might give the impression that rifampicin is a problem drug this would not be correct. For most people it is a safe and very effective treatment for itch, and it is our "go to" treatment once cholestyramine has failed. The other good news with rifampicin is that, unlike some drugs, the effect does not appear to "wear off" over time. We have patients who have been on the same dose of rifampicin, with complete control of their itch, for more than 20 years. In fact, the one thing we always tell people is, if the drug is working and there are no problems with it, DON'T FIDDLE WITH THE DOSE. We have seen several people who, after a long time on rifampicin with good itch control, wondered if the itch had in fact gone away and tried stopping the drug. The itch then comes back and appears to no longer respond as well to rifampicin.......

In our experience, most liver patients get good itch control with either cholestyramine, rifampicin, or a combination of both. There are, however, a small number of patients who do not get good control. We run a specialised service for itch so see patients from all over the country, meaning that we have more experience of this than most. If people are struggling with the simple therapies, it is worth revisiting the diagnosis and checking whether it really is liver itch. If it is, then this is probably the time to get expert advice.

## CHAPTER 12: **LIVING WITH MASLD**

### *The 2-Minute Version*

- At present, we do not have a cure for MASLD, although it is, in theory at least, controllable. This means that patients need to learn to live with their disease, understand the ways in which they can control it and ensure that it does not take over their lives. We call this "owning the disease" and it can be really empowering for people. If you own the problem, you can also own the solution.
- There are three critical aspects to "owning" your MASLD. The first is to understand it and the reasons why issues arise. You are reading this book so that's a great start!! The second is to not be shy about asking your doctors about your level of disease activity and making sure you get the best control possible. Do not die of not wanting to challenge your doctor.
- The third, and critical, aspect is that the most effective ways of controlling MASLD over the medium to long term involve lifestyle change. Diet and exercise. Remember that if you, as the majority of MASLD patients do, have metabolic syndrome as well as MASLD, then the lifestyle intervention will be effective for conditions such as type 2 diabetes. "Buy one/get one free" for disease control!
- Lifestyle change to control MASLD is what it says. A long-term change to what you eat and to your exercise habits. There is no "quick fix". Crash diets offering rapid weight loss seem highly attractive, but in reality, are probably the worst thing you can do as the metabolism changes make things worse not better in the long term.
- MASLD is a disease which typically "grumbles along" causing ever-accumulating damage to the liver over many years. What this means is that it really is a disease where it is important to bring it under control and then keep it under control. This maintenance of control is not just for a year or two but for ever. The person who has most to gain from good control, and most to lose if that control slips, is you, so make sure you know exactly where you are in terms of the activity of the disease and the aims of treatment. Own the problem and own the solution.
- The lack, in MASLD, of many of the acute features of liver disease that alert people to a significant problem means that it is easy to

under-appreciate the problem. "It's not that bad" can be an excuse to put off lifestyle modification until next year (or the year after). That can be the pathway to irreversible liver damage.

- It is important to know, and understand, the options for management, and the strengths and weaknesses of the various approaches and agents. MASLD (and the risk of MASLD) is a lifelong condition. Even if you do manage to fully control it, it is still "there" in terms of risk of recurring and what you need most of all is a management approach that works for you (both in terms of its effect on the disease and its acceptability to you in terms of side effects). It is worth putting the time and effort in, with your doctor or specialist nurse, early in the disease to find the optimal long-term approach for you. Get it right at the beginning and it tends to stay right in the longer term. Be very clear though, lifestyle modification is going to be a key part of it.
- The contribution you can make to fatigue control is enormous (much more so than any drug treatments). Steps you can take include learning to pace yourself (use energy wisely) and to arrange your days so important things are scheduled for the morning when energy levels are normally at their highest.
- It is critically important that you maintain your social networks. This includes carrying on working wherever possible. Cutting yourself off from the world can save energy, but it usually makes quality of life worse and is a false economy.
- Many things that people think are problems in MASLD are not at all. This includes pregnancy (with one or two important caveats) and taking most drugs for other diseases. There are a lot of myths out there so check these things with your doctor.
- Women get MASLD as well as men. The impact is slightly different. The treatment is the same for men and women.
- Across the world there are many patient support groups who do an excellent group supporting and advising liver disease patients and supporting the research efforts aimed at better understanding of the disease and improved treatments.
- DON'T FORGET TO LIVE YOUR LIFE!!!

MASLD is a condition that is not, currently at least, curable. It is also not a condition that resolves spontaneously. This means that, for most people diagnosed with MASLD, they will have the condition for the remainder of their lives. MASLD is, however, a condition that can be controlled, and potentially reversed with good and early lifestyle change, and with which people can, and do, live a completely normal life. Learning to live with MASLD, and the approach that you take to living your life is, therefore, of the greatest imaginable importance. In our experience it is quite simple. The patients who want to do everything that they can to control the condition and its impact are the people who do best; the people who live the longest and have the best quality of life. Doctors, nurses, and other healthcare professionals can help, but ultimately you yourself determine what happens to you. The many excellent patient groups who support people with liver disease, or associated problems like type 2 diabetes, can also provide valuable contributions. We did feel, however, that it was important to include this chapter to help people who are perhaps struggling to "get started". These are our purely personal views on the steps that we think people can take to make a difference for themselves.

## *OWN THE PROBLEM*

One of the most common phrases that we end up using in clinic with patients is "in life we have to play the hand we are dealt". What is meant by this is that if you have been diagnosed with MASLD there is nothing you can do about it other than get on with controlling it and living with it. Whether or not there was anything you could have done to prevent it is, in a way, immaterial as you cannot go back in time. All you can do is look forward and get on with dealing with it. "If only…." is a sentiment that really doesn't take you anywhere.

There are three ways of looking at it that are quite useful. The first is that although no one wants to be diagnosed with an illness, if you have MASLD, and it is not diagnosed, it doesn't mean that you don't have the condition! A tree that falls over in a forest with no one there does still make a noise. The good news about having the diagnosis is that it allows us to, collectively, get on with managing it, and we know that the earlier interventions are started the more effective they are. If you had MASLD and it hadn't been diagnosed it would actually have made things worse for you! The second, hopefully helpful, way of looking at it is, that if you have the symptoms of MASLD, and have been struggling to understand them, a diagnosis gives you an explanation. The symptoms are real, and the diagnosis of MASLD goes a long way to explaining them. Telling people this makes them realise that they are not alone, and not "going mad". The third helpful way of looking at it is that if you are going to be diagnosed with a condition, then at least be diagnosed with one which is reasonably well understood, and for which there is good evidence to suggest that you can improve it with lifestyle changes. It may not always feel an easy thing to do, but you have the opportunity, with knowledge and support, to be able to make a real improvement in your disease process.

One of the best life coaches we have heard talk to people about managing challenges is Paul McGee (if you haven't heard him talk or read his book then you should). He is also called the SUMO guy. His mantra is Stop, Understand and Move-On. This is perfect advice to take after a diagnosis of MASLD. Take a pause, understand what it is and what it means and take control of what you and your clinical team are going to do about it. Most of all, don't feel sorry for yourself. That will achieve nothing.

## *OWN THE SOLUTION*

One area where you can make an enormous difference to your care is by understanding what the level of disease activity is, and how it is responding to lifestyle changes and treatment of diabetes, if applicable. Increasingly this will include the use of the licensed drugs that are beginning to emerge.

One thing that is different about MASLD compared to other forms of liver disease is that, for many patients, they are not under the care of a liver doctor. Some people will have never even seen a liver doctor. The diagnosis may have been made by the GP, a hospital doctor from another specialty, or as part of related disease, such as diabetes surveillance. Some people are told they have MASLD, but given no further information, (other than to lose weight!) with no follow-up plan. Does that matter? Yes, it does, for several reasons. The first reason is that the level of disease activity should be assessed, and if severe enough to be progressing towards cirrhosis, then this needs monitoring by a liver team for the complications of cirrhosis. The second reason is that, without monitoring such as blood tests, it can be difficult to know whether any lifestyle changes are effective. This is so important, as it can help to reinforce the benefit of these changes. Another reason is that it may be possible to participate in drugs trials for MASLD, or to obtain newly licensed drugs, that may only be accessible if you are "in the system".

It doesn't particularly matter, therefore, where your monitoring happens, whether it is through the GP, diabetes clinic or hospital, but it is important that it does happen. It is equally important that you are kept informed of the results. Some people find it helpful to keep a record of the relevant blood tests or investigations that can give an indication as to how the disease is progressing over time. Ensuring ongoing follow-up and monitoring is therefore one of the key ways you can "own the solution". The fact that you are reading this book demonstrates that you are already well down that route!

We know that the quality of care for all types of liver disease can differ hugely between countries, and between centres within countries. This is not unique to MASLD, but typical of the challenge faced by everyone with liver disease. One of the challenges with liver disease is that it is a rapidly developing area, with increasing numbers of patients being diagnosed every year. This is particularly the case with MASLD which is, in practice, the most recently recognised of the major liver diseases (it has always been there, but we have only relatively recently recognised its importance). The scale of this effect often surprises people. PBC, the subject of the first book in this series, was first described in the 1850s. MASLD was first described, in contrast, less than 20 years ago. A recently described, fast developing disease area can challenge the knowledge base of non-specialist doctors. Depending on when they completed their training, many doctors may have received no training at all in relation to MASLD. Furthermore, given the time taken for medical textbooks to be published, they are in many ways out of date before they come out. All this combines to mean it can be very difficult for doctors to know what they should know about MASLD. Perhaps they should read this book!

Given, therefore, that the experience, level of interest and knowledge of both GPs and hospital doctors, and thus quality of care, can differ widely, how can you make sure that you get the best possible care? The answer is, don't be shy! Another of our sayings is that in a consultation with a doctor about your MASLD there are two people in the room, one of them with much more invested in the conversation than the other! Make sure that you get what you want and need out of it. In simple and stark terms **don't die from not wanting to upset your doctor.** We always feel that this is one area where the UK can learn from America. American liver disease patients are much more likely to push to get what they want. There are two important things that you can do to make sure that you get the best possible care. These are to understand your test results and what they mean, and to raise symptoms as an issue (if you have a problem with them) if the doctor or nurse doesn't ask about them.

Knowing your test results, and what they mean, is probably one of the most important bits of advice in this book. Ultimately, it is you and your loved ones that have the most to gain from good disease control, and most to lose by poor control. It is, therefore, in your interests to be aware of your disease state and to question actions taken. Ultimately, if things are not going well, the sooner you know the sooner you and your clinical team can make changes. In the worst-case scenario, issues are only recognised when it is too late to make a meaningful difference. Avoid this at all costs. Actually, understanding test results in MASLD is reasonably straightforward. The ones to be aware of (and understand) are blood tests and fibroscan. Whilst you are taking control of your MASLD, also take the opportunity to know and understand your blood tests that relate to heart disease risk (most obviously cholesterol) and diabetes (HbA1C)!

In terms of MASLD blood tests the most important to be aware of are your ALT, or the almost equivalent AST. If these are normal it is reasonable evidence to suggest that there is relatively little liver injury going on. Conversely, if one or both is elevated then it is likely that the disease is active and thought needs to be given to what more can be done to bring it under better control. If you have cirrhosis, then there are additional blood tests that you need to be aware of. These are bilirubin (elevated levels suggest issues with the function of the liver) and albumin (lower levels suggest issues). With all the blood tests in MASLD the link between them and what is happening in the liver is rather indirect. Watching trends over time is what matters rather than any particular value on any particular day. To plot trends many people find it useful to make a note of their tests or even to plot them out on graph paper.

The other test "number" to be aware of is the fibroscan value. This is a measure of how "solid" the liver is and, to a significant degree "solidity" equates to fibrosis or scarring. A normal liver has a value of around 4 whilst a cirrhotic liver will have a value of above 20. Values in between suggest some degree of fibrosis. Again, it is trends over time that matter rather than a one-off value. In many ways, for example, a value that jumps from 4 to 8 over the space of a year is a much more worrying finding than a value of 10 that has been unchanged for years.

A doctor who knows what they are doing will know the importance of tracking tests and will know the results of the tests (and have suggestions for the plan as to what to do). If you ask for your test values (and you should, every time you come to the clinic), that the doctor or nurse can tell you the answer immediately should reassure you that they have all aspects of disease management under control. The story one of us (DJ) always tells doctors in training is about the rock band Van Halen and the brown M & M sweets. It is part of rock and roll folklore (although on this occasion, and unlike much folklore, it is actually true!) that Van Halen required a bowl of M & Ms in their dressing room with all the brown ones taken out. This is always cited as the ultimate example of rock and roll decadence (and found its way into the film "This is Spinal Tap"). Nothing could be further from the truth. They were using it as a simple way of assessing attention to detail. If a concert venue had paid enough attention to detail to take the brown M & Ms out as instructed, then it is very likely they also paid attention to detail about stage safety and lighting; things that could put the band at risk if done incorrectly. The brown M & Ms are a "bell weather". In MASLD knowing a key test value is the equivalent of the brown M & Ms. If your doctor or nurse knows your value, they are likely to be doing other key things correctly as well.

The other thing to discuss with your doctor or nurse is symptoms. The issue of symptoms and their impact on quality of life is often underappreciated by doctors and nurses. The major issue is with fatigue, although mood problems can also arise. Fatigue is not directly treatable with a specific drug, but there is an approach that can certainly improve quality of life in relation to it.

## *DIET, EXERCISE AND MASLD*

The most obvious and important aspect of "owning the solution" in MASLD is through lifestyle management. We can't emphasise enough how critical this is. In early or mild MASLD you, quite literally, have your future in your hands. We have explained in **Chapters 3, 6** and **7** the reasons it is important, and the detail as to what you can and should do. In this chapter we are going to give a real-life perspective. We hope to give you some encouragement and practical help about things that aren't easy for most people. We know because we have been there ourselves.

Two of the most asked questions patients ask of their doctors are "why did I get this" and "what could I have done to prevent it". The answer to the first question is, in broad terms, for reasons completely beyond your control. Genes handed down by your ancestors are key in many diseases, but there is nothing you can do to change your parents (although our children frequently wish they could!). Fate also plays a big part. Wrong place at the wrong time. Sometimes people end up taking drastic steps to try and reduce their risk of things like infection (we saw this with COVID), but this too is full of risks to mental and physical health (we again saw this with COVID). It is an interesting observation that many doctors are risk takers. Drink too much, ski too fast etc. An element of this is fatalism. Ultimately, if you don't live your life now there is a risk you will never get to live your life at all. Morbid but true.

Even for many diseases that are avoidable by sensible adjustments to life there is a disconnect between the timing of the risk and that of the consequence. Lung cancer would be almost completely avoidable if people didn't smoke. The problem is that when you develop lung cancer it is too late to stop smoking. The damage is, sadly, already done and we can't go back in time. In liver disease we see this in the setting of hepatitis C infection. Many patients with hepatitis C were infected in the setting of iv drug abuse. Totally avoidable, but by the time you have the liver disease it is too late (although, of course, avoiding injecting drugs after it has been successfully treated will prevent you from getting it again……a lesson that some people fail to heed). And then we have MASLD………

Perhaps more than any other disease (with the exception of alcohol-related liver disease, although the issues around alcohol addiction are always in the background with this) MASLD is one where we know who is at risk with more than enough time to prevent it, and once it develops there is a significant time-window to reverse it. All those other people with all those other diseases are wishing that they could go back in time and do something different. **With MASLD you have that chance. DON'T WASTE IT.**

**Exercise:** We are going to make a very bold statement now. If you do an appropriate amount of exercise at least 3 times a week from now on, and lose a meaningful amount of weight then you WILL control your MASLD, you WILL significantly improve your type 2 diabetes and hypertension (if you have them) and probably reduce the number and the doses of the tablets that you take and you WILL feel much better (with less fatigue and more energy). **In simple terms you will get your life back.**

Many doctors will say these things (although usually with a few more ifs and buts put in than we have). We suspect that peoples' response to this is with two thoughts. The first is that it is "easy for you to say that". The second is "but what do you actually mean". In a way these questions approach the same issue from slightly different directions. When we talk about an appropriate amount of exercise, we mean at least half an hour three times a week (more if you can) and at a level that will change your body metabolism. As we discussed in **Chapter 7** you can gauge this in several different ways. One is through heart rate monitoring (simpler and cheaper than you may think; this type of technology is cheap and effective these days). Even simpler is to exercise to a level where you wouldn't be able to keep up a conversation with a person next to you. People often worry about the type of exercise. In fact, this probably matters less than you think, although a mixture of cardiac work (bike, walking, running etc) and resistance (weight training in its various forms) is probably ideal. There are two traps with exercise. The first is that, especially if walking is your chosen approach, the speed you walk at is a key issue. It is possible to walk all day and not change your metabolism if you walk slowly. Remember the rule about not being able to talk to someone next to you. Incidentally, this is also one of the reasons why golf isn't the best exercise option. Too much stopping and starting (and if you ride on a buggy, no use at all!). The second trap is that the more you exercise the fitter you get. This means that you need to exercise more or faster progressively to change metabolism. It may feel that this is making life hard but remember, it shows that it is all working! The way to avoid the 2 exercise traps is to work out your programme of exercise and then time yourself. As you get better, extend the programme. If you walk or jog, have a route that you do (not every time but every so often) that can act as your "benchmark" for speed. You will be amazed at how quickly you get fitter. This is a sign that it is all working!!

Perhaps the major challenge with exercise in the real world is not starting a programme (that can feel like a barrier but can be overcome) but sustaining it. Gyms are typically busy in January and empty by April when all the New Year resolutions have been broken. You are going to need to sustain it, however. It is going to be (literally) lifesaving for you. The other two things that get in the way, in our experience, are the weather, and work and family. Starting an exercise programme based on fast walking in June evenings can be a real pleasure. In December in the dark when it is cold and raining it is less attractive as a proposition. One way around this is to have a range of different exercise approaches (swimming and indoor cycling as well as walking) that allows you to swap based on the weather. At all costs keep going. Another way around is to reward yourself for each exercise session (not with food though!!). Put £5 in a jar and then treat yourself when the jar is full. It is your reward for working hard. One other tip is not to punish yourself if you have a week off. It isn't the end of the world. Just set a date, restart, and get it back in the groove. The other barrier is work. Shift work, working long hours and doing two jobs make exercise time a real luxury. One of the ways around this is to fit exercise into your daily life. As we mentioned earlier, one of our colleagues used the expression "movement as medicine". The fixed 30-minute exercise session is one way of doing it, but another is to do small chunks of exercise that all add up. Walk up the stairs, park the car a bit further away from the shops, get off the bus a stop or two early. It all adds up. An obvious question people ask with this is- how do I know I am doing enough exercise if I can't time it? This is where the step-counting technology comes in. If you do 10,000 steps a day for each of your exercise days then that counts (although remember the speed issue). We will give you an example of the use of this approach. One of us (DJ) used to fly a lot before the pandemic. A whole day of travelling involved a lot of sitting down on planes so how to do 10,000 steps? Simple, rather than go on the moving walkway I walked everywhere in the airport. 10,000 steps would come up in no time and I ended up moving through the airport quicker than I would otherwise have done. Instant exercise. Just like magic!

Our final comment on exercise is that there are lots of "instant experts" out there who will tell you what you must do, where you must do it, what expensive equipment you should buy and what specialised clothes. These are all just opinions. What you need to do is work out what works for you and your family, check that it is at the right level using our simple guide about being able to talk and/or heart rate monitoring, and get going.

**Diet:** We have gone into a lot of detail earlier in this book about diet, how it can drive MASLD and how change to the diet can control it. The types of food you eat (with culprits being trans-fats and fructose) and the timing and combinations are really important. There is, however, a simple and basic truth about diet, based on the laws of physics. These say, in simple terms, that matter (in this setting food) and energy (what powers your muscle) are essentially the same thing. Energy can only come from matter and once it is converted into energy it ceases to exist as matter. What this means in MASLD is that a balance between the energy you take in in the form of food, and the energy you consume through the function of the body ("ticking over" of body functions) and the increase in energy consumption with exercise needs to be struck. If you consume more energy than you burn, then the body will store it. Eventually this will be as fat, either directly in the liver itself, or as part of the other fatty tissues. Yes, genes come into it (are you a highly efficient energy "hoarder" who is therefore prone to lay down fat, or are you are an inefficient energy "burner" who can eat more and never put weight on), but fundamentally diet must come into disease management.

Does all this mean that if you have MASLD you should go straight onto a calorie-controlled diet then? Well, it isn't quite as simple as that. A long-term, sustained reduction in food intake, coupled with a change in the types of food that are eaten as outlined in **Chapter 6**, to minimise the degree of fat deposition in the liver and elsewhere in the body, is clearly an important part of MASLD management. Unfortunately, in the real world, people don't "work like that". We are bombarded with different diet types, often with a glossy book you can buy that explains them, and a (sometimes expensive) subscription meal plan. Rather as was the case for gyms at New Year, people embark on rapid weight loss full of good intentions. They are often rewarded by a rapid reduction in weight (although, sadly, this is usually initially just fluid and glycogen stores rather than fat). The problem is sustaining it week in and week out. You are working late and the only food available is chocolate from the vending machine……. We have all been there. The diet falls apart and all the weight goes back on.

This cycle can be very negative for two reasons. The first is the obvious psychological one. No one likes to feel that they have failed and for some reason a diet going wrong seems to be more negative for people than an exercise plan going the same way. The second aspect of the negative cycle is even more important. In the west we live in a world where energy- rich food is easily available, and in essentially limitless quantities. This was not the case even in the western world until the last few decades (and still isn't today in much of the world). We evolved as a species, however, over millions of years in a world where food was very limited indeed and had to be caught and killed or farmed without any labour saving tools. Food was therefore very valuable indeed. In (very) simplistic terms, if genetic variants arose that meant that people were much more efficient at using all the food they caught or farmed and could hoard every last bit of it in the form of fat which their body could then access when food wasn't easily available, it would give them a survival advantage compared to people whose metabolism was more "wasteful" of energy. In our simple model, a genetic pattern that was highly advantageous in past millennia (and was as a result enriched in the population), combined with a world where food is freely available is the fatal combination that gives rise to MASLD. It is telling that in a number of low- and middle-income counties that are developing (and thus becoming more affluent) very rapidly indeed, the rate of increase of MASLD is startling (and likely to present a significant future public health challenge).

What has all this got to do with dieting? In our simple model, we are genetically programmed to act like we are always on the point of having no food and, as a result, to hoard what we have. When we diet, this, in metabolic terms, mimics starvation through an absence of food and, in fact, augments the energy efficiency and hoarding responses. In essence, dieting makes the tendency to MASLD worse. This isn't an issue if energy intake continues to be restricted, but once you give up the diet there can be an overshoot, and you end up in a worse position than the one you started from. Basically, to diet and lose weight but then stop the diet and put the weight back on, leaves you worse off than if you hadn't dieted in the first place (and the more extreme the diet the more marked this effect is).

What is the answer? There are two simple and practical answers, a more involved one and then there is hope for the future. We will look at these in turn. The first practical answer is to try and get into a mindset that one bar of chocolate doesn't mean the whole diet "house of cards" must collapse. It isn't that bar of chocolate that is the problem (the direct effects of that will pass soon enough), it is what you do the next day and the day after that. If you are dieting, and have a bad day, don't hate yourself and give up, restart the diet the next day. Be positive not negative. The second practical answer is exercise. If the default mode of the genetic make-up of people with MASLD is to hoard food for the future, there is one thing that seems to stop that. Exercise and its energy requirements seem to trump energy hoarding. Presumably, in evolutionary terms, there was greater advantage conferred by being able to continue to hunt or forage for food than there was by conserving energy. What this means in MASLD is that you shouldn't think of diet and exercise as independent approaches to treatment. **It is the combination that is most effective**. Don't therefore think, when exercising, about the "number of calories that you burn". This can be rather dispiriting and misses the key point that exercise probably has its main actions through a switching effect on metabolism rather than simple energy consumption.

## *SELF-MANAGEMENT FOR FATIGUE*

In **Chapter 12** we discussed the approach to living with fatigue. A key component of this is the coping strategies to help minimise its impact. These are entirely in your hands and are helpful. These are the key things to think about

*1) Treat energy as a valuable commodity and use it wisely:* Pacing of your activity is a critical element of managing fatigue. It is important not to "wrap yourself in cotton wool". By the same token, however, using energy wisely allows you to make sure you do the most important things. Think of energy as you would do money. Save it when you can and make sure you get the best value for money when you do spend it.

*2) Understand and use the rhythm of the disease:* Fatigue in MASLD characteristically gets worse as the day goes on. This means that mornings are the best time to get things done. The corollary is that evening working, and, in particular, night shifts, can be very challenging indeed. If you have important meetings or engagements, try and organise them for mornings. If your work pattern involves evenings and nights, then speak to your employer about changing your work pattern. The other aspect to disease rhythm is to accept that there will be good days and bad days. If you are having a bad day, be philosophical, don't fight it and focus on the likelihood that tomorrow will be better. The same "tomorrow is another day" mindset is important when your diet slips, or when you can't exercise. You can pick it all up again tomorrow.

*3) Keep your social structures:* One of the really striking findings from our research on fatigue in liver disease is that being fatigued isn't automatically associated with poor quality of life. In fact, there is a group of people with significant fatigue who feel that their life quality is good despite their symptoms. What this group have in common is strong social networks. In contrast, people who have become isolated feel the symptom much more and their quality of life is worse. What does this mean in practice? What we often come across is people who try and save energy by changing their lifestyle, reducing or stopping their work, not going out and meeting friends etc. What our findings suggest is that this is almost always a false economy. This may save some energy, but there is a price to pay in terms of overall life quality. The message we give to patients is to keep doing things! Adapt what you do to your capability, but doing things remains really important. DJ knows a patient who used to go rambling with friends. She found this increasingly difficult with her liver disease, and that she was being left behind. What she did, however, was not to give up going but to meet people at the end of the walk, walk a short distance to meet them and then join them for coffee. A sensible compromise.

Many patients also get benefit from digital media based social networking. This can be of real use to people with profound fatigue and, of course, became a lifeline during self-isolation during the COVID-19 outbreak.

## *PATIENT SUPPORT GROUPS*
Around the world there are many patient support groups that do an excellent job in helping MASLD and other liver disease patients with the practical and emotional problems that can arise with their diagnosis. They are also great champions for research aimed at improving understanding of liver disease and its treatments and advocates for patients and their rights. We strongly encourage all patients to contact their own national or regional support group.

## *GENERAL HEALTH*
There are several other aspects of living with MASLD which are not well covered in medical textbooks (and certainly not on the internet!) and where people can, as a result, end up getting the wrong information. We will cover a number of these in this section.

*1) Are there any supplements I should be taking?* If you get the diet right this shouldn't be needed, except for vitamin D in times of low sun exposure. However, the natural antioxidants in the body, which reduce the impact of tissue injury, are reduced in chronic liver disease and many patients take an antioxidant and multivitamin preparation (easily available in pharmacies and supermarkets). The same effect can be achieved, however, by a healthy diet from a wide variety of plant, fish and animal products. In terms of supplements that are best avoided, our advice is to not take herbal medicines (in particular some of the unregulated traditional medicines). There have been cases of these being toxic to the liver.

*2) Can I take my other tablets now I have liver disease?* The issue of safety of medicines in people with liver disease is an area that causes real concern to both doctors and patients. There are, however, two potential sources of risk and not the single one that everyone worries about. The obvious risk comes from the possibility that, because of liver disease, the drug is handled differently (many drugs are cleared from the body by the liver), and this leads to either more toxicity from the drug or worsening of the liver disease. This leads to many doctors avoiding prescribing drugs to people with liver diseases such as MASLD. There is, however, and as we have already discussed, a counter-risk, which is that people end up not getting the right treatment for important illnesses because of a mild additional risk due to their liver disease. The other thing to be aware of is that the guides to prescribing, and patient information leaflets that come with drugs, very frequently talk about caution in liver disease. Sometimes this is based on examples of problems, but many times it is because we simply don't know whether there is a risk and, in the absence of being able to say there is no risk (and proving a negative is very difficult), drug companies are cautious. This can leave patients and doctors confused and worried. In our experience, issues with drug toxicity in MASLD are rare, and the risks of not getting the right treatment for another condition probably significantly outweigh the risks of a drug reaction.

Sensible practical advice would be to avoid unnecessary drugs and always keep the tablets you are taking under review with your doctor (this is general good advice; doctors have a habit of starting drugs and not getting round to stopping them, leading to over- and unnecessary treatment). Always remember, however, that not getting the right treatment can also be a risk. The other piece of general sound advice is that if you and your doctor suspect that a drug is causing significant side-effects, the first step should always be to stop it until it is clear what is going on. If the drug is for a life-threatening condition, then this decision clearly needs to be made quickly, but continuing with a drug causing significant side effects is a recipe for trouble. In our experience, where bad issues have arisen with drug side-effects it is because this basic rule has been ignored.

*3) Can I take HRT/Can I take the oral contraceptive:* HRT and the pill both contain female sex hormones. These hormones, both naturally in the setting of pregnancy and in tablet form in HRT (rarely) and the oral contraceptive pill (more commonly), can cause cholestasis with elevation of liver blood tests and itch. Cholestasis can, however, also occur in some people with MASLD. This leads to a perennial concern that HRT, or the pill might make MASLD worse. They are, however, completely different processes that aren't additive. HRT and the pill both have their risks, as well as their obvious benefits, and that balance of risk and benefit isn't particularly altered by having MASLD. Our only observation is that if HRT is being considered for osteoporosis risk reduction (as it sometimes is) there may be more effective treatments for you to consider. If it is for more general menopause symptoms, then it is something that we have seen be useful for improving overall life quality. As always, this is general advice and the pros and cons for you as an individual need to be discussed with your doctor.

*4) Is pregnancy safe?* The basic answer is yes, although there are important caveats and a need for care to be taken. It is important that having a condition such as MASLD does not rule your life. There are three areas where thought is needed. Getting pregnant in the first place, the impact of non-cirrhotic MASLD on pregnancy (and vice versa) and the issues around pregnancy and cirrhosis.

In terms of getting pregnant, MASLD can be associated with conditions such as polycystic ovary syndrome (PCOS) which is associated with reduced fertility. Advanced liver disease of all types can also be associated with fertility issues. Our standard advice for patients with liver disease applies just as much to MASLD as it does to other types of liver disease. Get the disease as close to being under complete control as you can before trying to get pregnant as that gives you the best chance (difficulty in getting pregnant can sometimes be your body's way of protecting you against the extra physiological stress of being pregnant if you are unwell and may therefore not be able to cope with pregnancy). Obviously, steps taken around getting diet and exercise right in advance of getting pregnant will also pay dividends in terms of coping with that pregnancy. One final important point is that people are, rightly, cautious about taking drugs and medicines in pregnancy. It is ideal, therefore, that the best way to control MASLD is through non-drug approaches such as diet and exercise.

In terms of disease activity and pregnancy there is some evidence of interactions. It has been suggested that the hormonal changes seen in pregnancy (release of high levels of oestrogen and progesterone) can worsen MASLD itself, although the importance of this (if any) isn't clear. Another, purely practical issue with late pregnancy can be a sheer lack of space in the abdominal cavity which contains both a pregnant uterus and, given the nature of the disease, a significant amount of fatty tissue. The other inter-relationship between MASLD and pregnancy is an association between fatty liver and both pregnancy-related liver disease and pre-eclampsia and related conditions. This area is a very complicated one, with several clinical manifestations of, essentially, the same problem, which is a failure of the placenta in late pregnancy causing issues for the mother and the baby. In terms of the baby, a failure of the placenta to provide enough nutrition for the baby is one of the causes of foetal distress and, in rare cases, loss of the baby. It is a major focus of antenatal care (and is one of the reasons why visits to the midwife increase in frequency as the due delivery date gets nearer). The failing placenta also has several impacts on the mother as the mother's body attempts to respond to the impact of the failing placenta. These include a rise in blood pressure (in essence the body tries to "squeeze" more arterial blood through the placenta and with that come risks of kidney disease and even stroke disease). The liver can also be injured with this with a number of linked conditions such as acute fatty liver of pregnancy and HELLP syndrome.

Please don't be worried about all this. None of it is a reason to think of not getting pregnant if that is the right thing for you and your family. Remember our earlier comment about not letting MASLD rule your life. Successful pregnancy in MASLD is absolutely the norm, provided three basic rules are followed:

1) Get into the best shape you can with lifestyle changes before getting pregnant and stay that way. The lower the level of fat in the liver and the degree of inflammation the less the placental stress. Getting into good shape is good for you and really good for the baby. This will also reduce the chance of developing gestational diabetes, which is a type of diabetes that develops during pregnancy. This occurs in people with the same risk factors as those

who have MASLD and type 2 diabetes and can have implications for the foetus and mother.

2) Take antenatal care seriously. All the problems outlined above can be identified in their earliest stages and managed. They can only be spotted, however, if someone is watching you carefully. This really matters.

3) Follow the old pregnancy and liver saying "if in doubt get it out" ……. What this means is that all the complications related to placental failure (be they pre-eclampsia, the impact on the baby and pregnancy liver disease) are improved by delivery. Clearly, the balance of risk and benefit in terms of early delivery will be influenced by how advanced the pregnancy is, however most of these complications accelerate towards the end of pregnancy meaning that the decision about early delivery normally becomes operative at the point where early delivery itself has the lowest risk to the baby………

The final aspect around pregnancy and MASLD (and indeed all chronic liver disease types) is the risk around cirrhosis and portal hypertension. Later in pregnancy the rise in pressure within the abdomen (a large baby in an abdomen with limited capacity to expand) can cause the pressure in the portal vein to rise. This can lead to a variceal bleed if varices are present. Standard practice is to do a routine endoscopy at around 6 months to check for varices.

*5) Can I smoke and drink alcohol?* NO and WITHIN REASON (BUT IDEALLY NOT) are the short answers here. There is no evidence to suggest that smoking is linked to MASLD. It's just that smoking is always harmful to everyone, and to people with metabolic syndrome, which is itself associated with cardiac risk, that risk is very real!! Everything we do in MASLD management is aimed at preventing the need for transplantation but if you ever did need a transplant, to be unfit for it because of smoking damage to your heart and lungs would be a disaster. Don't do it. E-cigarettes haven't been evaluated in liver disease and it is therefore difficult to give guidance. Our only practical observation is that whatever risk they may or may not have it is lower than cigarette smoking, although do themselves have health risks.

The answer regarding alcohol is more nuanced (and complex). Classical alcoholic liver disease is not related to MASLD, however, as we discussed in **Chapter 3,** alcohol can be a source of very high energy load which can drive liver fat deposition. Telling people to stop drinking just because they have liver disease is a knee-jerk reaction by doctors and serves to perpetuate the myth that there is some form of link between all liver disease and alcohol. Alcohol in small amounts is a normal part of life, and in a condition where disconnection from social structures can be an issue, it can have tangible benefits for people. Our advice for people with early MASLD (in essence people without cirrhosis) is that alcohol is fine, but the liver probably can't handle it in the same way that it can in people without MASLD, and it will certainly raise issues around nutritional load. We therefore advise no more than half the normal safe drinking limits. This effect is exaggerated in people with cirrhosis, and we would advise no more than one to two drinks per day, but ideally none. Many people with MASLD choose not to drink alcohol. That is what we would recommend to a friend with MASLD but it should be their choice.

# CHAPTER 13: AN INTRODUCTION TO MASLD IN CHILDREN AND YOUNG ADULTS

*The first book in this series, "PBC, The Definitive Guide for Patients with Primary Biliary Cholangitis" didn't have a chapter about children with the disease; PBC simply doesn't affect children (ever). The second and third books in the series, on autoimmune hepatitis (AIH) and primary sclerosing cholangitis (PSC) do impact on children and for this reason included chapters introducing the issues around childhood disease. MASLD is also a condition that really can impact on children and young adults. It is also important to note that this impact is growing very rapidly both in western countries and in rapidly developing economies, in parallel with rising rates of childhood obesity. In the AIH and PSC introduction to childhood disease sections we made an important point, that we will reiterate here. We are adult physicians and don't typically see or manage children, meaning that we don't have the experience to write a definitive patient and parent guide to MASLD in children. We do, as adult physicians, however, manage adults who first developed MASLD in childhood and we therefore know all too well the challenges that they experience. As with the earlier books we decided that it would be inappropriate to exclude childhood MASLD completely. This chapter is therefore what its title suggests it is; an introduction to the issues around MASLD in childhood from the perspective of adult care doctors to make sure that the whole spectrum of disease is discussed. If this catches your interest, there are far more qualified authors than us to provide the detail.*

Our paediatric colleagues always tell us that children are not just small adults. One scenario where this is true is in MASLD. MASLD is an important and growing cause of liver disease in children (important both because of its impact and because it is treatable by lifestyle changes (and potentially drugs, although it is important to note that resmetirom, the only as yet licensed therapy for MASLD, is not yet approved for use in children), making effective early diagnosis critically important). It also has important differences in its nature and impacts in children compared to adults. Some of these are the inherent differences of disease in childhood, and some are to do with the biology of the disease. In this chapter we will highlight the important specific issues around childhood MASLD in comparison to adult disease.

### *CLINICAL IMPACT AND THE GOALS OF TREATMENT*

At the global level, the goals of treatment for children with MASLD are the same as for adults - prevention of progression to cirrhosis and the maintenance of quality of life. At a practical level they are quite distinct and present their own unique challenges.

The first important difference is obvious; the duration of future life. A significant proportion of the patients we see with MASLD are in their 70s and above. Life expectancy even without MASLD would be around 85. MASLD management in this situation is, therefore, focused on a relatively short frame of time. A ten-year-old child developing MASLD (and shocking as this may sound it is not as uncommon as you might imagine) should have a reasonable life expectancy of 60+ years. It is essential, therefore, that the long view is taken regarding management. What does this mean in practice? The first implication is that it is maximally important to achieve and maintain disease control if possible. There can sometimes be a sense with liver diseases that there is no need to rush to bring them under control, that they take a long time to progress so we can "catch-up" with treatment at some point in the future. There is even a school of thought that fibrosis, and perhaps even cirrhosis, are reversible when you bring the disease under control. There is a final tendency for people to think that it doesn't really matter about controlling liver disease because you can "always have a liver transplant". These are all very short-sighted views indeed.

It is realistic to think of transplantation as a 20-year solution (if you do well). Towards the 20-year point more and more chronic health issues arise as graft failure begins. There is also a very real risk of disease recurrence. If the graft fails, then re-transplant is the only option. This is much more complex as a procedure (both surgically and in relation to immunosuppression) and the expected survival is less (say 10 years) with, again, a growing burden of ill health. What this all means in practice is two things. The first is that transplant is not "live saving" in the medium to long-term. In fact, it can be, compared to reversing the underlying disease, life-shortening. This is partly because of the risks of the operation and partly because of the metabolic risks of the immunosuppression tablets (remember that both tacrolimus and prednisolone worsen type 2 diabetes). The second is that, in many ways, it swaps one form of long-term chronic health problem for another. If you have a liver transplant for MASLD you don't stop coming to the hospital clinic, you just take different tablets and go to a different clinic. Sad but true.

You could ask why we are making all these points about disease horizons in a chapter on children with MASLD. It's simple. The compromises and consequences of treatment decisions vary depending on the age and the life-stage of the person concerned. For a 60 year old retired person a 20-year disease horizon may well be a very reasonable one. For a 20-year-old, with their life ahead of them, it absolutely won't be. What this means in practice is that the younger a person with MASLD is, the more important it is to address the underlying, root causes of the diseases and the less relevant "sticking plaster" solutions will be. In simple terms, just stopping advanced fibrosis evolving into cirrhosis is not enough. We must look to control the underlying disease process. This makes tackling fat through lifestyle modification essential. It is challenging in children but to not do it will condemn them to a shortened and reduced quality life with missed life chances. It's as simple as that.

## *THE BROAD IMPACT ON CHILDREN*

Whereas complicated cirrhotic MASLD is rare in children (although it does occur) the condition does have important impacts. There are two that are key. The first is that MASLD can, in all age groups, be symptomatic with, as we have discussed, fatigue as an important factor. The nature of the impact of fatigue varies, however, from person to person. It is also highly influenced by patient age. This gives rise to an important concept that we talk about which is the "function gap". In essence, the degree to which fatigue impacts on someone through the things that they are unable to do depends on what it is that they would like to, or expect to be able to, do. You don't miss things that you were never going to do. Although there are many 80-year-olds who are very active, most people would recognize that at this age people are typically slowing down and doing less. An 80-year-old who stayed at home reading a book rather than going on nights out because of fatigue would not look that different to most 80-year-olds. They may feel tired but the function loss from that tiredness may not be that great. The younger you are, however, the more you expect to be able to do and the greater the impact on life if you can't do things. A 20-year-old who can't go out and socialise is likely to really feel the impact on their life.

Depression is commonly associated with fatigue in liver disease, and many clinicians assume that people have fatigue because they are depressed. In our experience it is usually the other way around. People can get depressed because of the limitation that the fatigue places on their life; the "function gap" between what they can do and what they reasonably feel they ought to be able to do. If this gap is too large, at too early an age, then people can easily feel that their life is ebbing away. This phenomenon can reach its peak in children with MASLD, where inability to take part in the normal activities of childhood can have a real impact. This is both an impact around physical activity and one around social development, which is so important for children, but cannot be regulated or taught by adults. Due to fatigue and the hidden effects on mood and motivation, children can tend to be excluded from activities and thus social groups. Significant fatigue from MASLD in children can, therefore, impact on both physical and social development. A specific and important manifestation of this can be in lost education opportunity. Going back to the metaphorical 80-year-old we discussed earlier, the loss of social function in this setting has minimal or no impact on the future life chances. MASLD impacting on function in childhood is at the opposite end of the spectrum. The impact on education and thus life chances can be substantial. Lose out on schooling and social development through ill health and you may literally never catch up. Limiting the impact of MASLD in childhood can therefore very much be about protecting life chances.

The second important impact is through obesity. As with adults, although MASLD can occur without obesity most children with MASLD will be obese. This significantly adds to the life chance impact for children. Obesity causing MASLD is very much a "double whammy".

## *"TREATING" MASLD IN CHILDREN*

As has already been discussed, MASLD occurs due to a combination of genetic risk factors, and environment, in the form of the lifestyle factors of diet and exercise. This means it is likely that, if a child in the family is identified as having MASLD, the rest of the family will be at risk of, or already have, MASLD, due to sharing the same genetics and environment. This is one of the reasons why, unlike with other forms of liver disease, treatment of MASLD should be considered a matter for the entire family.

The second reason why treatment of MASLD should involve the whole family, is to make it effective. Without a change in lifestyle behaviour, once MASLD has got to a stage of being identified in a child, then it is very likely to progress to more serious stages of the disease. There are, at present, no drug treatments for MASLD that have been approved for use in children and, as described above, while transplant is a theoretical treatment option, this is not an option that would be anyone's choice.

Putting it bluntly, lifestyle change is the only treatment option that will improve the liver disease, potentially save the child's life, and certainly improve the child's quality of life. It is not an optional extra. Lifestyle change is something that must become a normal part of life, embedded into normal routine, so that it can be continued long-term. This is true of all patients with MASLD, but even more so for children, because they should be able to expect another 70 or more years of life. This is why it needs to involve the entire family, so that it becomes habit, without isolating one child as different. Unlike with many other forms of disease, this will enhance the health of all the family. One benefit of this approach is that seeing parents actively engage with improving their own health through lifestyle changes gives a positive example to the children of taking an active ownership of one's health. It will also signal that making these changes matter, that it's important. This attitude will then hopefully become a natural part of their own life.

Where to start? If you are reading this chapter and are a parent of a child with MASLD, you may have already had a shock with the diagnosis. Unlike with adults, where the diagnosis may have been made on routine bloods for a health check, or some other unrelated condition, children are unlikely to have fatty liver diagnosed unless they are already showing signs of related conditions, such as diabetes or obesity. This is likely to have been through a paediatric clinic, and you will hopefully have already been given some advice on lifestyle changes, and possibly some support for how to make them. As we have said, we are not paediatricians, and what follows below should be considered as, hopefully helpful, advice to be used in addition to what you have been advised by paediatricians and paediatric multi-disciplinary team members.

All the principles of lifestyle that we discussed in **Chapter 3**, the causes of MASLD, and **Chapters 6** and **7**, treating MASLD with diet and exercise, hold true for children with MASLD. The ***dietary guidance*** is just as relevant for children as it is for adults. There may be a perception that it is unsafe to restrict carbohydrate intake in children, with a low carbohydrate diet. However, the diet approach as suggested in this book, and in many of the links, includes many carbohydrates from minimally processed plant sources. It is not the case that children will come to harm from not having processed carbohydrates, as long as they are getting a good intake of varied unprocessed carbohydrates. Some of the suggested websites and links have family resources, with suggestions for things like school lunch boxes and snacks. A healthy diet for MASLD is a healthy diet for the entire family.

If you're a parent of a child with MASLD, or for older children themselves, there may be a concern that they will be stigmatised for being different; not able to eat the same foods as everyone else. There are two main reasons why this shouldn't be too much of a concern. Firstly, there are many children who follow some kind of restricted diets, some for medical reasons such as coeliac disease, some for religious reasons, and others for ethical beliefs. There is, therefore, an increasing tolerance and recognition that people have their own reasons for choosing a different dietary pattern. The second reason why it shouldn't worry you too much is, similarly to with adults, this is a lifestyle change for the long term, and an individual event or day, such as a birthday party with the inevitable pizzas, crisps, cake, and ice cream will not reverse the good that is being done the rest of the time. Having tried to provide healthy options when catering for children's parties, we know first-hand that birthday parties seem to end up with children choosing the lowest common denominator of nutritional value food, but also that birthday parties are an important part of childhood life, giving them fun, and a sense of community. Plus, a party bag that you probably wish they hadn't got…This is not the time to worry too much about what they are eating. Choose only the battles you can win.

Some of the tricks and good habits that are suggested around family eating include:
- Using smaller plates for children, so that the portion fills the plate in the same way that yours fill an adult plate.
- Eating meals at the table rather than in front of the television. Eating in front of the TV means that you are less aware of what you are eating, and more likely to overeat. Eating as a family at a table hopefully means the family will take note of the delicious home-cooked food and helps to develop an enjoyment of food. This is often the European way, where healthy food is very much enjoyed

- and appreciated, while at the same time giving family some time together to talk.
- If you are using processed foods or denser carbohydrates such as potatoes, weigh them so that you are aware of portion size. It can be surprising how little volume is required to meet the 'portion size' recommended, and how easy it can be to inadvertently overeat.

The principles of *exercise* outlined in **Chapter 7** also hold true in children. However, the implementation of exercise into children's lives needs to be done a bit differently to adults. Whereas adults will take up exercise to get fit, and we have talked about different forms of exercise and going to the gym, the emphasis is different with children. They should be exercising through a combination of activities, games, and sports, through school as well as clubs or family activity. All physical activity contributes to the health benefits of exercise. This should start from nursery onwards, when children run around the school yard playing tag, climbing up and down playground equipment, or kicking a football in the corner of the yard. Good schools will encourage this, and try and assimilate the (possibly already overweight) child who sits on a bench not joining in. One of the many devastating effects of the closure of schools during COVID was that children were deprived of this health, as well as social, requirement. As children get older, they are likely to spend less time expending energy during break time, but more time doing structured school sports. Again, a good school will provide a variety of sports in lessons, as well as extra-curricular clubs. Unfortunately, it is during school sports lessons that many children get put off exercise. Much of school sport revolves around team sports. If you are a child who is not naturally sporty or co-ordinated, being the one that "lets the team down", lets in the goal or comes last in the house running may turn a sport you don't particularly like doing into one that you hate. It can be particularly difficult for children who are already overweight. This may well limit their fitness and speed, but there is an added horror for them. Having to change for sports, or wearing a swimming costume or trunks may leave them feeling, literally, exposed, and vulnerable. They may be hyperaware of visible signs that make them stand out, such as stretch marks. All of this can lead to those children who are most at need of exercising, and developing a healthy enjoyment of it, to most dread it. If this is your child, it may be worth speaking to school to try and find a way for your child to participate in sports without them dreading it. There may be other options that don't involve team sports. Some schools may offer a variety of games options, which gives much more choice, and is likely to result in more enjoyment from sports. Which then results in more active participation and creates a virtuous cycle. We would strongly encourage you to try and help your child keep engaged with sports, it is important from a healthy liver perspective.

However, there is a third element to children's activity and exercise. The first is the playing around with other children, the second is the school sports. The third is you and your family. This is the element you have the greatest influence over. Being active as a family is invaluable for developing and maintaining health. What do we mean by being active? It may involve going for a swim at the weekend, not to do lengths as an adult would exercise, but to splash around. Go for a walk, preferably somewhere muddy, with sticks and stones and pinecones. Even grumpy teenagers tend not to stay grumpy for long when they are chasing each other with sticks or playing pinecone wars. Inviting a friend along can increase the activity exponentially. Go ice skating, walk along the beach or a river, cycle somewhere, bounce on a trampoline. As a family you can also do together more activities conventionally recognised as sport or exercise, such as doing Parkrun together, or playing badminton at a local leisure centre. Aim to build into every day an activity that gets them moving.

As children grow older, parents inevitably start to lose control over their children's activities, and their influence reduces, with greater influence coming from friends. You will not be able to stop your child from buying sweets on the way home, or a bag of chips, if that is what they choose to do. However, your influence will still go a long way, and may have more effect than you think. As long as you are still providing healthy, minimally processed food at home, and still keeping the family active, there will be liver health benefits. Being a teenager is a difficult time in life for those who have chronic disease, and trying to micro-manage your child's health is not good for either of you. Continue to provide a healthy and active family home, setting a good example yourself, and try not to worry about what happens between school and home.

We know it can be hard making changes in our own lives as adults, and for a whole family this can be even harder. For many reasons, family life can be disorderly or chaotic. There are the needs of other children to see to, other family members may have health problems too. There may be the juggle of parents' jobs, or multiple households and complex childcare arrangements. If it is your child who has MASLD, try and explain to adult members that diet and an active lifestyle isn't a burden to be imposed on the family, it is a way to an improved quality of life for all. For younger family members it won't even need to be considered as a 'treatment for MASLD'. It is just what becomes a normal routine and fulfilling part of childhood.

## *"THE SYSTEM" AND HOW IT IMPACTS ON CHILDREN*

What we see in young adults with childhood onset liver disease is a very consistent pattern. We see the same issues repeatedly. The next section is a very personal view about the issues and some thoughts (some hopefully useful ones) about what could do done better in the future. One thing we have heard many times is about the "system" and how it doesn't quite work for patients with liver disease. This is not to do with the care given, which is often exemplary, but the context and the environment. A peak time for the development of liver disease in the under 18s is in early adolescence, a difficult age at the best of times. The system manages them initially in a paediatric setting, which emphasizes young age. At a fixed point it then moves them to an adult hepatology service which emphasizes old age. One girl who was really struggling with her liver disease told DJ, vividly, about having one clinic visit in a children's clinic with Babar the elephant pictures on the wall, and the next one in a clinic where she was the youngest person in the waiting room by about 40 years, with all the patient literature talking about alcohol and the risk of viral hepatitis from IV drug use. At no point did she feel that she was looked after in an environment relevant to her or by people who "got" her. The art of adolescence is to learn to be an adult in a safe space. There are interesting examples of how to approach this in the health setting in relation to cancer management (the exemplary work of the Teenage Cancer Trust for example) and adapting and applying them to the teenage liver disease population would be a very helpful step.

Another important issue is frequent changes in the setting for care. As we write this DJ has been a consultant in the NHS for 24 years and is still looking after patients he met in his first year as a consultant, in the same clinic building. Consistency of care and familiarity with the care givers is, if there is confidence in those care givers, a recipe for good long-term care. Because of the age that children present with MASLD, and the need to move on into the adult care system at a time when people are still coming to terms with the disease, there can be real challenges. Some centres manage the transition in care very well with an overlap between paediatric and adult clinical teams, but this is probably the exception rather than the rule. One challenge can be that specialist children's care services are often based in different hospitals to those where adult care will be delivered. A healthcare system really focused on the needs of vulnerable patients would find a way to solve this issue.

The final issue we see is around the ownership of the problem. Parents naturally worry about their children (we worry about ours) and there is nothing they wouldn't do to protect them. In the setting of a long-term health problem such as MASLD, however, there can be a tendency to take over all aspects of the child's life. To overprotect. This is perfectly understandable, but it has its consequences. We see two in particular. The first is what could be called a "Peter Pan" state where the young adults coming to our clinic are still behaving like, and being treated as, children by their parents. This is an enormously difficult issue. This can lead parents to want to avoid mistakes by keeping hold of decision making and disease oversight. The problem is that this is unsustainable in the long-term as, eventually, everyone needs to take control of their own disease and its management.

Parents aren't around for ever. This issue needs to be handled in a sensitive way between the patient, the family, and the clinical team. The risk is always there so awareness of the need to avoid issues arising should be part of everyday thinking.

# CHAPTER 14: **THE FUTURE**

Sadly, none of us can see the future. If we could, we would be lying on the beach of our own tropical island wondering which yacht to take out today. Given our inability to see the future, why do we have a chapter entitled the future? What we are trying to do here is to outline how, in our view, the future needs to evolve over the next few years and how it might evolve (what needs to happen and what does happen being distinct things). We will also try to take a step back to take a broad view. To see the wood rather than the trees.

## *GETTING THE QUESTION RIGHT*

Without sounding over mystical the first and crucial thing we need to do is to work out what the question is that we are trying to answer. Without the right question we won't get a useful answer. MASLD is an area of an extraordinary amount of medical research; research that sets out to find answers. The scale of the research activity is completely appropriate given the scale of the problem, and the degree to which this is likely to grow over the next few years. Medical research doesn't just happen. It evolves and that evolution needs a starting point and a target endpoint. There are two broad approaches and directions. The first, and intuitive one, is to start with a problem and to work backwards to understand, and thus be able to address, the reasons why that problem arose. The alternative, academic, model is to start with developing an understanding of biology and use that knowledge to elucidate why a disease developed. Only then is that knowledge leveraged to develop a treatment. The limitation of the second approach is that it can end up answering the wrong question.

If you start with the science of MASLD and work from there to the clinical problem at the end of the path you reach cirrhosis. From this perspective, management of the complications of cirrhosis and preventing cirrhosis from developing in the first place are the entirely logical goals. This is very much the "traditional" model for hepatology - work out who has cirrhosis and book them in for endoscopy and an ultrasound (to look for varices and hepatocellular carcinoma respectively) and liver research (why does fibrosis develop and how can we block it).

If, however, you take the opposite approach of starting with cirrhosis as a clinical problem and working back to the beginnings of the disease to try and understand how you stop this from developing, you reach not fibrosis (which is actually a relatively late part of the pathway) or even inflammation, but fat in the liver. Much research of a very high quality has shown, beyond doubt, that many people with "simple steatosis" or fat without inflammation, will not develop significant liver disease (or probably more accurately will only develop progressive liver disease at a rate that is so slow as to be meaningless in life-risk terms). The converse, however, is that if you don't have fat in the liver, you don't have MASLD.

There are echoes of this dichotomy in how the clinical management of MASLD developed. Initially, management was focused around identifying who had advanced fibrosis or cirrhosis and managing them from a risk perspective. The nature of many of the clinical scores and tests developed in the early days reflect this. The issue was what was done with this information, and in particular how the people who were deemed "low risk" because they didn't have cirrhosis were managed. They were largely discharged from hospital care because the disease was too early to need hepatology input. The critical point was that this meant that this entirely focused on current risk (no cirrhosis means no cirrhosis complications and thus low risk) and the opportunity to reduce future risk (reverse the underlying process to prevent future cirrhosis) was missed. Even when the importance of lifestyle intervention to reduce that risk was recognised, the approaches used were cursory and put in the hands of family doctors/office physicians who were not really equipped to deliver those interventions in any meaningful way.

There is, of course, a third approach to the question which is the one that is critical to industry and that is how we can monetarise knowledge. What is the product that we can develop that we can sell? Traditionally this was drugs. More recently, tests have become big business. In recent years "apps", nutritional products, gym memberships and educational courses have become large earners. Companies with one of these products will naturally argue that this approach is the most important. Conversely, in the UK at least (this will be different in other health care systems) ordinary supportive clinical care and guidance is not monetarised. This includes most aspects of the management of cirrhosis complications. Surgical interventions (again in the UK) are mixed. Transplantation is not monetarised (you can't "buy" a donor organ) whilst bariatric surgery is available both on the National Health Service (with limitations to access and waiting times) and in the private sector (at a price but more freely available). This is not to criticise in any way commercially driven innovation (we have worked extensively and highly effectively with industry supporting the development of new therapies that have improved the lives of patients; changes that couldn't have occurred without industry involvement). It is just an important aspect that people need to consider.

Where does all this leave us? In essence we have two philosophical models. The first is developing and applying anti-fibrotic therapies which are used in patients who have inflammatory and pro-fibrotic disease (assuming that they can be identified). In this model it doesn't matter about the fat because the consequences are prevented. The second is that if you remove fat, you remove the whole problem, making the need for anti-fibrotic therapy disappear. One issue to bear in mind with these two models is that it remains far from clear what the drivers are for symptoms. Whereas developing cirrhosis is certainly associated with a worsening of symptoms, it is very likely that steatosis of the liver is also associated with some degree of fatigue. The anti-fibrotic model may leave this aspect of the disease under-treated to the disappointment of patients. It is also important to remember that interested parties will have vested interests in these two models that go beyond just what is best for patients. Governments and other reimbursement bodies who look at the numbers of patients with MASLD, and thus the potential costs of drugs, will naturally find the lower cost lifestyle interventions to reduce steatosis very attractive. In contrast, industry, who will wish to make a return on drug development costs, will find drug-based anti-inflammatory and anti-fibrotic models highly attractive.

Of course, it is not as simple as an "either/or" for the two models. This is for three main reasons. The first is that people are not usually diagnosed right at the beginning of the disease process. In practice, people can present anywhere in the pathway from simple steatosis all the way through to cirrhosis. The further along the pathway people are diagnosed the more anti-inflammatory and anti-fibrotic interventions become necessary. Clearly, anti-steatosis interventions remain important (otherwise the whole thing will recur), but the extent to which they will be sufficient in isolation becomes less and less. The second is the issue of how aggressive the disease is. We know that it can be very aggressive and rapidly progressive indeed (we have seen patients getting cirrhosis from recurrent MASLD within a year of liver transplant). By their nature, anti-steatosis interventions take time, and people with very rapidly progressive disease may not have that time. The final reason is that the logical conclusion of the "prevent and treat steatosis" model is not individual intervention but public health intervention (stopping steatosis at a population level). This is, of course, highly attractive to governments, especially if they will have to pay for health care consequences of disease. The problem is that these population interventions are, at best, limited in effectiveness and a worst counter-productive (the "nanny state"). A good question to ask is how many people who smoke don't know smoking is bad for them? We would suspect that the answer is very few, and yet people continue to smoke. The public health model around awareness and education rather fails when people know the advice already but choose to ignore it. The cycle escalates with legal restrictions with predictable consequences. In many ways COVID, and government responses to it, set this field back. Coercive public health controls imposed on the population which, it turns out, were not well thought through and were widely ignored by the lawmakers who imposed them does not help the next time we want to persuade the population to change behaviour…….

Ultimately, behaviour change will come when people truly believe that the guidance they are being given is correct and is directly applicable to them (think of all the drinkers who know alcohol is bad for them but assume it won't be them affected). This isn't usually enough, however, for long-term, even life-long behaviour change. This is why the concept of secondary gain introduced in **Chapter 7** (the benefits that you directly feel from an intervention so that you don't have to accept what a clinician says because you can see the effect yourself) is so important. In many ways, the message that "if you make this change you will feel better and be able to do more with your family in a few weeks' time" is a much easier sell to people than "if you make this change it may reduce your chances of cirrhosis in ten years' time". This is one of the reasons why the symptomatic angle to MASLD is so important. It is where the secondary gain is to be found.

## *TREATING MASLD*

Ultimately, the key questions around the aims of treatment need to be answered if we are to develop an effective treatment model to apply in practice. The over-arching concept needs to be, in our view, **early effective treatment to alter the natural history of the disease**. We believe that waiting for progression to institute treatment results in missed treatment opportunity, and is, ultimately, counter-productive for all. A second important concept will be **the right treatment given to the right patient at the right time**. There is an important concept in modern medicine which is personalisation. There is no single therapy for MASLD. Instead, there are likely to be a range of therapies which are given to different patients based on the nature of their disease. This will address the tension between anti-steatosis therapies and anti-inflammatory as both will be useful, just in different patients at different time points. Understanding this will also help with the issues of the competing liver biopsy endpoints which currently bedevil the field. Anti-steatosis, metabolic therapies should be judged in terms of their metabolic actions in clinical trials (which are, in their nature, relatively short term). Anti-fibrotic therapies should be judged in relation to fibrosis. In the Olympics we judge sprinters on how fast they run and throwers on how far they throw. The reverse would, to say the least, make no sense. This seems simple and logical but there are barriers in term of the acceptance by regulatory bodies. We suspect that this will change with time.

**Treating fat in the liver:** Reversing fat deposition must be the bedrock of MASLD treatment. Ultimately, if this is achieved early enough in the disease then there won't be a disease. There are also likely to be enormous knock-on benefits for patients in terms of reducing obesity, reducing type 2 diabetes risk and improving quality of life. It will be important to be clear in the messaging about "low risk" simple steatosis. As we have outlined in **Chapter 3** there are probably only faster and slower progression rates, with everyone with fat in their liver having some degree of progression risk. Given that the only way you would know you had a high progression rate risk would be to progress and observe the deterioration, the only logical approach will be treat all. There is, however, an important "elephant in the room". Given that significant elements of steatosis are lifestyle-related (dietary intake versus energy use) there will be, and should be, great concern about over-medicalising this and looking automatically to using drug therapy. Ultimately, steatosis is a physiological abnormality and needs to be managed physiologically (by a combination of diet and exercise). There are several arguments against making this a drug target. These include the risk of side-effects (and, as we have discussed, MASLD is inherently complicated as a part of the metabolic syndrome) and the sheer cost, which health care providers will blanche at. As therapies begin to emerge there will be an inevitable tension between health care providers and reimbursement bodies, who will be concerned about cost, and industry, who have a perfectly reasonable, but still vested, interest in therapies being used. A further aspect to this (another elephant if you like) is in relation to "ownership of the problem". Ultimately fatty liver is your problem as a patient and control is in your hands. If effective treatment depends on a drug prescribed by a doctor, then control is in their hands. This can, if we are not careful, end up absolving people of the control of their own health. Own the problem/own the solution. For all these reasons lifestyle modification should be a key intervention in all patients.

**Treating inflammation and fibrosis**: In a stratified model everyone would undertake a lifestyle programme focused on liver fat reduction, with specific therapy then being added in for higher risk patients. This is where we suspect many of the therapies in development will find their true role. Given the cardinal role of fat in the disease these second-line therapies would always be used in the context of ongoing lifestyle intervention. The critical issue will be identifying patients who need this enhanced therapy in a timely fashion (with all therapies aimed at fibrosis and its underpinning processes being much more likely to be effective if used early in the high-risk disease process). This will require the identification of biomarkers (in essence tests that allow us to identify high risk patients) that are accurate and easily available. Accuracy is key. The ideal test would identify all high-risk patients but would not lead to anyone who was not high risk being labelled as such. In practice tests are never perfect and compromise cut-offs need to be used. Get the cut-off wrong, and you either miss people who would benefit from treatment or identify and treat people who don't need it. There can be a tendency in medicine to set thresholds that ensure that no one is missed. If this is the case, and with a low accuracy test, it can be at the price of people being treated inappropriately with all the associated costs and risks. There is much focus in research on the development of new treatments for diseases. In practice it is just as important to develop the right tests to tell us how to use those treatments.

**Transplantation:** In an ideal world we would never need to transplant people for MASLD because our therapy approaches would be completely effective at preventing the disease ever progressing to cirrhosis. We don't, however, live in an ideal world. Treatments are ineffective in some people (or in the case of lifestyle change especially there can be resistance to taking them up). There is also the issue of late presentation and diagnosis. No matter how good our treatments are they won't be able to prevent cirrhosis in people who have already developed it by the point that the disease is diagnosed. We will, therefore, still be transplanting MASLD patients with cirrhosis for years to come. What future progress is therefore needed in transplant? The dominating answer is prevention of disease recurrence. MASLD frequently recurs post-transplant and often does so in a form that progresses far more rapidly than pre-transplant. The accelerated progression is likely to result from a combination of the actions of immunosuppression drugs (especially steroids and tacrolimus) combined with the increased appetite people typically have post-transplant (partly because of steroids again and partly because of the appetite suppressing effects of cirrhosis going) and the reduced mobility around the operation preventing exercise. It is critically important that we develop and apply very clear and bold lifestyle modification programmes for patients undergoing liver transplantation, ideally getting them established before the transplant (pre-habilitation). If we don't, we run the risk of "going round in circles" with people being re-transplanted for recurrent disease.

## <u>UNDERSTANDING WHY PEOPLE STRUGGLE WITH LIFESTYLE MODIFICATION</u>

It is an unfortunate reality that fatty live disease is one of the disease areas where there can be an element of patient "blaming" by doctors and others. The mindset that it is a patient's "fault" because they eat too much and don't exercise enough is an easy one to fall into (and one that, interestingly, doesn't seem to apply in other conditions where there might be regarded as a lifestyle element to risk such as COPD from smoking, or an anterior cruciate ligament knee injury from football!). We have discussed in **Chapter 3** the role played by genetic factors in MASLD risk and we don't think anyone would argue that genetic risk is something that a person brought on themselves..........It is far more positive to look forward and regard diet and exercise as areas where people can, in the future, improve their wellbeing (own the problem/own the solution). What we need to do is to try and do everything we can to support people making these lifestyle changes.

This leads to a key question which is: why, given the potential value, do people struggle with lifestyle intervention? This is not, of course, a question unique to MASLD. It could equally well apply to smokers not stopping smoking and drinkers not stopping drinking. The reality is that patients with MASLD really struggle to start diet and exercise programmes and, if they do manage to start with them, struggle to sustain them. In a "patient blaming" setting this is easy to explain. The same "weakness" that meant people got MASLD in the first place is coming into play. The patient's fault again.

We would like to put forward a different suggestion, and one that, potentially, points to a novel treatment approach. MASLD patients, in our experience, struggle to initiate and sustain behaviour change. They can't "get over the hump" and get going. The natural assumption in the "blame the patient" model is that this is the reason why they developed fatty liver in the first place. Mouse models of liver disease suggest a different picture altogether. There are several mouse models of MASLD that have been very useful in studying the impact and mechanisms of the condition as we look for treatments. It is becoming clear that, as part of the disease process, these animals also lose motivation to initiate behaviour that would previously have been normal for them (typically around looking for food if it isn't immediately obvious where it is). They have a go but quickly give up. Sound familiar? The pattern is exactly like a MASLD patient trying and failing with a diet or exercise programme. The point is that the mice were normal until they developed MASLD, and being mice, don't have any of the "personality" aspects that might lead them to behave differently. What the studies suggest is that it is the disease that is making them lack motivation, not lack of motivation making them develop the disease. Do we, in fact, have it the wrong way around?

What might this mean for patients? We know that exercise and diet prevent and treat the disease, but the disease prevents exercise and diet (in our new model at least). There is a vicious circle. Maybe this is where drugs that reduce steatosis have their use, to change the disease dynamic and allow people a window to begin their lifestyle change programme. It wouldn't be a case of drugs **or** lifestyle change, it would be drugs **and** lifestyle change, with the former facilitating the latter. In this approach drug use would be short term to help people get started. This is an unproven model now but one that is well worth exploring. If it were to be effective (and it is still obviously a big if) it would address the concern about over-medicalising the problem (drugs are the means to an end not the end itself) and the cost and side-effect risk of widespread therapy (we would probably be looking at 6 months to a year of drug therapy in people). MASLD is a condition where we feel some lateral thinking is needed, given the relative failure of the current treatment model (at the end of the day we have only one licensed therapy, only available in the

USA at the time of writing). Maybe this is one example that is worth thinking about.

### *A TREATMENT FOR FATIGUE*

We don't think it is particularly contentious to say that one of the biggest "needs" we have currently in MASLD is for an effective treatment for fatigue. This symptom blights peoples' lives and, at present, all we can do is support them to live their lives as best they can. This can be a real help for people, but it would be fantastic to make the approach entirely redundant by having a treatment that reverses fatigue in the first place. We think that a critical first step is to know what we are treating. This is partly to guide treatment development, and partly to make sure that in trials of new therapy (and new therapy won't get into clinical practice without trials) we are treating the right people. Almost certainly, fatigue comes in different forms in MASLD (central and peripheral being the obvious first split). It is likely that a treatment for one will not be a treatment for others. If we are developing and testing a treatment for central fatigue, then the trials need to be done in people with central fatigue. Central fatigue is certainly the area where we have made the most progress in terms of understanding the problem and, crucially, finding ways to measure the brain processes underpinning it in ways that can be incorporated into clinical trials. This is an area where we think there will be real progress soon. Peripheral fatigue is likely to be more difficult, and it may be that there is no specific treatment as such if it is all part of deconditioning. Exercise as part of a rehabilitation programme is likely to be key, and there needs to be progress in working out what type of exercise people need to do to help them to help themselves.

There is another major challenge regarding fatigue, however. We need to address the real issue of clinicians not recognising it for the problem that it is. It will be no good having an effective treatment if patients then do not receive it because their doctors think the problem is not real. The strong voice of patients and patient groups will be key here.

One obvious, but key, question is will this problem "go away" if we find an accessible, useable, and effective approach to treating the disease. At one level it feels self-evident that it will. Interestingly, in other liver diseases this has often proved to not be the case, with symptoms, especially fatigue, remaining as an issue even after effective control of the disease in terms of liver function. There are likely to be several factors at play. These include permanent change because of the disease that doesn't resolve when the disease is controlled, deconditioning and behaviour pattern change after a period of fatigue, and the side-effects of medicines. What we think will be important if we do develop effective disease control approaches will be the concept of rehabilitation. If anyone, for any reason, didn't do anything for a long period of time they would not expect to be able to immediately go back to what they were doing before. They would need to build themselves up. This is likely to be the case after fatigue in liver disease. The whole concept behind our fatigue management model is to take a medium-term view (a year) and set milestones towards that. "I don't feel any better" after a week of treatment can, all too often, lead to people giving up. They need to absolutely stick with it.

## *BETTER CARE FOR EVERYONE*

This may sound like an unambitious goal, but it is important. The data from the UK and all around the world have shown a pattern of inconsistent treatment for liver disease, with the quality of care varying often markedly across relatively small geographical areas. In the UK we talk about the concept of the "postcode lottery" but we suspect that variations of this exist around the world. Why is this? One reason is that liver disease is increasing in its frequency in the population very rapidly (and the growth in MASLD is a major factor in this), but the number of liver specialists has not grown at anywhere near the same pace. This means that in many hospitals even complex liver disease patients are managed by non-specialists. The increase in the level of education of current non-liver doctors, and medical students in training, in liver medicine has been even more glacial, meaning that non-specialists get little or no education in this area. This includes family doctors who wonder what to do with a patient with type 2 diabetes whose liver blood tests deteriorate, and anaesthetists wondering why an anaesthetic is going wrong in someone with undiagnosed liver disease. The scale of MASLD in the population means that specialist centres cannot possibly see and manage all patients. It is going to be essential that all clinicians are aware of the nature and implications of MASLD. Clearly one aspect of the change that is needed is **clinician education** at both the undergraduate (medical and nursing school) and professional level. The challenge with education initiatives like this is that they are most effective at reaching the people who are already thinking about the condition enough to want to find out more. We therefore need to find ways of information dissemination that are more uniform in their reach.

One such approach is through the development and use of **care pathways.** If we are driving somewhere and we don't know the route, we use satellite navigation. We used to use maps, but they were not as useful as we thought they were. Looking at a map before a journey explains the overall route, which at that point makes complete sense; the problem arises when you reach the end of the road and the options are left or right, with neither way being signposted for your destination. At that point the map isn't really very useful. The beauty of satellite navigation is that it tells you which way to turn when you reach that end of the road with the option of a left and a right turn (and at the turning after that and so on). We have the equivalent of maps for clinical care (guidelines which, like maps, aren't as useful in practice as you think they should be). What we need are care pathways that actively guide clinicians and patients through the whole disease journey from first diagnosis onwards. At each stage there would be simple options to guide you. Like turning left or right. There is much discussion of "apps" and other digital technologies and their potential value in patient care. Much of this is, to us, exaggerated. Where we think the technology may be hugely useful would be in just such a patient "sat nav".

A final approach is through what we call **"reverse education"**. Many patients we know describe consultations with doctors where they feel that they know more about the disease than the doctors do. Why do we not use this to help get information across to doctors? At the end of the day, the patient has more vested in the consultation than the doctor does. Maybe the way to get all patients on to the patient pathway in the future (the "sat nav" outlined above) is through empowering patients through the patient groups to ask for the approach to be used. In the UK at least we can sometimes be too polite for our own good……. The only way you can hold your doctor to account for how they are managing your MASLD is through you knowing and fully understanding your disease status. Reading this book is a great start!

# APPENDIX 1: *A DICTIONARY OF MASLD* (with INDEX)

*Aerobic Metabolism (128,139):* There are essentially two forms of energy generation that provide the power necessary for the function of the cells of the body. These are aerobic and **anaerobic**. They are utilised in different proportions, in different settings by different people with different physiology. Aerobic metabolism is characterised by being balanced between fuel and oxygen consumption. This distinguishes it from anaerobic metabolism, where there is disproportionate fuel consumption for the amount of oxygen consumption, building up an "oxygen debt". Because of its balanced nature aerobic metabolism is sustainable over long periods of time (physiologically at least). The enzymes that are responsible for aerobic metabolism are located within the **mitochondria**; something which has led to the alternative name for aerobic metabolism which is "mitochondrial metabolism". The importance to MASLD is that aerobic metabolism is inherently fat burning (**triglyceride** is in many ways the optimal mitochondrial fuel), meaning that increased aerobic exercise is a highly effective approach to reducing **hepatocyte** fat. This lies at the heart of the **exercise therapy** component of **lifestyle modification**.

*Albumin (12,17,20,75,87-89,92,95,147-148,190):* A protein made by the liver and released into the blood. It is the protein with the highest level of liver manufacture, meaning that the level (which is easily measurable in the blood) is a useful test of liver function (and as such forms part of the panel of **liver function tests**). The albumin in the circulation plays two important roles (neither of which is, paradoxically, the one everyone thinks of, which is as a source of nutrition). The first role is as a transporter for other molecules in the blood that are not soluble in water. One example, of many, is **bilirubin** which is transported to the liver in its insoluble form (prior to conjugation or "tagging" which renders it soluble) bound to albumin. The other important role is to help keep fluid in the correct place in the body. Although we think of the blood as the major fluid compartment in the body, the tissues themselves have fluid within them to help "perfuse" the cells (to carry nutrients to them). Where too much fluid gets out of the circulation and into the tissues, oedema or swelling can result (the classic example is swelling of the lower leg, swollen ankles). This can reduce the blood volume, causing blood pressure falls, and can cause damage to the swollen tissues (skin stretching and ulcer formation as well as "heavy legs" that can reduce mobility). The balance between fluid in the blood and in the tissues arises because of the net result of a number of processes. A key one is the pressure within the blood vessel (in the swollen ankles analogy the fluid is pushed out from the veins by the high pressure in the lower leg that occurs when people stand up). Although there is some degree of reverse effect by the pressure within the tissue, the main factor keeping fluid within the circulation is osmotic pressure; the tendency for fluids containing a large number of molecules to attract water and dilute themselves. Because albumin stays in the circulation due to its size (unlike ions such as sodium and chloride it cannot easily get across the blood vessel wall and out into the tissue) it is the key factor in exerting osmotic pressure to keep fluid in the circulation. This is why a low albumin (typically from liver disease but it can also occur with a very poor diet and through certain diseases of the bowel and kidney) is almost always associated with oedema or tissue swelling.

*__Alanine Transaminase (ALT) (66,69-75,80-81,86-87,92-94,96,147):__* A blood test that forms part of the normal *liver function test* panel. It is released predominantly by injured *hepatocytes* and is therefore associated with hepatocyte injury and hepatitis in its various forms. Because the level of release from hepatocytes relates, to a degree, to the level of hepatocyte injury, ALT has use as a marker of disease activity in MASLD and, as such, its measurement forms part of the normal clinic follow-up. Typically, higher levels of ALT suggest more active disease with lower levels indicating better control. In the setting of possible **MAFLD**, measuring a second transaminase (*aspartate aminotransferase; AST*) is also very useful. In the **MASH** form of MAFLD, AST increase is typically seen at the same time as ALT elevation (with the value for AST usually being around 0.8 times the ALT value) and reflects the presence of *steatohepatitis*. Occasionally, distinguishing MASH from steatohepatitis related to excess alcohol (alcohol-related liver disease) can be a clinical challenge (although the alcohol history usually allows easy distinguishing). The relative values of AST and ALT can help in alcohol-related steatohepatitis as the AST level is frequently twice as high as the ALT (contrasting with the slightly lower AST than ALT in MASH).

*__Alkaline Phosphatase (ALP) (64,66,69-70,75,94-95)__*: An enzyme released by the *biliary epithelial cells* (the cells lining the *bile duct*). Release of ALP by bile duct cells is a marker of stress or injury and is classically thought of as an indicator of *cholestasis*. It can be released (in slightly different forms) by other tissues, in particular the bone, so caution must always be taken in automatically ascribing its elevation to liver disease. If in doubt, the level of the specific liver form can be measured or, alternatively, the presence of cholestasis can be cross-checked by also measuring *gamma-glutamyl transferase (GGT)*, another enzyme released by stressed/injured bile duct cells. ALP forms part of the standard *liver function test* panel. Although MASLD is principally one of hepatocyte injury, with ALT elevation predominating, alkaline phosphatase (and GGT) elevation can be seen and in some patients is the dominant change. This possibility should always be born in mind when investigating liver disease.

***Anaerobic Metabolism (127-128,194):*** There are essentially two forms of energy generation that provide the power necessary for the function of the cells of the body. These are ***aerobic*** and anaerobic. They are utilised in different proportions, in different settings by different people with different physiology. Anaerobic metabolism is characterised by disproportionate fuel consumption for the amount of oxygen consumption, building up an "oxygen debt" (sugars are converted into lactic acid which then must be re-metabolised at the end of the period of exercise). Because of its unbalanced nature, anaerobic metabolism is not sustainable over long periods of time. The importance of aerobic metabolism for fat use means that ***exercise therapy*** approaches are geared towards promoting this form of energy consumption in MASLD. With fitness training, the anaerobic threshold, the level of exercise where the body changes from aerobic to anaerobic, can be increased, therefore further increasing the capacity to exercise. This is what happens when people feel that they are getting fitter with exercise.

***Anti-Nuclear Antibody (ANA) (63-64,82,96):*** An antibody that recognises the body's own cells (***autoantibody***); in this case the nucleus of cells. These antibodies are seen, at a low level, in a significant number of **MASLD** patients, and the presence of them can cause confusion as to the diagnosis (the autoimmune liver disease ***autoimmune hepatitis*** is characterised by these autoantibodies and also typically has elevation of ***alanine transaminase*** just as MASLD does). It is most likely that the presence of these autoantibodies is a consequence of ***steatosis*** (oxidant stress caused by fat deposition altering the structure of nuclear proteins so that the immune system can recognise them) rather than a reflection of an autoimmune component to the disease process. Certainly, the use of steroid therapy (the standard approach for autoimmune hepatitis) is completely counter-productive in MASLD patients with ANA, because there is typically no improvement in any immune element, and steroids worsen insulin resistance and the metabolic syndrome.

***Antioxidants (54,117,149,153,219):*** A class of drugs and vitamins that prevent or reverse tissue damage from ***oxidant stress***. Given the apparent role of oxidant stress in the disease process they have, very reasonably, been explored as potential treatments in **MASLD**. The results have largely been unimpressive, and they are therefore not recommended as standard therapy. A number of people can, however, end up with depletion of the natural antioxidants that the body needs to prevent tissue injury and therefore an antioxidant vitamin supplement can be an appropriate thing to take. It shouldn't, however, replace consideration of other, potentially more effective, therapies.

***Apoptosis (15,36,60-61,77):*** A process of programmed cell death, and one of the three key mechanisms by which the body loses functioning cells in disease (the others are necrosis and ***senescence***). Necrosis is where a cell literally falls apart. This happens in situations such as ischaemia (where the blood supply is cut off to a tissue) and burns. As well as the loss of the cell itself, necrosis is a harmful process because cell contents are leaked which can themselves stimulate more inflammation and tissue damage. Apoptosis is a "cleaner" way for a cell to die. In essence, it turns in on itself, neatly packaging itself up for disposal. This avoids the harmful consequences of necrosis. The cell is, typically, "told" to undergo apoptosis by an external signal, usually sensed through a receptor on the surface. The stimulus can come from a ***T-cell*** or other form of killer cell. Apoptosis appears to be a key process for cellular injury in ***MASLD***.

***Aramchol (153):*** (icomidocholic acid). A bile acid-based therapy that is currently under investigation in ***clinical trials*** in ***MASLD***. It is a partial inhibitor of an important enzyme in the pathway of synthesis of unsaturated ***fatty acids***, so should theoretically reduce fat manufacture. In its phase 2 trial it showed significant reduction in liver fat levels. In terms of the conventional ***MASH*** trial ***endpoints*** it showed MASH resolution without fibrosis worsening and fibrosis improvement without MASH worsening, as well as significant improvement in ***LFTs***. Although these effects were significant, they were only seen in a minority of patients. Further trials are now under way and suggest that longer treatment duration is associated with even greater benefit. This is a very promising therapy for MASLD.

***Ascites (12-13,17,20,70-71,147,161-162,164-167,180,190):*** Collection of fluid in the abdominal cavity leading to swelling of the abdomen. It can be caused by a number of processes, including heart failure and the presence of tumour cells in the abdominal cavity in the setting of cancer. The commonest cause by a long way is, however, ***cirrhosis***. The mechanisms by which fluid accumulates are complex and include ***portal hypertension***, low ***albumin*** levels in the circulation and retention of the steroid hormone aldosterone. Ascites is only ever a feature of advanced disease in ***MASLD***, and it is an important prognostic sign. If the fluid volume is very high it can restrict movement and compromise breathing through pressure on the diaphragm. Ascites can occasionally become infected by bacteria from the gut to cause ***spontaneous bacterial peritonitis***. This is a potential cause of further deterioration in liver function in people with cirrhosis. When ascites is a problem, it is usually controlled with diuretics ("water tablets" such as furosemide and spironolactone). Occasionally it needs to be drained through the abdominal wall using a needle and plastic drain.

***Aspartate Transaminase (AST) (66,69,70,73-75,80,86-87,92-94,212):*** A blood test that often forms part of the normal *liver function test* panel. It is released by injured *hepatocytes* and is therefore associated with liver injury and hepatitis in its various forms. It can also be released by damaged muscle cells as well and is therefore a little less specific for liver disease than the other widely measured test *alanine transaminase (ALT)*. Because the level of release from hepatocytes relates, to a significant degree, to the level of hepatocyte injury, AST is a useful marker of disease activity in **MASLD** and, as such, its measurement forms part of the normal clinic follow-up. Typically, higher levels of AST suggest more active disease with lower levels indicating better control. One caution is that in very severe disease the levels can fall, not because the disease is well controlled but because the remaining number of hepatocytes which can be injured in the disease, and thus release AST, is falling. In the **MASH** form of the disease AST is typically seen at the same time as ALT elevation (with the value for AST usually being around 0.8 times the ALT value). Occasionally, distinguishing MASH from *steatohepatitis* related to excess alcohol can be a clinical challenge (usually the alcohol history allows easy distinguishing). The relative values of AST and ALT can help. In alcohol-related steatohepatitis the AST level is frequently twice as high as the ALT (contrasting with the slightly lower AST than ALT in MASH).

***Autoimmune Hepatitis (AIH) (1,2,63-64,75-76,80-82,96):*** A form of chronic liver disease in which the immune system recognises the liver, erroneously, as being harmful and tries to attack it. AIH can sometimes be confused with **MASLD** because one of the important features of AIH, *antinuclear antibody (ANA)* can also be seen in MASLD. Other features such as the presence of *fat* in the *hepatocytes* are not seen in AIH meaning that, in practice, distinguishing the two is not difficult. Making the diagnosis is, however, essential as the standard treatment for AIH, steroids, can make MASLD worse.

***Autoantibody (63,82,96):*** Antibodies that react with the body's own proteins (and other molecules such as DNA). Antibodies are a key part of the normal immune response to foreign proteins. They are themselves proteins that are both present on the surface of immune cells (the **B-Cells**) and free in the circulation. They bind to specific proteins (the protein that they match up to which triggered their production in the first place) blocking their function and helping the immune system to clear them. Normally, antibodies are specific for proteins that are foreign to the body. As part of the mistargeting seen in autoimmune disease, however, they can end up reacting with the body's own proteins. Antibodies of this type are known as autoantibodies (from "auto", the Greek for self). Autoantibodies are seen reasonably frequently in **MASLD**, although there is no real evidence to suggest that an autoimmune response contributes to liver damage. The most commonly seen autoantibodies in this setting are ***anti-nuclear antibodies.*** These are frequently accompanied by anti-smooth muscle antibodies (SMA). Perhaps the most important aspect to autoantibody presence in MASLD is the potential for the diagnosis to be missed, and an erroneous diagnosis of ***autoimmune hepatitis*** made (AIH is characterised by ANA and SMA). Given that the therapy for AIH is ***prednisolone***, which drives fat deposition in the liver, it is important to get the diagnosis right.

***Banding (159,160):*** A technique used at ***endoscopy*** to control bleeding from oesophageal ***varices***. The wall of the bleeding vessel is sucked up into the end of a special banding tube which has preloaded rubber bands on it. The band is then applied around the sucked up vessel wall thus blocking it (and thus stopping the bleeding). The bands will tend to come off after around one to two weeks and can leave an ulcer behind which can itself, paradoxically, bleed. Repeat endoscopy with banding every three to six months is an effective approach to achieving complete control of varices. Banding has entirely replaced an older endoscopy approach to variceal bleeding of varices injection with a scarring solution which irritated the vessel walls causing them to stick together, but which also had significant side-effects.

***Bariatric Surgery (101,103-104,122-123):*** A generic terms for a number of different surgical and other physical interventions which are designed to facilitate weight loss. They are increasingly being used in **MASLD**. All are based around the principle of distorting the normal capacity to ingest food and/or the flow of food through the gut. They range in invasiveness from minimally invasive approaches such as intra-gastric balloons which reduce the intra-gastric volume, meaning that a sense of being full arrives much earlier in a meal than would normally be the case (thus reducing overall food intake), to invasive surgical bypass procedures, altering the pattern of flow through the gut. Given the value of weight loss for the management of **MASLD** it is unsurprising that bariatric surgery can be very effective, although the surgery can also have clear downsides. There is emerging evidence to suggest, however, that the benefits actually outweigh those that might be predicted simply from the degree of weight loss seen. It has been postulated that these interventions can have an additional beneficial effect over and above the direct reduction in food intake, potentially through alteration in the ***faecal microbiome***, the bacterial micro-environment present in everyone's gut, and which plays a key role in natural food metabolism. There is emerging evidence that over the longer-term bariatric surgery can actually worsen liver fibrosis in MASLD though.

***"Batteries Running Down" (193,259):*** The term patients frequently use to describe the peripheral type of ***fatigue*** that is a common symptom in **MASLD**. In this type of fatigue, people know what they want to do, and can clearly plan it, but the power in their arms and legs lets them down. The imagery is very powerful. This is never severe enough to be mistaken for complete non-function (if there was a fire in your house you would be able to run outside just as fast as anyone else) but it can have a major impact on day-to-day function and quality of life.

***B-Cell (177,178):*** A key part of the immune system responsible for antibody production. B-cells are lymphocytes (the cells that generate specific immune responses (i.e. those targeted at specific molecules/cells rather than acting more generally)). The role of B-cells is to produce antibodies; proteins that are released into the circulation where they can bind to and help eliminate bacteria and viruses in a targeted fashion. Each B-cell produces a single antibody of a unique specificity. Although antibodies are typically directed against proteins foreign to the body (viruses, bacteria, fungi, vaccines etc) mistargeting can occur, giving rise to antibodies specific for one of the body's own proteins. These are known as ***autoantibodies***.

***Belapectin (154):*** A novel anti-fibrotic drug which has been evaluated in **MASLD**. Animal studies suggested a significant anti-fibrotic effect in **MASH** models. Human studies have been less convincing. Trials are ongoing.

***Beta Blocker (159,197):*** A family of drugs developed to treat hypertension (high blood pressure). They work by a combination of slowing the heart rate, reducing (slightly) the strength of the heartbeat and, to a degree, dilating the blood vessels. Their main relevance in liver disease is that they can reduce the level of ***portal hypertension*** and, therefore, lower the risk of ***variceal bleeding***. Whereas the heart action is most important for arterial hypertension (the classical "high blood pressure") it is the vessel effects that are most important probably for varices protection. ***Propranolol*** was the original beta blocker and for many years the one with the greatest effect on portal hypertension. It has largely been replaced by ***carvedilol*** which is probably more effective and has fewer side-effects. All beta blockers can, by their nature, drop arterial blood pressure and, if given at too high a dose, cause blackouts.

***Biliary Epithelial Cells (BEC) (13,61,75):*** The cells that form the lining for the ***bile ducts***. These cells are the target cells for injury in ***primary biliary cholangitis***. Bile duct injury is a relatively infrequent finding in ***MASLD***; however it does occur and can contribute to the development of itch, which is a relatively uncommon, but important, symptom in the condition.

***Bile (6,9-11,13,18,75,87,94-95,175,203-204):*** The drainage fluid of the liver. It is actively produced by the ***hepatocytes***, and then modified by the cells of the ***bile duct***. It performs two key functions. The first is to facilitate outflow of the by-products of metabolism by the liver. The second is to transport ***bile acids*** into the bowel, where they perform their critical normal function of helping the uptake of fat from the diet into the body by making it soluble.

***Bile Acids (6,10,13,204):*** Cholesterol-based molecules synthesised by the ***hepatocytes*** and actively transported into the ***bile canaliculi,*** where they form an important component of ***bile***. The physiological role of bile acids is to act as a detergent, emulsifying lipids or fats in the bowel to make them water soluble. This allows them to be taken up across the bowel wall. Bile acids are, therefore, key for normal nutrition. There is emerging evidence to suggest that bile acids have, however, a broader additional role, regulating metabolism in the body. Bile acids, although natural to the body, have the potential to be irritant to cells. They do, however, vary in the degree to which they can have this effect. The role played by bile acids in metabolism and energy regulation has underpinned the exploration of bile acid modifying therapies as treatments for ***MASLD*** (which is, at the end of the day, a disease of disordered metabolism).

***Bile Canaliculi (9):*** The space between the sheets of ***hepatocytes*** where the constituents of bile form together. The bile canaliculi, which represent the upper-most part of the biliary tree, drain into the small ***bile ducts.***

***Bile Duct (6,7,9,10,62-65,75,94,175):*** The tubular system that drains bile from the liver into the bowel. Bile constituents are actively transported into the ***bile canaliculi,*** where flow towards the gut begins. "Downstream" of the canaliculi, the bile enters a structure of increasing size tubes, all lined by ***biliary epithelial cells.*** The bile duct drains into the ***duodenum*** (the part of the small bowel immediately after the stomach). The traditional way of describing the bile duct network is as the biliary "tree". The bile ducts start as very small structures equivalent to the twigs to which the leaves are attached. Follow the twigs down and you get to branches that eventually join together to form two or three main branches which join the tree trunk.

***Bilirubin (6,11,75,87-88,95,147-148,166):*** The pigment chemical that gives rise to ***jaundice*** (the yellowing of the skin seen in advanced liver disease of all causes). Bilirubin is produced naturally as part of the recycling process for red blood cells that have reached the end of their useful life (at around 150 days). Ageing red cells lose their shape and function and are taken up and broken down by the ***macrophages*** in the spleen. Haemoglobin, the complex structure that carries oxygen within the red blood cell, is partly recycled and partly disposed of. The actual oxygen carrying part of haemoglobin is called haem and contains the iron essential for oxygen transport. The iron is stripped out to be recycled, but the rest of the haem group cannot be used and must be disposed of. It is this that goes on to form bilirubin. At this initial stage it is not water soluble and needs to be carried to the liver for disposal by *albumin*. In the liver, the insoluble bilirubin is taken up by the *hepatocytes* and is "tagged for disposal" by a process called conjugation, in which another chemical group is attached to it. It is then actively transported out into the *bile canaliculi* and carried out in the *bile*. In *MASLD*, raised serum bilirubin is usually because of a failure of the hepatocytes to process bilirubin (to conjugate it and then transport it out into the bile). Occasionally, liver swelling because of inflammation can end up putting pressure on the bile canaliculi and can add an obstructive element. If bilirubin is elevated and falls very rapidly with therapy this is usually the explanation. The serum bilirubin level is an important and useful marker of disease activity in any liver disease. The goal of treatment must be to achieve and then maintain a normal bilirubin level.

*"Brain Fog" (194,198,202):* A term frequently used by patients to describe *cognitive symptoms* and central *fatigue*; two of the key symptom types in *MASLD*. The imagery is very powerful and describes the sense that people have to actively think their way through problems.

*Carvedilol (159,197):* A drug used to lower *portal hypertension* and reduce the risk of *variceal bleed*. It is one of the *beta blocker* family of drugs. It is now the mainstay of drug-based varices protection, having largely replaced the older *propranolol*, which is probably less effective with more side-effects.

*Cholangiocytes (13):* The alternative name for the *biliary epithelial cells*. They line the *bile duct* from the small intra-hepatic bile ducts all the way to the bile duct outflow into the duodenum. They are damaged in a minority of *MASLD* patients who have features of impaired *bile* flow (*cholestasis*), exemplified by *pruritus* (itch).

*Cholestasis (82,151,203,205,220):* A state of impaired *bile* production and/or bile flow and its consequences. The term does not imply the mechanism responsible, which can range from blockage of the bile duct through a *gallstone* or pancreatic tumour, all the way to a failure of the transporter molecules in the liver which produce bile in the first place. Cholestasis is seen in a minority of *MASLD* patients. Cholestasis has characteristic clinical features including itch and jaundice. In terms of investigations, *liver function tests* tend to show elevation of *alkaline phosphatase* out of proportion to any elevation in *alanine transaminase*. *Bilirubin* will only be elevated in more severe forms of the condition.

***Cholesterol (6,10,12-13,51,53,105):*** A form of lipid or fat present in the body. It is used as a fuel source and as the precursor for ***bile acids*** and steroid hormones such as cortisol, oestrogen, and progesterone. The association between elevation of cholesterol and risk of atherosclerosis and heart disease (an important issue in the metabolic syndrome and thus in MASLD) has led to a widespread perception that cholesterol is a "bad thing". It is, however, essential for life and is only an issue if it is at the wrong level, in the wrong form or is in the wrong place. Cholesterol forms a key part of lipid transport complexes called lipoproteins. These shuttle lipids between the gut (where they are absorbed from the diet aided by the dissolving actions of ***bile acids***), the liver where they are modified and synthesised (the focus on diet control for high cholesterol rather misses the point that most of the cholesterol present in the body is in fact created in the body) and the cells of the body where the lipids are taken up and used. It is the nature of the lipoproteins that determines the risk they pose to the blood vessels. Very low density lipoprotein (VLDL) and low density lipoprotein (LDL) at elevated levels do result in blood vessel damage and atherosclerosis and are termed "bad cholesterol" in the lay press. High density lipoprotein (HDL), in contrast, is protective for the blood vessels ("good cholesterol" which actually removes cholesterol from the cells of the vessel wall). An absolute cholesterol number is, therefore, difficult to interpret on its own. You should ask for the total cholesterol and HDL cholesterol measurements. A good result is where HDL comprises at least a quarter of the total cholesterol. Exercise leads to in an increase in "good" HDL levels, and improving diet e.g. Mediterranean diet, results in a reduction in "bad" LDL cholesterol.

***Cholestyramine (204-206):*** The first-line treatment for itch in ***cholestasis*** and an old-fashioned treatment for high cholesterol. In use since the 1960s, it is thought to bind bile acids in the gut and remove them from the body (they pass through and out of the bowel bound to cholestyramine). Some patients respond well to it, but it is very much towards the milder end of the spectrum of treatments for itch in cholestasis. One issue with it is tolerability. It has an unusual texture that many patients struggle to tolerate. Adding fruit juice or chilling it in the fridge overnight before taking it can help.

***Cirrhosis:*** A pathological term describing the end state of chronic liver injury of all causes. It arises when there is a combination of significant ***fibrosis*** (scars developing like a lattice work across the liver) occurring at the same time as ***hepatocyte*** regeneration. The development of cirrhosis has three clinical sequelae. The first is that the function of the remaining hepatocytes is impaired, putting the patient at risk of liver failure over time. The second is that the increased pressure caused by liver regeneration within a scarred liver leads to a rise in pressure in the ***portal vein*** leading to ***portal hypertension***. The third impact is the increased risk of ***hepatocellular***

*carcinoma* resulting from poor regulation of hepatocyte proliferation. The risk of portal hypertension and its complications, and hepatocellular carcinoma following cirrhosis development, guides our clinical screening protocols. It is the end-stage of all forms of liver disease, whatever the cause.

***Clinical Trials (91-92,143,144):*** The bedrock of the testing of new drugs and approaches to treating any disease. Clinical trials allow us to understand the extent to which a drug is helpful, and also the potential side-effects that it may cause. From this, the risk and benefit can be determined. Regulatory bodies such as the Food and Drug Administration (FDA) in the USA, the Medicines and Healthcare products Regulatory Agency (UK) and the European Medicines Agency (EMA) in Europe use this information to decide whether a drug is safe and effective enough to be granted a licence (i.e. be approved to be prescribed by doctors). In diseases, or versions of diseases, with no current treatment the drug under investigation will normally be compared with a dummy treatment or *placebo*. If the question is whether a drug improves on the current best treatment (or "standard of care") then it is this that the new drug is compared with. One of the critical issues in clinical trial design, and particularly an issue in **MASLD**, is that of trial *endpoint*. This is the aspect of the disease that you are measuring before and after the use of the treatment in order to demonstrate change. The challenge in trial design is the tension between endpoints that really matter to patients (avoiding death, avoiding the need for liver transplant etc.), but which would need a trial with very long follow-up to show change; (a real issue in a trial with a dummy treatment or *placebo* arm given that participants are likely to have concerns over taking a dummy rather than active treatment for many year), and those, like blood tests, that are easy to measure, and may show change over a shorter period of time, but which may have a limited direct clinical significance. This is important as issues around endpoints have been a major contributor to the slow progress in drug development in MASLD.

***Cognitive Symptoms (186,191,202,204):*** Symptoms of reduced short-term memory and/or concentration. People often struggle to follow plots in books or films or to do puzzles. This symptom set is seen in around 20% of **MASLD** patients (although it has not been very well researched). If severe, it can cause real problems for people at work (especially if information processing is a key part of their job). As is the case with *fatigue*, the cognitive symptoms can be seen at any stage in the disease process and are NOT a feature exclusively of advanced disease. There is often confusion between these symptoms and those of *encephalopathy* which also exhibits memory and concentration problems. Encephalopathy is a feature of advanced cirrhotic disease, and in cirrhotic **MASLD** patients the impact of the generic cognitive symptom process, and that associated with encephalopathy can be additive, increasing patient impact. Liver disease patients with cognitive symptoms often worry that they are developing dementia. We suspect that this is a reason people often do not discuss their memory problems in clinic.

**_Cytokine (23,30,59,61-62,191):_** The chemical mediators of the immune and inflammatory response. They are produced by activated ***T-cells, macrophages,*** and other inflammatory cells. They can activate immune cells to function, or even cause ***apoptosis*** directly. Targeting cytokines such as TNF-alpha has been an effective approach for the treatment of a number of inflammatory and immune diseases and has been tried in small numbers of ***MASLD*** patients (without any clear evidence of benefit). This approach also has the disadvantage of changing the immune system, probably permanently, and thus opening patients to long-term risks.

**_Drug-Induced Liver Injury (DILI) (82-83):_** Many drugs can cause liver injury in a small number of patients, and avoiding liver toxicity is a major focus in the development of new drugs. Too high a risk of injury to the liver is one of the main reasons why drugs end up not being licensed for use in patients. The reason the liver can be particularly injured by drugs is two-fold. The first is that, as most drugs are taken by mouth, they are taken up into the ***portal vein*** and transported directly to the liver. The liver is, therefore, exposed to the highest level of such drugs (the same issue is not seen with drugs given as injections, ointments, patches, or inhalers). Given that higher doses are more likely to cause injury, this places the liver in pole position for damage. The second reason is that the liver plays a key role in modifying and getting rid of chemicals (such as drugs) from the body. This active handling of drugs means that the liver cells take them up and are thus exposed. There are many different forms of DILI. The relevance to ***MASLD*** is twofold. Firstly, DILI can, in terms of ***liver function test*** and ***liver biopsy*** appearances, mimic ***MASLD***. Indeed, DILI is one of the forms of ***specific aetiology SLD*** that are recognised in the new classification of ***steatotic liver disease***. In other words, the drug itself directly causes steatosis in a way that is unrelated to ***MASLD***. There are a number of drugs that are well known to do this and the possibility should always be thought of in people taking them. These include amiodarone (a drug for controlling abnormal heart rhythms), sodium valproate (an anti-epilepsy drug) and tamoxifen (a breast cancer treatment). Anyone in whom steatotic liver disease is a possibility should have a full drug exposure history taken and any drugs with a particular risk of causing DILI should be stopped immediately of possible. The other way in which drugs can contribute to ***MASLD*** is through an augmentation of the metabolic dysfunction that drives the process. The classic example of this would be steroid therapy. In this setting it is not a DILI as such, rather an exacerbation of the ***MASLD*** process.

***Duodenum (10):*** The first part of the small bowel, immediately down from the stomach. The ***bile duct*** drains into the duodenum.

***ELF (Enhanced Liver Fibrosis) Test (91):*** A blood-based test for the estimation of liver ***fibrosis***. When scarring develops in the liver the scar tissue isn't fixed and unchanging. Rather, it is constantly "re-modelled" (i.e., existing scar tissue is broken down and replaced by new scar). It is possible to measure the parts of the scar tissue that have been broken down and released into the blood. In simple terms, the higher the levels of these breakdown products the more scar tissue there is in the body. It is a more direct measure of the amount of fibrosis than clinical scores such as ***FIB-4*** and the ***NAFLD fibrosis score (NFS)*** which would more properly now be called the MASLD fibrosis score but is still universally available under the old name; the perils of a name change!). It is an alternative to (and probably more accurately thought of as being complementary to) ***fibroscan*** as both approaches attempt to quantify the amount of fibrosis tissue. It is less widely used in the UK than fibroscan. It is very useful for risk stratifying patients at disease outset (i.e., ascertaining whether there is already advanced fibrosis at the point of ***MASLD*** diagnosis) and for following up to identify progression to ***cirrhosis***. At present, it isn't clear whether it is a useful dynamic treatment marker or not (i.e., does improvement in ELF score with therapy reflect a reduction in fibrosis and is this a disease improvement or not). One thing to be aware of with ELF is that it is a marker of degree of fibrosis in the body as a whole and not just the liver (unlike fibroscan where the assessment is directly of the liver). Excessive fibrosis in other parts of the body could therefore conceivably give a high false positive value for ELF.

***Encephalopathy (11,16,21,32,160,163-165,189-190):*** A blanket term for a state of toxic brain dysfunction. In the context of ***MASLD***, this is an abbreviation for hepatic encephalopathy. This state occurs in advanced cirrhosis when the liver fails to effectively clear the toxic by-products of metabolism. These can then build up and cause a reversible toxic state affecting brain function. This can range from minor changes in memory, concentration, personality, and sleep pattern, through to coma. This can be a very disabling (and distressing) complication of ***cirrhosis***. When it occurs in ***MASLD*** it should be a trigger to begin considering liver transplantation as a treatment option. It is important to treat it to maximise quality of life. In the past, first line treatment was with the laxative ***lactulose*** which reduces bowel transit time (the time taken for bowel contents to flow through the bowel) and is said to reduce uptake of bowel contents, including the breakdown products of bacteria, that worsen encephalopathy. More recently the non-absorbable antibiotic ***rifaximin*** has begun to be used to good effect in the treatment of encephalopathy (further supporting the idea that bacterial load in the bowel may contribute to encephalopathy).

***Endoscopy (93,159,160,222,233):*** Known colloquially as a camera or "telescope test". Flexible endoscopes are one of the key medical technology inventions of the last 50 years, transforming the management of bowel and bladder disease. Upper GI endoscopy is the examination of the oesophagus (gullet), stomach and duodenum under direct vision. The endoscope is a flexible tube with a fibreoptic light source that allows the doctor or nurse to directly examine the inside of the bowel. An instrument port allows biopsies to be taken if needed and to pass instruments down. These allow, for example, the direct treatment of **varices**. Guidelines recommend that patients with ***cirrhosis*** of all aetiologies have regular endoscopies to check for the presence of varices. This is a minor procedure normally done with just an anaesthetic throat spray. It takes a few minutes at most.

***Endpoint (141,144,146-147,150-154):*** A critical aspect in the design of ***clinical trials*** in **MASLD** (and any other disease for that matter). The endpoint of the trial is the aspect of the patient and their experience that will be measured and compared in the different trial "arms" (the groups receiving different types of treatment). A trial will typically have one "primary endpoint" which is the main headline comparison, and a number of secondary endpoints which will shed further light on the nature of the response. Concepts of trial success, or otherwise, hinge on the primary endpoint, which must always be specified before the trial starts. The perfect trial has an endpoint which is unequivocally relevant to patients (whether you die or not or need a transplant for example). The challenge in liver disease, however, is that even if you don't have treatment, the risk of death or need for transplant remains low over a few years. It is therefore very difficult to see a therapy "signal" (evidence that the drug you are interested in is changing this endpoint value).

There are several ways around this. One is to do very long trials so that you capture the long-term effects. These are difficult to do for a number of reasons, including the cost. One of the main issues, however, is that long-term ***placebo***-controlled trials in particular (ones where the active drug is compared to a dummy or placebo) are very unattractive to patients. Imagine a 5 year trial which you have taken part in because of the risk of your liver disease, after which you discover you were taking a dummy tablet all along. This is compounded by the fact that by taking part in a trial you are "locked-out" of other changes being made to your treatment.

Another "short-cut", often taken to address this challenge, is to restrict the trial to people who are at very high risk of reaching the endpoint. If that endpoint is a really hard one, such as death or transplant, then it means that only people with already very advanced disease will be able to participate. This may, of course, be the group in who the disease has progressed to the point where it doesn't respond to therapy, thereby negating the point of the trial.

It was to try and "square this circle" that the concept of the "surrogate marker" was developed. This was an endpoint that wasn't itself a definitive one, but one that accurately predicted the future development of a "hard" endpoint. There is a spectrum of such endpoints in liver disease which give rise to an accompanying spectrum of problems. The concerns of the regulators in relation to the use of these endpoints have been a major factor in the slow progression in therapy development in **MASLD**. At one end of the spectrum there are features of clinical progression that would certainly indicate risk, such as the development of *varices*. If variceal bleeding is a hard endpoint, then the development of varices themselves in the first place is risk predictive (not everyone with varices will bleed, but in order to bleed at all you must have first developed varices). The problem is that, again, varices development is a relatively late-stage process. At the other end of the surrogate marker spectrum are blood tests such as *alanine transaminase* and other *liver function tests*. These are all markers of disease and, across the population as a whole, the higher the values the more aggressive the disease. Does, however, reduction in ALT values in an individual suggest the disease has improved? Possibly, possibly not (values can reduce for reasons other than a reduction in liver injury). Does reduction on its own justify the approval of a drug with potential side effects and, given the frequency of MASLD in the population, significant additional health care costs? Probably not. We need to be certain that the ALT improvement reflects a genuine improvement in disease severity.

In the middle of the spectrum of surrogate endpoint values comes *liver biopsy* and its own surrogate, *fibroscan*. Given that the process of inflammation in the liver drives the development of *fibrosis* or scarring of the liver, and it is the progression of fibrosis that drives the development of *cirrhosis*, is liver biopsy a useful surrogate endpoint? The answer is probably, and this has been the endpoint most frequently used in clinical trials in **MASLD** to date. Even with this there is complexity as the two aspects of liver biopsy finding, inflammation and scarring, represent distinct processes which might be expected to respond differently to different drug types. A therapy that treated both aspects of **MASLD** would be highly attractive but, at the moment, feels like an unachievable goal. Most trials go for an either/or approach to biopsy, with an endpoint of inflammation resolution (without worsening of fibrosis) or significant improvement in fibrosis.

Biopsy, of course, has its own issues, in particular cost and its deterrent effect on patient participation (in simple terms people don't like having biopsies). It can also have issues with disease patchiness (are the changes seen in one area reflective of the liver as whole). In normal practice, of course, we don't typically use biopsy any more to assess disease progression to cirrhosis. We use fibroscan which is cheaper, non-invasive and, of course, surveys more of the liver. It is a useful surrogate trial endpoint. At the moment it is not being accepted as a surrogate endpoint by the FDA in particular. More work is needed on validation (understanding what certain values actually mean) but it seems to us very likely that its day will come as a trial surrogate endpoint.

***Exercise Therapy (125-139):***  A key part of the ***lifestyle modification*** approach to the management to the treatment of ***MASLD*** . Exercise has three very clear benefits in this setting, which go far beyond the simple aspect of calorie burning. The first and most important of these is the impact that it has on the metabolism. Exercise training at an appropriate intensity is highly effective at promoting ***aerobic metabolism*** which is inherently ***fat*** burning. It is thus effective at reducing the elevated ***hepatocyte*** fat levels which lie at the heart of MASLD. The second is that it lies at the heart of the concept of "owning the problem and owning the solution" which we return to throughout this book. Exercise is something that you can decide to do right now, and which will begin to make your liver better almost immediately! The third reason is that exercise gives rise to a sense of wellness, reducing levels of ***fatigue***. This, of course, becomes a virtuous circle as reduced fatigue levels allow you to do more exercise which in turn further reduces fatigue. What is not to love about it?

***Fat:*** A general term for a family of water-insoluble molecules that are taken up in the diet (they are an important source of energy for the body) or made by the body to allow energy storage. It is widely assumed by people that the fat that is laid down in the body when people are overweight represents the actual fat that they have eaten. This, in fact, largely isn't the case, with fat in the diet being broken down in the liver and "new" fat made for storage. If the storage is in the liver, this is ***MASLD***. There are two main types of fat, ***cholesterol,*** and ***triglyceride.***

***Fatigue   (70,71,99,191-202,217-218,226,240-241):***   The commonest symptom described by ***MASLD*** patients, and one that is often underappreciated by doctors. At least half of all MASLD patients will experience noticeable fatigue at some point in their disease, and half of these will have significant fatigue (fatigue that is bad enough to have an impact on day to day living and quality of life). There appear to be two "types" of fatigue in MASLD, although it is important to understand that we do not, as yet, fully understand the causes of fatigue, meaning that the relationship between these two "types" may be a lot more complex than we currently appreciate. Peripheral fatigue is a sensation of weakness in the muscles which affects a person's ability to carry tasks out, the motivation to do something is there but the arms and legs let people down; people often describe the sensation as being like their ***"batteries running down"***. Central fatigue is a sensation of difficulty in initiating activities. People just cannot get going. They also feel like their thought processes are slowed down, and often use the term ***"brain fog"***. This type of fatigue overlaps with the ***cognitive symptoms*** which are increasingly being recognised in MASLD. Fatigue can cause significant reduction in the quality of life of MASLD patients. A systematic approach to reducing its impact can have real benefits. It is really important for patients to "own the problem" and find ways to adapt and minimise the impact of fatigue. One really important thing is to avoid social isolation which can be one consequence of energy-saving lifestyle modifications. These can improve fatigue but often do so at the cost of worsening of overall life quality.

***"Fatty Liver Disease":*** An old and now rather redundant term to describe liver diseases that are characterised by the deposition of fat within the **hepatocytes**. The term has now been replaced by ***steatotic liver disease***. One of the main forms of steatotic liver disease is **MASLD**, the subject of this book.

***Faecal Microbiome (248):*** The population of bacteria and other micro-organism that naturally populate our large bowel. This is what is called a symbiotic relationship with the host (us) providing a warm, safe environment for the bacteria, and a constant stream of nutrition, and the organisms playing important roles in the handling and metabolism of our diet. The spread of organisms making up the faecal microbiome varies significantly from individual to individual with factors such as the maternal microbiome in early life, local environmental influences, diet and antibiotic use all playing a role. It is also increasingly possible to manipulate the microbiome in individuals through the use of probiotics, and even faecal transplant. It is highly likely that variation in the faecal microbiome, and thus impacts on nutrition and metabolism, between individuals, may help explain individual variation in **MASLD** risk. ***Bariatric surgery*** may exert some of its beneficial effects on MASLD through alteration in the faecal microbiome.

***FIB-4 (92):*** A clinical score that includes the values for patient age, ***platelet count, alanine transaminase*** and ***aspartate transaminase***. It is easily calculated using widely available on-line tools and, because it uses every day clinical test data, is universally "available". Across the whole population it is very effective for identifying groups of people with advanced fibrosis and cirrhosis in MASLD. At the individual level, however, other factors that cause the value to be abnormal (most obviously a low platelet count for reasons other than advanced liver disease) can make it less accurate. It is not a definitive test but very useful for screening people to assist with decision making about further investigations to assess risk.

***Fibroscan (90-93,211-212):*** An important technology in liver disease that allows us to examine for the likely presence of liver ***fibrosis*** or ***cirrhosis*** without needing to do a ***liver biopsy***. The technique, actually called liver stiffness measurement (Fibroscan is a trademark albeit one that is in universal use) is a variant of ultrasound. The principle is very much like sonar on a submarine. A "ping" is sent out and the machine measures how much is returned. The more of the ping that returns the more solid (i.e. fibrotic) the liver is. The test can be done in real time as part of a clinic review and is painless. It has almost completely replaced biopsy in the monitoring of ***MASLD*** patients for cirrhosis development. It cannot, however, determine the level of inflammatory activity of disease. There are more challenges undertaking fibroscan in MASLD than in any other type of chronic liver disease because of the impact of fat in the liver and, in particular, under the skin, on the signal. This can be compensated for to a degree by increasing the size of the probe (the part of the machine that sends out the "ping" through the skin and measures how much is returned).

***Fibrosis:*** The development of scar tissue. The natural response of the body to injury is to attempt to repair the injury and return the tissue to a normal structure and function. Where this is not possible, scar tissue forms to at least retain the physical integrity of the tissue. An example is the skin where a burn, if shallow, will normally heal, returning the skin to normal appearance and function. If the burn is very deep, then it cannot heal and instead a scar forms. This is not as effective as normal skin, but at least keeps the integrity of the body surface intact. Similarly, following most forms of acute liver injury the liver will recover to normal size and structure. If the injury is chronic, as in ***MASLD***, the rate of injury can exceed the capacity to repair, meaning that chronic injury builds up. The response of the body to this is to form scar tissue. Once scarring becomes extensive the state of ***cirrhosis*** develops.

***Frusemide or furosemide (161):*** A diuretic (or "water tablet") that increases the volume of urine that is passed (it changes the way that the kidney handles both water and salts). It can be a useful treatment for fluid retention. In the case of ***MASLD*** this is usually ***ascites*** developing in the context of ***portal hypertension*** in ***cirrhosis***. It is normal practice in the UK to give it in combination with another form of diuretic called ***spironolactone***. Caution always needs to be used with diuretics in liver disease as they can worsen kidney function and can deplete salts from the blood. If kidney function begins to be impacted by diuretics it is really important the dose is reduced or stopped. This needs to be done in discussion with your doctor.

***Gallstone:*** Accretions that form in the ***bile duct*** and/or gallbladder from the crystallisation of ***bile*** contents. These soft "stones" are typically formed from either ***cholesterol*** or ***bilirubin*** ("pigment stones"). Gallbladder gallstones are the commonest type and usually cause no problems (the days of automatically having your gallbladder removed because stones had been found have, thankfully, long gone). They can cause intermittent pain ("biliary colic") which, if severe and frequent, is in indication for gallbladder surgery. Occasionally, gallstones form in, or move from, the gallbladder into the bile duct. These are much more problematic, potentially causing obstruction of the bile duct (characterised by pain and *jaundice*). Infection can develop in the obstructed bile duct because the bile can no longer drain. This is a medical emergency. In this situation the first step is to treat the infection with antibiotics, drain the bile duct (either through an *endoscopy* approach called ERCP or through a drain inserted into the liver and through into the bile duct). Then the bile duct stone is removed at ERCP. It is almost always appropriate to later remove the gallbladder to prevent recurrence. A gallstone blocking the very bottom of the bile duct, just as it joins the *duodenum*, can also block the duct draining the *pancreas* (which usually joins the bile duct very low down). This can cause an acute inflammation of the pancreas called pancreatitis which is, again, an acute medical emergency. Gallstones can impinge on *MASLD* care in several ways. Firstly, pain from gallstones (which are seen in MASLD patients at a higher frequency than in the general population) and capsular stretch pain in MASLD can be mistaken for each other. Over the years many MASLD patients have ended up having their gallbladders taken out unnecessarily (just because you have gallstones on a scan and abdominal pain it doesn't mean that the pain is caused by those gallstones). Secondly, some of the drugs that are being trialled or considered for use in MASLD can increase the risk of gallstone development.

*Gastroenterologist:* A doctor who is a specialist in the prevention, diagnosis and management of diseases of the gastrointestinal tract (the bowels) and related organs, which includes the liver, gallbladder, bile ducts and pancreas. For the purpose of this book, the word will be used to refer to both *hepatologists* and gastroenterologists, who also look after people with liver disease.

*Glitazones (152):* A family of drugs that have been explored as therapy for *MASLD*. They reverse *insulin resistance* in fatty tissue. Given the importance of insulin resistance to the biology of MASLD this gives an obvious potentially valuable mode of action. As with many of the other drugs explored in MASLD, they improve *liver function tests*. They also improve liver biopsy features of hepatic steatosis (and to a lesser extent fibrosis). There is no evidence, however, in relation to directly relevant clinical endpoints of more significant effects. There have also been concerns about their safety in MASLD. There is a particular concern with regard to worsening of pre-existing heart failure. Furthermore, patients can describe weight gain, which is logical given that it is making tissues more responsive to insulin, which means they are then able to take up and store nutrition. The benefit is that it is being stored as fat in safer places than in the liver. They are not *licensed* for MASLD use and are, accordingly, not used, other than for people who are already receiving them for type 2 diabetes, for which they are licensed.

***GLP-1 Agonist (151):*** An emerging class of drugs, originally licensed for type 2 diabetes, showing real promise for the treatment of **MASLD**. This is also a class of drug that has caught the popular "zeitgeist" as weight loss drugs such as Wegovy or Ozempic, and Mountjaro. ***Semaglutide*** is a weekly injection. This is the version that has been widely taken up as a weight loss therapy. These drugs mimic the action of a natural peptide called glucagon-like peptide (GLP-1) which appears to have two important actions that are relevant to MASLD. The first is that it stimulates the islet cells of the pancreas to produce increased levels of *insulin*. The second is that it seems to act on the brain to give sense of "satiation" (i.e. people feel full and therefore don't feel like eating). Experience of the drugs in the clinic is that they reduce *insulin resistance*; one of the cardinal biological process of MASLD, and help with weight loss through reduced dietary intake. Both are very attractive effects in MASLD management. In terms of specific clinical trial outcomes they significantly improve liver function tests and promote resolution of MASH on liver biopsy, with preliminary trial data showing they may also reduce *fibrosis*. There are words of caution, however, before we label them as MASLDs "wonder drugs". They can cause injection site discomfort, and nausea is a common issue. More significantly they can, rarely, be associated with cancer risk and pancreatitis. Finally, there is some evidence that although they can give rise to dramatic weight loss (at face value a good thing), this is actually more marked for muscle than it is for fat tissue. Given our desire to build muscle for metabolic reasons in MASLD, this may be somewhat counterproductive.

***Glucose:*** The archetypal sugar molecule and, as such, the basis of all carbohydrates. The balance between glucose levels, *insulin* levels, and carbohydrate underpins almost the whole of cellular energetics, type 2 diabetes, insulin sensitivity and resistance and thus **MASLD**.

***Glycogen (11,16,27,43,57,128):*** A physiological carbohydrate storage form of *glucose*. Immediately after a meal, glucose levels rise rapidly in the *portal vein,* triggering the release of *insulin*. This insulin stimulates those cell types that can make glycogen (the *hepatocytes* of the liver and muscle cells) to take up the glucose and convert it into glycogen. This reduces the blood sugar level. In between meals the portal vein glucose levels fall, switching off insulin production. In the absence of an insulin effect (and in the presence of a second hormone called glucagon which promotes the opposite effect) the cells break down glycogen, releasing glucose into the blood stream. This shuttling backwards and forwards of glucose into a rapidly accessible storage form helps to smooth out the blood glucose peaks and troughs that would otherwise be seen with intermittent food consumption. In insulin resistance, and thus **MASLD**, this whole pathway fails. The hepatocytes fail to "sense" insulin correctly and instead of converting excess glucose into glycogen they convert it into *fat*. Because muscle cells can also convert glucose into glycogen under the influence of insulin, and because they can't synthesise fat as an alternate pathway for storage, they represent an alternative metabolic pathway for glucose in insulin resistance. Boosting this muscle glycogen storage boosts whole body insulin response. This is one important reason why **exercise therapy** works.

*Hepatologist:* A doctor who is a specialist in the prevention, diagnosis and management of diseases affecting the liver, bile ducts and gall bladder. For the purpose of this book, the word will be used to refer to both hepatologists and **gastroenterologists**, who also look after people with liver disease.

*HbA1c (212):* A blood test that is the standard way of diagnosing type 2 diabetes, a condition where there is usually too much insulin but with lost responsiveness, and monitoring response to treatment or lifestyle control. The haemoglobin in your red blood cells can be modified by the attachment of glucose molecules. This is perfectly normal, happens in everyone and has no impact on the way that the cells work. The amount of glucose that is attached, however, depends on the glucose level in the blood. Just measuring glucose itself is useful but it naturally goes up and down depending on what and when you have eaten. The amount of HbA1c is a measure of the "average" blood glucose level over a prolonged period of time (about 90 days). This makes it a really useful clinical test to understand what is happening with regard to diabetes control. Given the important association between type 2 diabetes and **MASLD** this is a frequently used test in MASLD patients.

*Hepatic Artery (9,10,72,174-175,183):* One of the two sources of blood flowing into the liver (the other is the *portal vein*). This dual perfusion type is unique to the liver. In fact, the majority of the blood flow into the liver actually comes from the portal vein, although all the blood supply to the *bile duct* comes from the hepatic artery. Hepatic artery problems typically only arise in **MASLD** after *liver transplant* when thrombosis of the artery can be an early complication.

*Hepatic Vein (9,18,77,85,160):* The vein (actually usually several veins) that drain blood from the liver out into the *inferior vena cava* for return to the heart. It is not to be confused with the *portal vein* which is one of the sources of blood flowing into the liver (the liver has two sources of blood flowing in, the portal vein and the *hepatic artery* but only a single outflow, the hepatic vein).

*Hepatocellular Carcinoma (HCC) (21,28,32,98-100,160,162,233):* A cancer of the *hepatocyte*. Most cancers in the liver are metastases or secondary cancers arising from elsewhere in the body (commonly the colon or large bowel). Primary cancer of the liver can, however, arise and it is growing in frequency. It typically arises in an already injured liver. This is usually *cirrhosis*, but in the case, in particular, of viral hepatitis it can be in pre-cirrhotic liver. HCC is therefore, correctly, viewed as one of the complications of cirrhosis. It is, worryingly, a growing problem in **MASLD**, which is now one of the commonest underlying liver diseases seen in HCC patients. It is likely that the rise in HCC in MASLD reflects the growing numbers of MASLD patients who have now progressed to cirrhosis. The risk of HCC in all liver diseases is greater in men than women as testosterone appears to favour its growth. We screen everyone with cirrhosis, or probable cirrhosis, with a specific blood test called an alpha-fetoprotein and an *ultrasound* scan on a 6-monthly basis. If HCC is suspected, a second type of imaging, usually a CT or an MRI scan, will be used to confirm it. HCC management is a complex and rapidly developing area, and as such a detailed consideration of it is beyond the scope of this book. As is the case with all complications of cirrhosis, HCC is something that is far better managed by the prevention of the development of cirrhosis by effective disease treatment, than it is by being treated once it develops.

*Hepatocytes:* The cells of the liver. A normal adult male will have up to 1.5Kg of liver cells. Each hepatocyte performs all the functions of the liver (i.e. there is no sub-specialisation of the cells). Liver failure arises when there is an insufficient mass of functioning hepatocytes to undertake all key functions. The hepatocytes are at the heart of the biology of **MASLD**, storing fat within themselves and being the target for inflammatory injury. Reducing, reversing, and preventing that injury is at the heart of our treatment approach. One property that hepatocytes have is that they can regenerate when the liver is injured (the cells themselves can divide to create more hepatocytes, and stem cells in the liver can turn into hepatocytes). This property of regeneration is really important for recovery of the liver after injury, and plays a key role in the process of cirrhosis development.

*Immune Response (15,29-30,61,62,80-83,163,174,176-177,184):* The system in the body that mounts targeted response to foreign proteins and other molecules. It is the second part of the response to infection (after *inflammation*). It is more targeted (that is its nature) with **T-cells** and **B-cells** arising that are specific to the foreign protein or infectious organism. The specific nature of the response means that it takes longer to develop than inflammation (which is non-specific in nature and therefore acts as a "holding response" to fight infection until the immune response develops). Specific immune responses give rise to immunological memory whereby a particular response type is "archived" for future access. This reactivation of a memory response is much quicker than a new immune response and underpins vaccination. Inflammation appears to be a much more important part of the disease process in **MASLD** than the specific immune response.

*Immunoglobulin G (IgG) (64,96):* The immunoglobulin fraction in the blood is a technical term for all the antibodies of all types measured as a protein level (i.e. including both ordinary antibody and *autoantibody* and includes antibody of all specificities). The IgG fraction represents the mature, finely-tuned antibodies that are produced long-term after an immune stimulus. IgG is normally elevated in *autoimmune hepatitis* (AIH) but not in **MASLD**. This makes the IgG a useful test in patients with *anti-nuclear antibody*; (the classic autoantibody seen in AIH and frequently seen in MASLD, causing diagnostic confusion) for distinguishing AIH and MASLD.

*Inferior Vena Cava (9,172):* The large vein that takes blood from the lower half of the body back to the heart to be re-oxygenated in the lungs. The *hepatic vein* drains into it. The inferior vena cava actually passes through the liver, meaning that in liver transplant surgery a section of it has to be removed. Current practice is to use bypass to connect the portal vein and the inferior vena cava below the liver with the venous circulation above the liver, to allow normal venous drainage during surgery.

*Inflammation:* A critical part of the disease process in the more aggressive forms of **MASLD**. In essence it is the presence of inflammation that turns *simple steatosis* into *metabolic-dysfunction associated steatohepatitis (MASH)* which is the disease form that can progress to *fibrosis* and eventually *cirrhosis*. Inflammation is part of the body's natural response to threat or injury. It is typically the initial response to any injury and is "non-specific" in the sense that inflammation is activated by patterns of common molecule types seen on infectious organisms rather than the specific molecules of the infection (that is the hallmark of the *immune response*). The cells of the inflammatory response include *neutrophils* and *macrophages* which normally "patrol" the tissues and can be attracted in larger numbers by stress signals released by damaged tissues. These calls can phagocytose ("eat") bacteria and debris from damaged tissues and can release chemicals into the tissues that can also kill. Inflammation and the immune response are, in fact, closely linked because it is the actions of the inflammatory response that can activate the immune response. Inflammation followed by immunity is the normal sequence. In MASLD, inflammation is activated not by an infection but by the irritant properties of fat. The process of inflammation therefore "comes from within". Because of this absence of an infection against which an immune response would be mounted, the progression from inflammation to immunity is very limited. The only specific immune responses that are seen are against nuclear proteins (**anti-nuclear antibodies**) that have been altered by the effects of inflammation causing their structure to be changed and thus allowing them to be "seen" by the immune response. There is no evidence that these immune responses add significantly to the process of tissue damage in MASLD and the main importance of ANA is that their presence shouldn't be misinterpreted as reflecting the presence of *autoimmune hepatitis*.

*Insulin:* A hormone that plays a key role in controlling the handling of components of the diet taken up into the ***portal vein*** after meals, especially glucose and amino acids. It is the failure of the ***hepatocytes*** in particular to respond to insulin that underpins the process of ***insulin resistance*** that lies at the heart of both MASLD and ***type 2 diabetes.***

*Insulin Resistance:* A critical factor in the pathogenesis of **MASLD** specifically, and the ***metabolic syndrome*** in general. The key step in the body's handling of nutrition is the release of ***insulin*** by the ***pancreas***, and the action of insulin on the cells of the body, stimulating them to take up ***glucose*** and amino acids. In simple terms it promotes the healthy storage of "spare" nutrition that can be returned to the circulation in between meals, thereby keeping blood glucose and amino acid levels stable. An effective insulin response, therefore, needs the combination of insulin release, and the capacity of target cells (especially liver, muscle and fat cells) to respond appropriately. If the cells don't respond appropriately to an insulin signal this is a state called insulin resistance. When people become insulin resistant, glucose that cells don't take up because they aren't "listening" to insulin remains in the circulation and, if high enough, results in ***type 2 diabetes.*** In the liver, glucose taken up from the blood under the instruction of insulin is converted into a storage version called ***glycogen*** which can be rapidly manufactured from glucose in response to insulin directly after a meal, and equally rapidly converted back into glucose between meals, when the glucose level drops again. In insulin resistance glycogen is not made, and as a fall back response the ***hepatocytes*** turn glucose into ***fat*** which is then stored within the cells. This is the origin of the liver fat in MASLD and explains the very strong link between type 2 diabetes and MASLD. Insulin resistance develops for a number of reasons. It can be genetic, arise in response to obesity and be worsened by infections and treatments such as steroids. In most people, it develops after a prolonged period of high insulin levels (hyper-insulinaemia), when insulin secretion has been chronically raised as a response to high dietary intake, in particular to excess carbohydrate intake. After a while of being exposed to high insulin levels, cells lose their sensitivity to the signal i.e. they become "resistant" to it. Reversing insulin resistance is, very logically, an attractive potential approach to treating MASLD. This can be achieved by weight loss (reducing the amount of body fat) and exercise (the cells of the muscles need to take up amino acids to strengthen themselves and thus become insulin sensitive, taking on some of the burden that the liver is not carrying (muscle is the only other tissue after the liver that can synthesise glycogen)). This explains why *lifestyle modification* is such an attractive treatment option in MASLD. The simplest way to think about it is that chronically high carbohydrate intake causes chronically high insulin levels, which have less and less response. To reverse the insulin resistance, the best way is to turn off the tap. When carbohydrate intake in particular is reduced, insulin levels drop, and the cells start to regain their sensitivity to the insulin response again. This has the double benefit of less dietary carbohydrate needing to be stored, and more liver cells that are able to store it as glycogen rather than fat, rebalancing the liver glycogen to fat storage in favour of glycogen.

*Interface Hepatitis:* A form of inflammation seen in the liver. The term describes an inflammatory reaction reaching into the plates of **hepatocytes** adjacent to the *portal tract*. It is one of the less commonly seen patterns of liver inflammation in **MASLD** (*lobular inflammation* is much commoner) and its presence usually indicates a more aggressive form of the disease. Interface hepatitis is most classically associated with **autoimmune hepatitis (AIH)** and if significant levels of interface hepatitis are seen, the possibility of AIH should always be considered.

*Itch (64,192,203-206):* An occasional symptom in **MASLD** patients, especially when *cholestasis* is present. It is certainly not the commonest symptom seen in MASLD (fatigue is much commoner) but its importance lies in the fact that it is one of the more easily treated symptoms. The characteristics of itch in liver disease are different to those of allergic skin reactions. In liver disease the sensation is very much one of irritation deep under the skin (a sensation of "creepy crawlies" under the skin is commonly described) whereas allergic itch is more superficial in nature. The distribution of the itch is also characteristic, often affecting the palms of the hand and the soles of the feet, the scalp, and the back. It is not associated with the presence of rash (other than as a result of scratching). It is often worse at night and can disturb sleep, thereby contributing to fatigue. It is relatively easy to treat with *cholestyramine* used as first line treatment and, in most centres, *rifampicin* as second-line. Effective treatment of itch is one of the major contributions clinicians can make to quality of life in liver disease.

*Jaundice (11,16,70-71,83,87-88,95):* The clinical consequence of elevated *bilirubin* levels. Clinically, it is a yellowing of the skin. Initially this is very subtle and usually only visible in the whites of the eyes (it is easier to see in the only truly white tissue in the body). Bilirubin levels can rise because of liver disease itself (a failure to conjugate and transfer bilirubin into the *bile duct*). It can also occur if the flow of bile is impaired (it backs up into the *hepatocytes* and leaks back into the blood). Jaundice can also occur if the breakdown of red blood cells is greater than normal in a haemolytic anaemia. Thus, although jaundice is usually a feature of liver disease, it does not have to be. In *MASLD*, jaundice is seen in two settings. The first is as part of a very acute inflammatory process in non-cirrhotic disease. This is actually uncommon in MASLD as the level of inflammation is rarely severe enough to cause such a severe acute hepatitis picture. The second setting is as a consequence of a failing liver in cirrhosis. As with hepatic *encephalopathy* and bleeding from *varices*, the advent of late jaundice is a significant event in MASLD and should always lead to consideration as to whether transplant might be appropriate. There is one significant trap with jaundice in MASLD (as in any other liver disease). This is the phenomenon of Gilbert's syndrome. This is a genetic variation in one of the transporter molecules that carries bilirubin out into the bile duct. It leads to a less effective transporter, which leads to a higher background bilirubin level. It is not an illness (it is best thought of as a variant of normal) and does not cause problems, but it does mean that the bilirubin level is elevated, and jaundice can be seen. To make it even more complicated, the bilirubin level can go up even further if people are stressed or ill. The important point is that if we use bilirubin and jaundice level as a risk marker in a liver disease, then the presence of Gilbert's can make people look like they have more severe disease than they actually do. This is why we do not only look at bilirubin and jaundice as severity markers, but look at the whole picture.

***Kupffer Cells (11,12,17):*** The population of ***macrophages*** found in the liver. The scavengers of the immune system, the Kupffer cells play a key role in eliminating bacteria that get across the bowel wall and into the ***portal vein.***

***Lactulose (68,163,189):*** A liquid form of laxative that is widely used for the prevention and treatment of hepatic ***encephalopathy***. This is a manifestation of liver dysfunction, typically seen with ***cirrhosis***, which is characterised by ***cognitive symptoms***. It seems that build-up of colon contents can drive the process, probably through increased levels of bacterial breakdown products overloading the failing liver. Lactulose speeds up bowel transit, reducing the levels of potential toxin build-up. The dose of lactulose needs to be adjusted upwards and downwards to achieve the optimal stool frequency (around 2 bowel motions per day). Obviously, too much lactulose can result in diarrhoea. The non-absorbed oral antibiotic ***rifaximin*** is an alternative approach which is increasingly being used for the prevention and treatment of encephalopathy.

***Licensing (143-154):*** The process by which a new drug, or an old drug being used in a new disease setting, is approved for use in patients. The licensing process ensures that new treatments are both safe for use in people and are likely to be effective. Different parts of the world have different licensing bodies. In the USA it is the Food and Drug Administration (FDA), in the UK it is the MHRA (Medicines and Healthcare products Regulatory Agency) and in Europe the European Medicines Agency (EMA). All such bodies use the data from ***clinical trials*** to decide whether drugs should be licensed. In many ways, safety is the primary concern as the licensing process in its current form arose in response to drug injury scandals, such as that linked to thalidomide, where unsafe drugs were made available to vulnerable patients. Effectiveness is clearly important as well, as a safe but ineffective drug would indirectly harm you by not treating the disease. Drug licensing implies that a high bar has been cleared for both safety and effectiveness; something which should give patients confidence. A licence per se does not mean that a drug will be available to all patients, however. Depending on the health care system there will typically be a second stage of assessment of a drug by the body that will pay for it if the patient isn't paying directly (the NHS through NICE in the UK and the insurance companies in the USA). In this second stage the licensed drug will be assessed as to whether it is effective enough to justify the cost. Clearly, both the level of effectiveness and the cost enter into this assessment of balance.

The process of evaluating drug effectiveness and safety in clinical trials involves several stages or "phases". In Phase 1 trials the drug is given to healthy volunteers to assess blood levels for given doses (starting with very low doses), and to ensure that there is no toxicity (in cancer Phase 1 trials are sometimes done in patients). Phase 2 trials are where the drug moves to patients. These are small trials with a short duration, principally to show that the drug is safe in patients who might be very different in their age and physical status to healthy volunteers. We are also looking, in Phase 2, for evidence that the drug is effective for the disease, typically through improvement of an aspect of the disease which is meaningful and measurable (such as blood tests in the setting of ***MASLD***). If a drug is safe, and there is evidence to suggest that it is effective, then it moves to Phase 3. These are the larger and longer clinical trials with an endpoint, or trial question, that is highly relevant to patients (ideally survival or avoidance of a major and meaningful endpoint such as, in the case of liver disease, liver transplantation). A typical Phase 3 trial might still only involve the patients getting the drug for a couple of years, so it is common to have what is called a long-term safety extension where the drug is, if participants in the trial want it, available for, typically, another 5 years during which time the longer term effects are monitored.

One issue which is integral to the design of trials, and one which has been especially challenging in MASLD, is the concept of the trial **endpoint**. This is the aspect of the disease or patient progress that is being measured. This needs to be both meaningful (so that any change in its value is likely to reflect real patient benefit) and attainable (within the plausible time frame for a clinical trial). The challenge in all liver diseases is that they tend to be slowly progressive so that a really meaningful trial endpoint (such as death, need for transplant or varices development) will need a long study (people take many years to reach these advanced disease states). This does mean that a trial that apparently doesn't show any benefit in terms of these endpoints may in fact just have been done for too short a period of time. This is something important to remember in MASLD where demonstrating benefit in trials has been a real challenge.

In all good quality trials the effect of the new drug needs to be compared directly with either a dummy or placebo (if there is no currently available treatment in the space) or with the current most effective treatment ("standard of care") if such a treatment is available. Trials include a high level of monitoring of participants. This is partly to ensure safety but also to ensure that all the possible evidence to support the drug being licensed is collected (it would be a disaster if a drug clearly works but the tests collected don't manage to show it because they are the wrong ones; it happens!). To license a drug the FDA, MHRA or EMA will typically want to see that the drug is safe and that it is effective in a minimum of two Phase 3 trials.

Once a drug is licensed it will be provided with a "label". This is a description of the situations in which it is approved for use (the disease area, the types of that disease and, importantly, the situations when it shouldn't be used). If a drug is licensed and labelled for use in a disease, and the patient meets all the conditions for use (typically around kidney function being normal/acceptable, pregnancy, breast feeding etc) then a doctor can prescribe it with full legal protection (the issue of whether the health authorities or insurance companies in their country will pay for it and thus "allow" it to be prescribed is a slightly different question). At the other end of the spectrum, an unlicensed drug can only ever be used as part of a clinical trial that has gone through all the approvals to check for safety and which is being monitored closely (the route to the drug becoming licensed). The grey area is where a drug is licensed for use in another disease area but not MASLD (i.e. licensed but not labelled for use in MASLD). This is important because a number of the drugs increasingly being considered for use in MASLD fall into this category.

Research and clinical care in MASLD reached a major milestone in spring 2024 with the USA licensing of the first drug specifically for use in MASLD; **resmetirom**.

***Lifestyle Modification:*** A blanket term for the changes in way of life when used as an approach to treating a condition such as ***MASLD***. In MASLD there are two main components to lifestyle modification - diet change and ***exercise therapy***. These synergise, which is why we think of them as a pair rather than each individually. Lifestyle modification can be very effective in MASLD. The challenge, however, is in getting started and then keeping up the diet changes and exercise programme in the "real world". An important concept in this is that of secondary gain. This is the situation that arises once you as an individual feel the benefits of the change. Doctors and nurses can encourage and support you, and you will, to a greater or lesser extent, accept what they say and change your lifestyle. This is all, however "on trust" and it is human nature to limit the amount of trust that you put in the advice given by clinicians. Once you feel the benefit however, it becomes far easier to stick with the change.

***Liver Biopsy (76-78,90,176):*** The technique by which a very small sample of liver tissue is taken to examine under the microscope. These days it is done either under ultrasound control through the skin, or via the hepatic vein through a line inserted in a peripheral vein, usually in the neck. There is often great concern about biopsy amongst patients, however some of these concerns are perhaps a little overstated. In reality, it is a simple process. There can be a little bit of discomfort, and there is a small risk of bleeding, but it is actually very safe and well tolerated. Liver biopsy is an important test in MASLD as it allows us to differentiate the milder forms of disease (such as ***simple steatosis***) from the more aggressive forms such as ***MASH***. In the past, liver biopsy was an important tool for investigating for the presence of ***cirrhosis***. There are now effective non-invasive tests that can provide the same information without the risk of a biopsy (***fibroscan, ELF*** etc). There are, as yet, however, no reliable tests that can distinguish simple steatosis from MASH. Given that the goal of therapy will be, increasingly, to prevent disease progression to fibrosis in the first place, over-focus on tests to show that fibrosis is there, rather than tests to identify those at risk of developing fibrosis, will be to rather miss the point.

***Lobular Inflammation:*** Sometimes also called lobular hepatitis. One of the forms of liver ***inflammation***. In lobular inflammation the cells of the inflammatory response infiltrate into the sheets of ***hepatocytes*** that make up the bulk of the liver. This is the type of inflammation that is most frequently seen in more aggressive forms of ***MASLD*** and reflects the inflammatory cells responding to the signals being released by hepatocytes that have been injured by ***fat*** deposition.

***Macronutrients (42,113):*** The molecules that make up the bulk of food intake, providing energy. The main macronutrients are carbohydrates (which also includes fibre), protein and fat. MASLD is generally associated with an excess of macronutrients.

***Macrophage (10,15,61):*** The scavenger cells of the inflammation and immune system that are critical for mopping up bacteria and cellular debris in the context of infection or tissue injury. Macrophages in the spleen are responsible for the breakdown of red blood cells which have reached the end of their useful life, generating ***bilirubin***. Macrophages in the liver are called ***Kupffer Cells*** and play a key role in protecting the body from bacteria that have leaked out from the bowel and entered the portal vein.

***Maintenance:*** An important part of effective long-term treatment for any condition. Once a condition is diagnosed the first goal of treatment is to achieve ***remission*** (i.e. bringing the disease under control). The second goal is then to keep it under control. This is maintenance. Typically, higher treatment levels are required for achieving remission than for maintenance. It is too early in therapy development for these concepts to be relevant in ***MASLD***. It may be, however, that the role of ***lifestyle modification*** approaches to treatment in MASLD may be more effective in maintenance than in remission induction, other than for the early stages of changing from steatosis to healthy cells, with initial control of the disease for more severe stages being with drug therapy. Time will tell.

***MASH:*** The universally used abbreviation for ***metabolic dysfunction-associated steatohepatitis***. As such it refers to the inflammatory form of ***MASLD*** which is associate with an increased risk of progression to ***cirrhosis***. The abbreviation can, however, sometimes be used incorrectly to refer to all forms of MASLD. Care is needed because the term actually has a very specific meaning.

***MASLD:*** The widely used abbreviation for ***metabolic dysfunction-associated steatotic liver disease.***

***MASLD and Increased Alcohol Intake (MetALD)(54,79):*** The clinical features of MASLD in the setting of excess alcohol consumption. This is a newly defined entity in the setting of the renaming of steatotic liver disease which acknowledges the role played by the calorie load in ethanol in driving MASLD. Given the role played by energy contained in ethanol in driving steatosis, reducing, and ideally completely eliminating, ethanol consumption is an important approach to lifestyle modification in MASLD.

***Metabolic Dysfunction-Associated Steatotic Liver Disease:*** The new term to describe the condition formerly known as ***non-alcoholic fatty liver disease (NAFLD)***. The old condition name is still widely used, and will be visible for a long time on the internet and in legacy publications. It is important to realise that we are talking about the same thing. The name change came about to avoid defining a condition in terms of what it wasn't (i.e. "non-alcoholic"), to avoid the use of the term alcoholic with its often negative connotations and to avoid the term "fatty" which, again, people felt was negative ("steatotic" is a technical term for the same thing). The two main forms of MASLD are *simple steatosis* and *metabolic dysfunction-associated steatohepatitis (MASH)*. Both these entities are characterised by fat deposition in the *hepatocytes.* The difference between them is that in simple steatosis all that is happening is fat deposition, whilst in MASH it is accompanied by *inflammation.* This more complex process is key for the subsequent development of *fibrosis* and, ultimately, *cirrhosis*. The progression of disease can be summarised as:

healthy cells ↔ steatosis ↔ steatohepatitis ↔ fibrosis → cirrhosis

*Metabolic Dysfunction-Associated Steatohepatitis (2,5,28,32,34,85,87, 99-100,154):* Frequently abbreviated to *MASH* this is the form of *MASLD* in which the fat deposition in the *hepatocytes* is accompanied by significant *inflammation.* The presence of inflammation significantly increases the level of *hepatocyte* injury, which can reduce cell numbers and trigger the development of *fibrosis*. The step by which *simple steatosis* comes to be accompanied by significant inflammation is a really critical one in understanding MASLD, as progression of the disease to *cirrhosis* almost always goes via it. Many of the treatment approaches under development in MASLD target this inflammatory disease component.

*Metabolic Syndrome:* A term for the combination of disease states linked to obesity and *type 2 diabetes*. These include type 2 diabetes itself, *MASLD*, elevation in *cholesterol*, hypertension and vascular disease. The presence of one of these disease states significantly increases the chances of one or more additional ones. What this means in practice in MASLD is that patients are also at significantly increased risk of ischaemic heart disease and its own specific risk factors. In fact, patients with MASLD are more likely to die of heart disease than they are of liver disease……This is one of the reasons why *clinical trials* design and, in particular *endpoint* identification, are so important. If we only look at a liver endpoint in a trial in MASLD (*liver biopsy* or *liver function tests*) we could potentially miss a worsening in heart disease risk for example; a potential disaster.

*Metformin (152,153):* A drug that is widely used in the treatment of *type 2 diabetes*. It has a number of actions around appetite reduction but appears to mainly function through restoration (to a degree) of insulin sensitivity. Unlike other oral diabetic therapies it does not cause weight gain (indeed it can result in weight loss). Given its mode of action there has been a great deal of interest in it as a potential therapy in **MASLD**. The data from the numerous, frequently small, clinical trials suggest that although *liver function test* improvement is seen (especially *alanine transaminase* and *aspartate transaminase*), and weight loss is consistently seen, there is no apparent improvement in *liver biopsy* abnormalities. Metformin can also have significant, albeit rare, side-effects such as lactic acidosis. It is not licensed for use in MASLD and therefore shouldn't be used purely for this indication. In people who also have type 2 diabetes it is a logical agent to use.

*Micronutrients (42,49,54-56,58,106-108):* The molecules or chemicals that make up a very small part of the diet, but which support important functions within the body. These include vitamins and minerals. Deficiency in some of these may contribute to the development of, or be a consequence of, **MASLD**. See **Appendix 3** for more details.

*Mitochondrion (128,133)*: A specialised structure within the cytoplasm of the cell that plays a key role in energy generation. Mitochondrial energy generation is typically *aerobic* in nature, meaning that there is a balance between fuel and oxygen consumption. *Triglyceride*, a key form of *fat*, is a very effective fuel source for mitochondrial energy generation meaning that increase in this form of energy generation is fat-burning. *Exercise therapy* is an effective way of increasing the level of aerobic metabolism through, amongst other mechanisms, an actual increase in mitochondrial biogenesis (an increase in mitochondrial numbers).

*NAFLD Fibrosis Score (92):* A clinical risk score that includes the values for patient age, *platelet count, alanine transaminase, aspartate transaminase*, albumin, body mass index and presence or absence of diabetes. It is easily calculated using widely available on-line tools and, because it uses every day clinical test data is universally available. Across the whole population it is very effective for identifying groups of people with advanced fibrosis and cirrhosis in **MASLD** (although, perhaps counter-intuitively, the name change from NAFLD to MASLD hasn't, as yet, reached as far as the score!). The fact that, in contrast to *FIB-4*, it was derived in NAFLD/MASLD and includes metabolic factors known to be associated with fibrosis/cirrhosis risk probably makes it a more sensitive marker for risk assessment in MASLD. At the individual level, however, other factors that cause the value to be abnormal (most obviously a low platelet count for reasons other than advanced liver disease) can make it less accurate. It is not a definitive test but useful for screening people to assist with decision making about further investigations to assess risk.

***NASH (34):*** The universally used abbreviation for ***Non-Alcoholic Steatohepatitis*** before the change of name to ***metabolic dysfunction-associated steatohepatitis (MASH)***.

***Neutrophil (77):*** A type of white blood cell, and one of the key cells responsible for ***inflammation***. Neutrophils are made in the bone marrow, and then released into the blood where they "patrol" the body. Injured tissues send out signals which attract them to help fight the cause of the injury. The pus in an abscess represents white cells attracted into an area with infection, for example. They release chemicals such as cytokines and induce ***oxidant stress***, both processes that contribute to liver injury in ***MASLD***.

***Non-Alcoholic Fatty Liver Disease (NAFLD) (2,5,34,79):*** The old term for ***MASLD***. It is likely to appear in information and online for a long time until the name transition is fully embedded.

***Non-Alcoholic Steatohepatitis (2,5):*** Frequently abbreviated to ***NASH*** this is the old term for ***metabolic-dysfunction-associated steatohepatitis (MASH)***.

***Nucleus (63):*** The structure at the centre of all cells (other than red blood cells) which contains the genetic material of the cell (the DNA formed into chromosomes). Where ***autoantibodies*** are seen in MASLD they are directed against nuclear structures. These are termed ***anti-nuclear antibodies***.

***Obeticholic Acid (OCA) (150,151):*** One of the most intensively studied therapies in ***MASLD*** and one that exemplifies the challenges. It is a drug that has a number of potentially key actions relevant to MASLD. These include reducing both ***inflammation*** and ***fibrosis*** and a number of metabolic actions. It also significantly reduces ***cholestasis*** by suppressing bile acid production and, on that basis, has been licensed for use as a second-line therapy in primary biliary cholangitis (PBC). In MASLD it has a clear effect on improving ***liver function tests*** and there is some evidence to suggest it improves liver fibrosis. As is the case with all therapies for MASLD there is, as yet, no data on improved survival. The FDA ultimately deemed, however, that the risk/benefit ratio was unfavourable and it was not approved for use in MASLD. As a result all development work has stopped for this indication.

***Osteoporosis (220):*** A process of bone thinning that can leave the patient at risk of fractures (especially of the hip and spine). It is a process that happens naturally with age and is worsened by female sex, low body weight, smoking and poor diet. There is also a significant familial component (the daughters of mothers with osteoporosis have a significantly higher level of the process themselves). Its risk is significantly increased in all chronic liver disease patients, with the greatest increase in risk being seen in men (although the absolute risk always remains highest in women). There are now effective screening tools and treatments for osteoporosis and with their widespread use the risk of fractures for **MASLD** patients has decreased significantly in recent years.

***Oxidant Stress (30):*** A key part of the pathway of tissue damage in ***inflammation***. Inflammatory cells produce free radicals (activated toxic atoms and molecules) as part of their pathway to killing bacteria and viruses (think of how we use hydrogen peroxide as a disinfectant). The same process of inflammatory cell activation occurs in higher risk **MASLD**, probably as a direct consequence of the presence of fat. These free radicals cause oxidant stress tissue damage which contributes to liver cell damage. The importance of oxidant stress explains why there has been interest in **antioxidants** as potential therapies in MASLD. This treatment approach has not been hugely successful and it isn't used routinely in practice. This is probably because it does nothing to correct the fat-induced inflammation that drives the process, just the downstream manifestations of it.

***Pancreas (10,11,27,152):*** The gland that produces most digestive enzymes. It drains through the pancreatic duct which joins the ***bile duct*** just before it joins the ***duodenum***.

***Placebo:*** A "dummy" tablet given in ***clinical trials*** to one group of the participants. Placebos are designed to fully match the actual drug being investigated in terms of shape, size and colour, but to lack the active ingredient. The inclusion of placebo in trials is essential if we are to demonstrate that an effect seen with a new drug is a direct result of the actions of the drug, rather than the extra clinical care (as well as the patient positivity) that can come with a clinical trial.

***Platelets (17,88-89):*** The very small blood cells (or more accurately fragments of cells) that are responsible for blood clotting. Their importance in **MASLD** is that they are a useful blood test measure of whether there is ***portal hypertension***. In portal hypertension, the spleen swells and pools blood cells including platelets. This leads to a reduced platelet count. A value below 150 is a strong suggestion of the presence of portal hypertension and thus ***cirrhosis***. This value in terms of clinical prediction is reflected in the fact that the platelet count is part of the main predictive scores for MASLD such as ***FIB-4*** and ***NAFLD fibrosis score***.

***Portal Tract (10,18,31-77):*** The structures within the liver that contain the ***hepatic artery*** and ***portal vein*** branches as well as the small ***bile duct*** branches. These structures are integral to the functional anatomy of the liver and have been likened to 3-core electric cable because of the triple structure. Portal tract inflammation is less common than ***lobular inflammation*** in

***MASLD***, but where present seems to be associated with a more aggressive disease type.

***Portal Hypertension (19,20,90,159,161,172,180,197):*** A state of increased blood pressure within the ***portal vein***. This can arise as a result of injury or obstruction to the portal vein early in life, but is most commonly seen in adults in chronic liver disease. The vast majority of liver disease patients developing portal hypertension do so as a result of ***cirrhosis***. The combination of liver regeneration within a constricted space resulting from ***fibrosis*** formation puts pressure on the liver sinusoids (the very small blood vessels in the liver fed by the portal vein and hepatic artery that bathe the ***hepatocytes*** in blood). Occasionally, portal hypertension can arise in the absence of cirrhosis. The most important complications of portal hypertension are ***varices*** and ***ascites***. Portal hypertension is detected in practice by a finding of varices on ***endoscopy*** and strongly suggested by the presence of cirrhosis on ***liver biopsy***.

***Portal Vein (9-11,17,20,27,32,89,160,172,190):*** The large blood vessel that drains blood from the bowel. It enters the liver and all the blood draining from the bowel is therefore "filtered" through the liver. This allows the ***hepatocytes*** to take up nutrients for processing and the ***Kupffer cells*** to remove any bacteria or fungi that have crossed the bowel wall to get into the portal vein blood. The portal vein is also an important source of oxygenated blood for the liver, as the level of arterial blood flow into the bowel wall is so high that even the blood draining out through the portal vein is oxygen-rich. The pressure within the portal vein is typically very low (as is the case in all veins); much lower than in arteries. The pressure can, however, rise in chronic liver disease causing complications. This state is known as ***portal hypertension***.

***PPAR agonist (152,153):*** A family of drugs, some of them licensed for other indications and some still unlicensed, a number of which have been explored as therapies in ***MASLD***. These include bezafibrate, fenofibrate, seladelpar, elafibranor, lanafibranor and the ***glitazones***. The different variant drugs have slightly different patterns of action in terms of which of the family of PPAR receptors they activate. In MASLD terms they share the pattern of improving liver biochemistry but not, as yet, (with the possible exception of lanafibranor), showing any improvement in either liver fibrosis or inflammation or survival. They have not, therefore been ***licensed*** for use in fatty liver and are not used in normal clinical practice for MASLD.

***Remission (114):*** An important part of effective long-term treatment for any condition. Once a condition is diagnosed the first goal of treatment is to achieve remission (i.e. bringing the disease under control in the first place).

The second goal is then to keep it under control. This is *maintenance*. Typically, higher treatment levels are required for achieving remission than for maintenance. It is too early in therapy development for these concepts to be relevant in MASLD. It may be, however, that the role of *lifestyle modification* approaches to treatment in MASLD may be more effective in maintenance than in remission induction, with initial control of the disease being with drug therapy. Time will tell.

***Resmetirom (1,63,143,149-151,154,224):*** The first therapy *licensed* for use in *MASLD*. The approval of this first therapy is a major milestone in the history of MASLD. The licensing decision reflects clear evidence of patient benefit in the context of acceptable patient safety. Resmetirom has, amongst MASLD therapies, a unique mode of action, mimicking the actions of T3 (the active form of thyroxine, the hormone released by the thyroid) on liver cells. Thyroid hormones regulate energy usage and cell metabolism (it is for this reason that the thyroid is often talked about as the "body's thermostat"). There is evidence that *hepatocytes* in MASLD are under-responsive to T3, meaning that although the levels of thyroid hormone in the body are normal, the liver acts as if the body is under-producing the hormone. This leads to a state of energy under-use in the liver; something that contributes to energy storage in the form of *fat* in liver cells. Resmetirom specifically activates the liver T3 receptor, boosting thyroid-driven metabolism in the liver cells. This targeted action boosts liver metabolism, increasing fat utilisation and reducing fat deposition without any of the side effects of boosting thyroid function throughout the body. Complete resolution of fat and inflammation in the liver (i.e. MASH) was seen in 29.9% of people taking resmetirom compared with 9.7% of the *placebo group*. A significant reduction in *fibrosis* was also seen. Importantly in terms of the balance of risk and benefit, a significant reduction was seen in the levels of blood *cholesterol* associated with heart disease. One of the limitations of other drugs that have shown promise for the treatment of MAFLD is that they worsen cholesterol; an important issue when heart disease is associated with MAFLD in the context of the *metabolic syndrome.* At the time of writing, resmetirom has only been licensed for use in the USA.

***Rifampicin (205-206):*** An agent sometimes used to treat moderate or severe itch in chronic liver disease. Rifampicin probably works by increasing metabolism of the molecule causing the itch or blocking its production. Rifampicin can sometimes cause nausea and, more significantly, *liver function test* abnormality (typically elevation in *alanine transaminase*). For this reason, liver function tests should be measured between 2 and 4 weeks after rifampicin is started (and if the dose is increased). If the ALT has increased it should be stopped (after which LFT typically return rapidly to normal). The starting dose is 150mg daily increased to a maximum of 600mg daily if needed (and if tolerated).

***Rifaximin (68,163,189):*** A treatment that is increasingly being used for the management of hepatic ***encephalopathy***. It is an antibiotic that is taken in tablet form but not then absorbed from the gut, meaning that it only acts within the gut. The fact that it is so effective for the treatment of encephalopathy would support the view that bacterial growth/overgrowth in the bowel plays a role in the pathogenesis of this complication.

***Selonsertib:*** A drug with a mechanism that is aimed at the ***fibrosis*** component of ***MASLD*** and which, as a result had real early promise for the disease. The key trial showed, however, that the improvements in fibrosis seen were no better than with placebo and the drug is no longer being developed for ***MASLD***.

***Senescence (15,60-62,77):*** One of the ways in which a cell responds to injury. Probably a key process in many forms of liver disease, including ***MASLD***. Given the importance of ***hepatocyte*** and stem cell proliferation in the body's response to liver injury it may play an important role and, potentially, be a treatment target for the future. The key point is that proliferating cells can rapidly run out of the ability to replicate and can enter a state called senescence. This has been described as the "zombie cell" state, where cells don't die but also don't function. They do, however, send out a distress signal in the form of cytokines and chemokines; the chemicals that attract ***T-cells*** of the immune system. This is probably a protective mechanism of the body to recognise and eliminate the no longer functioning cells. In a disease such as MASLD, however, this clearly has the potential to compound and exacerbate the disease.

***Semaglutide (123,151):*** A member of the ***GLP-1 agonist*** family of drugs (more familiarly known by its trade names of Wegovy and Ozempic), currently licensed for type 2 diabetes and obesity, which shows real potential in MASLD, with reductions in both fibrosis and steatosis (MASH). Beneficial effects include an insulin re-sensitising effect, as well as a brain action to reduce appetite and thus food intake. Semaglutide is given as a weekly subcutaneous (under the skin) injection. This may get licensed for use in MASLD in 2025. As with many drugs, there are rare serious side effects.

***SGLT2 inhibitors (152,197):*** (sodium glucose co-transporter inhibitors) This is a new group of drugs for type 2 diabetes, known as the gliflozins. They cause the kidneys to lose glucose into the urine. They are also increasingly being used in the treatment of heart failure, even for people without diabetes. There has been some interest in whether it could be beneficial in ***MASLD***, reversing insulin resistance and reducing liver ***fat***, but at present it is too early to know to what extent this will be true, and the actual impacts on hard disease endpoints. It can cause a dangerous condition known as diabetic ketoacidosis if people take it when they are unwell or fasted, for example before and immediately after surgery. They can also cause urinary tract infections, because of the increase in glucose in the urine.

***Simple Steatosis:*** The most benign form of **MASLD**. In this form, **fat** deposition within the hepatocytes is not accompanied by ***inflammation***, meaning that there is much less injury to them (although large deposits of fat alone can cause some injury). The steps by which inflammation develops in simple steatosis, leading to **Metabolic dysfunction-associated steatohepatitis (MASH)** are the target of a great deal of research activity (and drug development). Although simple steatosis per se is relatively benign it does strongly suggest the presence of ***metabolic syndrome*** which brings its own health risks. A diagnosis of simple steatosis, therefore, should trigger a review of overall health, and consideration of lifestyle change to prevent progression.

***Specific Aetiology Steatotic Liver Disease (79,81):*** Although the vast majority of ***steatotic liver disease (SLD)*** is either related to excess alcohol consumption or metabolic dysfunction (***metabolic dysfunction-associated steatotic liver disease (MASLD)*** there are a number of other much rarer causes. These give rise to what is called specific aetiology steatotic liver disease. Of these the commonest cause (albeit one which is still rare) is a reaction to certain drugs. The reactions are rare and the drugs that cause it (such as tamoxifen and sodium valproate) are only used in specific situations by clinicians who should be aware of the risk, meaning that confusion about diagnosis shouldn't usually happen. As with all potential drug toxicity, if there is any concern that a drug might be causing the problem it is imperative to stop it if possible. Given the specialised nature of the drugs that can cause this this should only be done under the supervision of a doctor.

***Spironolactone (161,190,197):*** A diuretic (water tablet) that is widely used in the management of ***ascites***. It is particularly useful in ***cirrhosis*** because its mode of action (on the aldosterone pathway) specifically counteracts an effect which is abnormally elevated in cirrhotic patients. It can cause elevation in the blood potassium level (which can, if high enough, cause cardiac rhythm problems meaning that blood tests need to be monitored carefully). It is frequently used in combination with ***furosemide***. Given that furosemide naturally drops blood potassium levels (and thus "protects" against the potassium rising effect of spironolactone) the combination is a very useful one.

***Spontaneous Bacterial Peritonitis (SBP) (21,162-163,172,180):*** A bacterial infection arising in pre-existing ***ascites***. Ascites is a warm, nutrient rich fluid that is relatively inaccessible to the immune system. It is, therefore, unsurprising that bacteria that get into it thrive and reproduce, leading to active infection. SBP is a recognised complication of ascites in all chronic liver diseases and can contribute to temporary worsening of the liver disease ("disease decompensation" in ***cirrhosis***). The bacteria probably enter the ascites from the bowel, helped by the general leakiness of the bowel wall seen in advanced liver disease. The reduction in the effectiveness of the immune system in cirrhosis also contributes to infection becoming established. SBP should be considered in any patient with ascites if the ascites gets worse quickly, becomes painful, or is accompanied by a worsening in liver function. SBP is diagnosed by taking a small sample of the ascites using a syringe and needle which is then cultured to identify bacteria and analysed for the number of white blood cells. Treatment is with antibiotics.

***Steatohepatitis:*** The combination of fat deposition in the liver cells ("steatosis") and ***inflammation***. This is the pathological process seen in the higher risk **MASH** form of **MASLD**. The combination of inflammation and fat deposition triggers the development of ***fibrosis***, the progression of which can result in ***cirrhosis***.

***Steatotic Liver Disease (SLD):*** The overarching term for all forms of liver disease which are characterised by fat deposition ("steatosis") in the ***hepatocytes***. The term itself does not imply any specific aetiology. Aetiology is linked to the names of the subtypes. The subtypes are

1) ***Metabolic dysfunction-association steatotic liver (MASLD,*** formerly known as ***non-alcoholic MASLD (NALD)*** and the subject of this book
2) Alcohol-associated (alcohol-related) liver disease (ALD or ArLD)
3) MASLD and increased alcohol intake (MetALD) where people have features of and risk factors for both MASLD and ALD
4) ***Specific aetiology steatotic liver disease***; conditions where fat deposition is related to other specific disease processed such as drug side effects and a result of genetic disorders
5) Cryptogenic SLD where there is steatosis without any apparent cause

***Systemic Lupus Erythematosus (SLE or lupus)(96):*** An autoimmune condition which can involve a number of different organs (it is an example of a "non-organ specific" autoimmune disease). These can include the joints, skin (with a characteristic facial rash), brain and kidney. The issue in relation to **MASLD** is that the characteristic autoantibodies of lupus (***anti-nuclear***

*antibody*) can also be seen in MASLD, leading the unwary doctor to diagnose SLE when in fact the patient has MASLD.

***Tacrolimus (174,179,184,225,238):*** A powerful immunosuppressive drug which is the mainstay of rejection prevention after liver transplantation. One of the issues with tacrolimus is tolerability and side-effects, and the drug needs to be carefully monitored by measuring blood levels. Side-effects associated with blood levels that are too high can include neurological issues such as tremor, kidney impairment and, importantly in the context of recurrent ***MASLD*** risk after transplantation, diabetes.

***T-cell (60,61):*** A key part of the immune system. T-cells are lymphocytes (the cells that generate specific immune responses (i.e. those targeted at specific molecules/cells rather than acting more generally)). They split into 2 broad types: helper T-cells and cytotoxic T-cells. The role of helper T-cells is, as their name suggests, to assist the production of targeted immune response by both ***B-cells*** (producing antibodies) and cytotoxic T-cells. They do this both by directly interacting with the cells they are helping via receptors on their surface and by the action of ***cytokines*** (chemicals released by cells which act indirectly to activate or change the nature of other cells of the immune system). Cytotoxic T-cells are the killer cells of the immune response and are the main candidates for ***hepatocyte*** injury in immune-mediated liver disease. They normally recognise cells that are infected with viruses and other pathogens (as well, probably, as cancer cells) and induce them to die through ***apoptosis***. The effect is highly specific (they only kill in response to recognising a particular viral or other "foreign" protein). They are highly potent, so have checks and balances to prevent inappropriate activation (this is at both the level of their recognition of target cells and the need for T-cell help which is itself specific and targeted).

***Terlipressin (Glypressin) (160):*** A drug used to control bleeding from ***varices***. Variceal bleeding is one of the major complications of ***portal hypertension*** which itself is an important complication of ***cirrhosis***. Variceal bleeding can be, if not controlled, a life-threatening event. The standard approach to management is currently intravenous terlipressin therapy to control the bleeding, followed by ***endoscopy*** with ***banding*** to give a more definitive degree of control. By stopping an acute bleed, terlipressin therapy can be, literally, lifesaving. It can also, however, cause spasm of the cardiac arteries causing worse heart muscle ischaemia in people with already restricted cardiac blood flow. Terlipressin is only a short-term therapy given its intravenous mode of delivery. If long term medical therapy is thought to be appropriate, it will normally be in the form of ***beta blocker*** tablets.

*Triglyceride (40-41,43):* One of the key natural forms of *fat* and a key player in the pathophysiology of *MASLD*. The term in fact refers to a whole family of molecules which share a common structure consisting of three fatty acid molecules all linked to a molecule of glycerol. The different physical characteristics of the triglyceride (e.g. solubility) relate to the properties of the free fatty acid component. Triglyceride has an important physiological role as an energy source fuelling **aerobic metabolism**.

*Type 2 Diabetes:* The strongest disease association of MASLD. In fact the condition is perhaps best thought of as the "other side of the coin" of MASLD. Both are conditions of **insulin resistance**. Treatment approaches are similar for the two conditions. Many of the non-liver disease risk associations of MASLD (with ischaemic heart disease for example) reflect the complications of type 2 diabetes.

*Ursodeoxycholic Acid (UDCA) (64,153-154,177):* A hydrophilic (i.e. non-toxic) **bile acid** which can be given as a medicine in tablet form. It is the first line treatment for primary biliary cholangitis and is used in all disease settings where **cholestasis** occurs (including a minority of **MASLD** patients). It has **antioxidant** effects and may be **apoptosis** reducing. It has been trialled as a therapy in MASLD and, although very safe, has only limited beneficial effects (restricted to **liver function test** improvement).

*Ultrasound:* A quick and easily available approach to imaging the body. An ultrasound finding of fat in the liver (often described as a "bright" appearance) is often the first investigation test that points the way to a diagnosis of **steatotic liver disease** (*"fatty liver disease"*). It is important to be aware that there can often be significant fat deposition in the liver before it becomes apparent on ultrasound, so the absence of fat (or "brightness") on ultrasound does not exclude the possibility of **MASLD** as a diagnosis. It is also important to remember that ultrasound cannot distinguish between the different forms of MASLD (between, for example, **simple steatosis** and **MASH**). Ultrasound is useful in general for assessing the liver and bile ducts as it allows accurate assessment of liver and spleen size, liver texture (including the presence of any masses) and the integrity of the **bile duct**. It forms part of the regular assessment for the presence of **hepatocellular carcinoma** undertaken in all patients with cirrhosis. Ultrasound is also used at the time of **liver biopsy** to ensure that the procedure is safe.

*"Upper Limit of Normal":* The vast majority of blood tests carried out in the clinic have a range for normal values that reflect normal variability in the population (they are not "black or white", normal or abnormal as, say, a genetic test might be). To complicate things slightly, the assays used by

different hospitals can vary, meaning that the range for normal values can be slightly different from centre to centre. For this reason, when looking at whether a test is abnormal or not in liver disease, we use the concept of the "upper limit of normal" for tests which are abnormal if elevated such as ***alanine transaminase, bilirubin*** or ***alkaline phosphatase.*** The reverse applies with use of "lower limit of normal" for tests such as ***albumin*** where a lowering in the value is the abnormality that causes concern. A test value would be described as a multiple of the upper limit of normal. For example, if your alanine transaminase was 120 and the upper limit of normal for your local laboratory was 40, then your alanine transaminase is three times the upper limit of normal (3x uln). The cut-offs used to signify disease control have changed over time as the significance of abnormality becomes better understood. They also differ from centre to centre and country to country which is an unhelpful source of confusion for patients. Over time, it is likely that the target values for treatment will be lowered.

***Varices (20,147,159-161,180,222):*** One of the complications of ***cirrhosis*** of all aetiologies. ***Portal hypertension*** is a common feature of cirrhosis (and very occasionally chronic liver disease that isn't cirrhotic) because of the impaired flow of the blood in the ***portal vein*** through the distorted anatomy of the cirrhotic liver. The increased pressure can open up residual blood vessels left over from the fetal circulation present in utero, and which shuts down, but doesn't completely disappear, when you are born. This can lead to the development of, often high pressure but weak-walled, blood vessels in places where the old fetal and current adult circulations meet. This is most typically in the bowel (although they can also be seen in the abdominal wall which is one of the reasons why abdominal surgery in patients with cirrhosis is often high risk). Within the bowel, the commonest site is the lower oesophagus. They can also be a problem in the rectum (sometimes being mistaken for haemorrhoids) and stomach. Oesophageal varices can be a particular problem because the passage of food over big varices in a relatively narrow space can probably increase the risk of bleeding through surface trauma. If varices bleed then it is a medical emergency as the blood loss can be significant (because of the relatively high pressure within the vessels). In the setting of an acute bleed the first key step is to give fluid intravenously to support the circulation. After this, we use medicines (such as glypressin/terlipressin) to lower the portal venous pressure to reduce or stop the bleeding to allow the definitive short-term treatment which is done at ***endoscopy***. The commonest treatment in current practice is to ***band*** the varices (to put small rubber bands on them to constrict them and seal them off). If someone does develop varices, but those varices haven't bled, then the approach is to lower the pressure in the portal circulation typically using drugs such as ***propranolol*** or ***carvedilol***. ***MASLD*** patients in whom cirrhosis is suspected should undergo regular check endoscopy to see if propranolol or carvedilol are needed.

***Viral Hepatitis (82):*** Acute inflammation in the liver caused by a viral infection such as hepatitis A, hepatitis B, hepatitis C, hepatitis D and hepatitis E. It can cause a similar pattern of ***liver function test*** abnormality to that seen in MASLD and is therefore one of the important alternative diagnoses to exclude. Positive test results for the presence of a virus, and the absence of any evidence of liver fat deposition on ***ultrasound*** with viral hepatitis mean that the two conditions shouldn't be confused in practice.

***Vitamin E (153,204):*** Vitamin E is an antioxidant vitamin which has shown some benefits in clinical trial in non-diabetic patients with non-cirrhotic ***MASH***. It is thought to work through reduction in ***oxidative stress***. Vitamin E levels are seemingly low in MASH patients suggesting an element of consumption. The vitamin E trials suggest both ***liver function test*** and biopsy improvement but there is no evidence to show any survival improvement.

***White Blood Cells:*** The cells in the blood (lymphocytes, neutrophils and monocytes) responsible for fighting infection. Levels are elevated in an acute infection. In hepatology, a raised white cell count in ***ascites*** is an important sign that ***spontaneous bacterial peritonitis*** has developed and is complicating cirrhosis. This can cause an acute deterioration in liver function and requires antibiotic therapy.

# APPENDIX 2: *THE NEWCASTLE APPROACH....*
## ......*TO MANAGING FATIGUE IN MASLD*

This is a really important issue for patients and a key part of our work in the clinic. It is an area of MASLD management where taking a structured, long-term approach is really key. There are, regrettably, no specific therapies for MASLD fatigue at present. There are, however, many things that we can, and do, do to improve quality of life from fatigue. This needs a comprehensive approach, however, not just a prescription.

**Step 1:** *Explain, reassure & support:* The first key step is to explain to people that fatigue is part of liver disease (for some people), that it is "real" and that they are not alone. There are lots of other patients just like them and that we are there to help. We don't sympathise (people don't want our sympathy) but we do empathise; try to understand what it must feel like and to commit to try and help. Most people presenting with liver disease fatigue have had, by the time they reach us, a very negative experience of not being believed by clinicians, and told that they do not have a "proper problem". For some reason, fatigue is an area where doctors feel the need to share and equate their own experience. A fatigued liver disease patient is not particularly helped by hearing that you were on call last night and are very tired!! Explaining the current understanding of the mechanisms of fatigue is often really useful for patients. This is partly because it helps people to understand the disease process and partly because it reinforces the view that the problem is "real".

**Step 2:** *Get treatment for MASLD right:* Probably the single most important step in the management of fatigue in MASLD is to put lifestyle modifications in place. We can't emphasise this enough. Both weight loss and exercise have a positive benefit on fatigue that is over and above their potential to improve the liver disease process in MASLD. It really is a "win/win" situation. Weight loss has both a simple and a more subtle benefit. The simple one is that the lighter you are, the less energy your body needs to consume to move. Given that fatigue is, in essence, a relative shortage of energy, the benefit is obvious. The more subtle action is through reduction in inflammation. As we discussed in earlier chapters, fatty tissue is pro-inflammatory in terms of its actions, with adipose or fat containing cells releasing inflammatory cytokines. These have both direct and indirect actions on the brain which lead to fatigue. They can also modify the actions of energy generating enzymes within cells. For all these reasons, if you lose weight through diet modification you will reduce the amount of fat in the body and thus fatigue. Own the problem and own the solution.

Exercise likewise has several effects. The first is that it assists with weight loss or optimisation. If weight gain is a result of too much energy in the diet not being balanced out by the amount of energy expended through exercise, then higher energy expenditure through exercise than energy intake through the diet will support weight loss. In terms of biology, however, exercise has a couple of important actions that change cell function. Firstly, it is a major contributor to restoring insulin sensitivity. Given the importance of insulin resistance in MASLD this is really important. Secondly, exercise changes the biology of muscle cells so that they can cope with the metabolic results of exercise better. Think of athletes training. The more they train the more exercise they can do before running out of energy.

What this means in practice is that whereas a diet and exercise programme is important for the treatment of MASLD, it is crucial for the treatment of fatigue in MASLD. We aim for simple and practical guidance that people will be able to actually follow "in the real world". Overall calorie intake is almost always important. What is usually equally important, however, is to look at the nature of the calorie intake. We talk to people about moving away from carbohydrates as the principle source of calories, with an increase in protein intake and, perhaps paradoxically, fat (remember that the fat that is deposited in the liver cells in MASLD isn't fat that was eaten in the diet, but fat made by the liver largely from the excess glucose in the diet, glucose that comes from carbohydrate……). In terms of exercise the key thing is to do it. There is much debate about the "right sort of exercise". In reality as long as you stick to the following basic rules it will be right for you. You need to exercise for long enough (30 minutes a time), frequently enough (three times a week as a minimum) and at a sufficient intensity (enough to make yourself a little short of breath). If you start to develop a passion for it then do look to combine different exercise types, alternating cardiovascular exercise (swimming, walking (fast) and cycling) and resistance exercise (weight training). In reality, however people are much more likely to fail in their exercise programme because they don't stick with it than because they go for the wrong exercise type.

In terms of drug therapy in the area of getting treatment right for MASLD, there is almost no data. Our suspicion is that even if effective drug treatments are identified that slow disease progression, lifestyle modification will still remain at the centre of fatigue management in practice.

**Step 3:** *Treat treatable causes:* MASLD patients frequently have other conditions that are themselves also associated with fatigue, and which may be easier to treat than liver fatigue. These should be thought about, looked for and, where found, treated. Examples include:

- Other components of the metabolic syndrome. This is most obviously type 2 diabetes and its complications such as chronic kidney disease, but also includes heart failure from ischaemic heart disease.
- Age-related conditions (i.e. those that are not specifically associated with MASLD, but which are common in the population) these include anaemia of various causes and conditions such as hypothyroidism. Menopausal symptoms and vitamin D deficiency can also be easily addressed.

**Step 4:** *Treat things that make the fatigue worse:* There are a number of clinical processes or problems which are not a direct feature of liver disease, but that are seen at an increased frequency in liver disease patients and which appear to contribute to the severity of the fatigue. Reducing their impact can lessen the severity of fatigue. These include:

- *Sleep disturbance:* Poor sleep is very common in fatty liver and contributes to fatigue the following day. This is sometimes, but not always, a feature of obstructive sleep apnoea. Assessment of sleep by the affected individual is notoriously difficult, so the observation of partners is very helpful. If there is a question of poor sleep, then the input of a specialist sleep clinic is often really helpful. This is especially the case if obstructive sleep apnoea is suspected, as airway support interventions will require their input. Simple things that patients can do is to avoid simulants (tea, coffee, energy drinks etc) after around 5pm in the day and, wherever possible, avoid sleeping tablets and alcohol. These superficially seem to help sleep but the sleep that you do get is almost always poor quality and therefore of low value.
- *Autonomic disturbance:* Blood pressure regulation seems to be a real issue in MASLD, with significant ups and downs, especially in older patients or those who have progressed to cirrhosis. This blood pressure can, in particular, fall when people stand up suddenly. These blood flow changes probably result in poor muscle perfusion (and maybe even altered blood supply to the heart) reducing function. This is commonly, in our experience, linked to excessive blood pressure lowering treatment (a common challenge in MASLD because of the metabolic syndrome association). Re-assessing blood pressure treatment is therefore a very useful thing to look at. DON'T STOP BLOOD PRESSURE TREATMENT WITHOUT DISCUSSING IT WITH YOUR DOCTOR! The things that should make you think about blood pressure regulation as a factor in fatigue in MASLD include dizziness when standing up quickly.

- *Depression:* A complex issue. Depression can be a cause of fatigue in MASLD, with issues around body image compounding those related to having a chronic and currently difficult to treat disease (as well, of course, as liver-disease unrelated issues). Anti-depressants such as sertraline can help. They don't make the fatigue better, but they can help people cope with it.

**Step 5: *Coping Strategies:*** This is really key. At the moment it is not possible to cure fatigue. It is perfectly possible, however, to live a perfectly normal life despite it. The capacity to do this lies IN YOUR HANDS! We can help you cope effectively but, fundamentally, the desire to do so comes from within. Here are some important things that we discuss with patients:

- *Owning the problem so you can own the solution:* This is about accepting the reality of the situation. We have several sayings ("you are where you are" and "in life we have to play the hand we are dealt"). There is no point wishing it had not happened or blaming the world. The problem is yours; it is here, and you have to get on with making the most of it. It is okay to be fed up for a little bit but after that, make a plan and get on with it. The ultimate example of "owning the problem and owning the solution" is, of course, lifestyle modification interventions which are so very important for MASLD in general and fatigue in MASLD in particular.
- *Set realistic time scales:* Whatever you do, you will not beat this in a day or a week. We always suggest to people that they take a fixed point in the calendar one year (Christmas, summer holiday, birthday etc) and set the same day next year as the target to be doing more and coping better.
- *Help others to understand:* In the same way that doctors sometimes struggle to understand this, so can family members. MASLD patients with fatigue don't typically look any different to other people, which means that others do not understand how you can look well but feel awful. It is just the way the disease works. Explain to partners, children etc what you can and can't do and the importance of their understanding and help. Have a way of being able to flag that you are struggling and need a bit of help without having to go into detail.
- *Understand the rhythm of your day:* Liver disease fatigue is characteristic in getting worse as the day goes on. People are usually better in the morning than in the afternoon. Use that information to plan your day. Do important things in the morning. If you are working and struggle later in the day, discuss with your employer about moving your hours around. These simple changes can make a huge

difference without impacting on your effectiveness. One thing that is really critical is to avoid doing night shifts if at all possible.

- *Accept there will be good days and bad days:* Again, this is just the way the disease works. If you have a good day enjoy it (but don't overdo it). If you have a bad day, then be philosophical. The next day is likely to be better.
- *Avoid getting isolated:* THIS IS REALLY IMPORTANT! People can sometimes withdraw from normal activities to save energy (work, social activities etc). This is always a false economy. What you gain from conserved energy you lose in overall life quality. The secret is to keep doing things but to adapt what you do to take account of the limitations.
- *Stay positive:* Treatment is on its way!!

# APPENDIX 3: *MICRONUTRIENTS*

## *Water soluble vitamins*

| Water soluble vitamins | Source | Biological function | Deficiency | Interactions, comments |
|---|---|---|---|---|
| Thiamine (vitamin B1) | Pork, poultry<br><br>Peas, nuts, dried beans, soybeans<br><br>Whole grain cereals, lentils, legumes, rice<br><br>Yeast | Helps the breakdown and release of energy from food.<br><br>Nervous system function<br><br>Heart function | Beriberi – heart failure, nerve damage and muscle weakness<br><br>Wernicke-Korsakov syndrome – temporary or permanent damage to the brain function, particularly memory | Deficiency occurs in people with a poor dietary intake, especially when their body has increased requirements e.g. emergency bowel surgery.<br><br>Also associated with chronic alcohol dependence, Crohn's disease, eating disorders<br><br>Dialysis, certain water tablets e.g. furosemide and excess tea and coffee also reduce levels |
| Riboflavin (vitamin B2) | Milk and dairy products<br><br>Eggs<br><br>Red meat<br><br>Salmon, tuna<br><br>Almonds, spinach | Breakdown of fat, protein, and carbohydrate | Involved in processing nutrients, deficiency can lead to other nutrients and anaemia | Increased risk of deficiency in pregnancy and with vegan diet |
| Niacin (vitamin B3) | Meat, fish, eggs<br><br>Dairy products<br><br>Nuts | Release of energy from food<br><br>Skin and nervous system | Pellegra.<br><br>Skin rash or discolouration, red tongue<br><br>Vomiting, constipation, diarrhoea<br><br>Fatigue, memory | Increased risk of deficiency with chronic alcohol dependence, eating disorders and gut malabsorption disease e.g. Crohn's disease |

| | | | loss | |
|---|---|---|---|---|
| Pantothenic acid (vitamin B5) | Chicken, beef, eggs<br><br>Many vegetables, including tomato, broccoli, legumes.<br><br>Whole grains | Release of energy from food<br><br>Making blood cells | Vague symptoms, may include headache, fatigue, irritability, impaired muscle coordination, bowel function disturbance | |
| Pyridoxine (Vitamin B6) | Poultry, pork, sirloin steak<br><br>Halibut<br><br>Bananas, avocados, baked potato with skin, raw red pepper, prunes, lentils | Protein metabolism<br><br>Essential for the liver to break down fat and glycogen to make glucose.<br><br>Helps the immune system.<br><br>Nervous system function | Skin rashes (dermatitis)<br><br>Cracked and sore lips<br><br>Sore glossy tongue<br><br>Anaemia, fatigue, and tiredness<br><br>Depression<br><br>Seizures<br><br>Neuropathy – tingling and numbness | Deficiency commonly goes along with deficiency of other B vitamins, such as folic acid and B12.<br><br>Deficiency is more likely in people who are obese, chronic alcohol dependent, pregnant, have coeliac or inflammatory bowel disease, or bariatric surgery, autoimmune or kidney disease |
| Biotin (vitamin B7) | Made by the gut bacteria.<br><br>Food sources include – yeast, soybeans, eggs, peanut butter, mushrooms | Fatty acid and glucose metabolism | Hair loss<br><br>Rashes, mouth sores, dry skin<br><br>Nausea and vomiting<br><br>Depression, lethargy | Deficiency is rare but can occur with very restricted diets |
| Folate (Vitamin B9) | Green vegetables, beans, legumes, whole grains<br><br>Lesser amounts in fruit | Essential for all cell replication | Megaloblastic anaemia<br><br>Spina bifida | |
| Vitamin B12 | Meat, fish<br><br>Milk, dairy | Making red blood cells<br><br>Release of | Anaemia<br><br>Nerve and spinal | Deficiency may occur due to impaired absorption from the stomach e.g. |

| | products

Eggs | energy from food

Needed for folate use | cord damage

Impaired mental function | pernicious anaemia, or lack of intake from vegan diet |
|---|---|---|---|---|
| Ascorbic acid (vitamin C) | Fruit and vegetables, especially –

Raw red and yellow peppers

Guava, blackcurrants, kiwi fruit, lychee, lemon, orange, strawberry

Broccoli | Vital for a range of metabolic 293unction

Protein metabolism

Collagen synthesis

Nervous system function | Scurvy, impaired wound healing

Fluid swelling

Fatigue, depression

Poor immunity | Low vitamin C levels have been seen with central obesity, but it's not clear whether this is a cause or effect.

Commoner in people with poor diet, chronic alcohol dependent, smokers |

## *Fat soluble vitamins*

Deficiency of fat-soluble vitamins is associated with fat malabsorption e.g. cystic fibrosis, chronic pancreatitis, coeliac disease, cholestatic liver disease, Crohn's disease.

| Fat soluble vitamins | Source | Biological function | Deficiency | Interactions, comments |
|---|---|---|---|---|
| Vitamin A (retinol) and carotenoids | Liver, dairy products

Yellow, red and green (leafy) vegetables, such as spinach, carrots, sweet potatoes, and red peppers

Yellow fruit, such as mango, papaya, and apricots | Function of the immune system

Night vision

Health of the skin and body linings e.g. nose and mouth | Xerophthalmia (drying out of the tear ducts of the eyes, if prolonged this can lead to corneal damage and impair vision)

Impaired immunity (immunosuppression)

Diarrhoea | Absorption is reduced in people with fat malabsorption |
| Cholecalciferol | Oily fish – salmon, sardines, | Regulates calcium and | Rickets in children | Sun exposure allows the skin |

| | | | | |
|---|---|---|---|---|
| (vitamin D) | herring, mackerel  Red meat  Liver  Egg yolks | phosphate.  Promotes bone formation.  Immune system function | Bone weakness in adults  Decreased muscle strength.  Poor immunity and wound healing  Fatigue, poor sleep | to make vitamin D.  Deficiency is very common in the UK, as there is inadequate sun exposure in the winter, and for many people all year round |
| Tocopherol (vitamin E) | Vegetable oils  Nuts, seeds, whole grains | Maintain cell membranes | Nerve damage,  Ataxia (difficulty with coordination of walking)  Muscle weakness  Red blood cell breakdown  Impaired vision  Poor immunity | Vitamin E is fat soluble, which means it needs to be absorbed with fat. People at risk of deficiency include those with fat malabsorption, e.g. chronic pancreatitis, cystic fibrosis, Crohn's disease, short bowel syndrome |
| Vitamin K | Green leafy vegetables  Vegetable oils  Cereal grains | Blood clotting  Wound healing | Prolonged blood clotting | Warfarin is given to reduce blood clotting by creating vitamin K deficiency |

## *Minerals and Trace Elements*

| Minerals and Trace Elements | Source | Biological function | Deficiency | Interactions, comments |
|---|---|---|---|---|
| Calcium | Dairy products, tofu, sardines, green leafy vegetables | Muscle contraction, including heart and blood | Bone weakness (rickets in children, osteoporosis in adults) | Absorption is reduced in vitamin D deficiency.  Some foods (spinach, |

|   |   |   | vessels. | Impaired blood clotting | rhubarb, soy) reduce calcium absorption. |
|---|---|---|---|---|---|
|   |   |   | Nerve conduction | Impaired heart function |   |
|   |   |   | Blood clotting |   |   |
|   |   |   | Bones and teeth |   |   |
| Iodine | Sea fish | Essential for thyroid function | Those of an underactive thyroid - Fatigue, weakness, weight gain, dry skin, hair loss | Common deficiency worldwide, and particularly with vegan diet |   |
|   | Shellfish |   |   |   |
|   | Fortified salt |   |   |   |
|   | Seaweed (depends on location it comes from) |   | Goitre (enlarge thyroid gland in neck) | Caution with using seaweed for replacement as may cause toxicity |
| Iron | Red meat | Red blood cells | Iron deficiency anaemia – fatigue, breathlessness, lethargy | Iron in meat is more readily absorbed that the iron in plants |   |
|   | Beans, peas, broccoli, nuts and seeds, green leafy vegetables |   |   |   |
| Magnesium | Leafy green vegetables, grains, legumes, some fish, nuts, seeds, chocolate | Many metabolic functions throughout the body | Muscle weakness, tremors, or cramp | Some diuretics (water tablets) such as Bendroflumethiazide cause magnesium to be lost in the urine |   |
|   |   |   | Cardiac rhythm disturbance |   |
|   |   |   | Altered mental function. |   |
|   |   |   | Seizures |   |
|   |   |   | Abnormal absorption or vitamin D |   |
| Phosphorus (phosphate) | Fish, poultry, meat, and dairy products | Essential for release of energy in cells throughout the body | Bone weakness and pain | May be caused by vitamin D deficiency, as this helps with absorption. |   |
|   |   |   | Muscle weakness, stiff joints |   |
|   | Nuts, seeds, whole grains (less easily | Necessary for |   | Other causes – poor intake from diet, |

| | | absorbed) Transports nutrients into cell Bone and teeth strength | cell replication | Anxiety, fatigue Breathing problems and heart failure | malnutrition, particularly in people with chronic alcohol excess and eating disorders. May occur when recovering from diabetic ketoacidosis, or starvation from any cause (refeeding syndrome) |
|---|---|---|---|---|---|
| Potassium | Fruits – especially bananas, citrus fruits, raisins Beans, nuts, grains Vegetables – potato with skin | Essential for the electrical activity in muscle cells, particularly the heart | | Heart rhythm abnormalities, cardiac arrest Muscle weakness | May be lost in bowel disorders causing vomiting or diarrhoea, or from the kidneys with water tablets |
| Selenium | Fish, shellfish Content in grain and vegetables depends on the soil content | Supports the action of vitamin E and thyroid function | | Cardiomyopathy Weak hair and nails Nausea and vomiting Neuropathy (nerve damage) | |
| Sodium | Salt | Fluid and acid regulation Electrical activity of nerves | | Weakness, fatigue, confusion, seizures | Inadequate intake is rare. Sodium loss may occur from sweat due to exercise in hot weather, from vomiting or diarrhoea |
| Zinc | Shellfish Red meats Legumes, nuts | Many enzyme systems, including immune function | | May contribute to MASLD. Impaired immune function, wound healing, sense of | Dietary deficiency is common as the daily requirement is high |

|  |  |  | smell and taste |  |
|--|--|--|--|--|

## *Phytonutrients (plant pigment chemicals):*

**Sources**: Skin of brightly coloured fruit and vegetables e.g. citrus fruits, berries, grapes, peaches, tomatoes, red cabbage, onion, peppers, beans, sage. Soy, dark chocolate, green tea, red wine

**Biological functions**: Reduce risk of vitamin C deficiency. May improve cardiovascular health, reduce blood pressure, and reduce cancer risk.

**Deficiency**: increased risk of scurvy

## ABOUT THE AUTHORS

Professor David Jones has treated people with liver disease for over 30 years. He has a particular interest in the management of the symptoms of liver disease and runs a dedicated symptom clinic at the Freeman Hospital in Newcastle upon Tyne in the UK. He was awarded an OBE in the 2018 Queen's Birthday Honours List for services to patients with liver disease.

Dr Vanessa Linnett is a consultant anaesthetist and specialist in intensive care medicine at the Queen Elizabeth Hospital in Gateshead in the UK. She has a particular interest in diet and the impact that it can have on chronic disease.

www.ingramcontent.com/pod-product-compliance
Lightning Source LLC
Chambersburg PA
CBHW052241220526
45471CB00001B/140